NEW DEVELOPMENTS IN MEDICAL RESEARCH

BILE DUCT

FUNCTIONAL ANATOMY, DISEASE AND INJURY CLASSIFICATION AND SURGICAL MANAGEMENT

NEW DEVELOPMENTS IN MEDICAL RESEARCH

Additional books in this series can be found on Nova's website under the Series tab.

Additional e-books in this series can be found on Nova's website under the e-book tab.

NEW DEVELOPMENTS IN MEDICAL RESEARCH

BILE DUCT

FUNCTIONAL ANATOMY, DISEASE AND INJURY CLASSIFICATION AND SURGICAL MANAGEMENT

MIGUEL ÁNGEL MERCADO, M.D.
EDITOR

New York

Library of Congress Cataloging-in-Publication Data

ISBN: 978-1-63321-771-3

Library of Congress Control Number: 2014948045

Published by Nova Science Publishers, Inc. † New York

Contents

Preface

The treatment of bile duct benign pathology demands a multidisciplinary approach, involving a team of both specialized physicians and solid infrastructure. Radiologists, endoscopists, and surgeons are all involved in the treatment of these kinds of patients. This statement is also true for the diagnosis and treatment of the catastrophic results of bile duct injury.

Cholecystectomy is one of the most common surgical procedures done either openly or through laparoscopy. The presence of bile duct injury is one of its most severe complications. The solution for this unfortunate event poses a technically demanding approach that involves an array of alternatives comprising surgical and radio-interventional procedures.

This book focuses on benign bile duct diseases, mainly related to iatrogenic bile duct injury. The reader will find a complete and profound review of bile duct anatomy and function, a thorough explanation about the type of bile duct injuries and how to approach them, beautiful descriptions of both the surgical and radiological techniques used in the management of bile duct injuries, a compilation of the experience of a high-yield center of this kind of diseases, and logical techniques to lower the incidence of these injuries.

This text is aimed at an audience composed of health care professionals involved in the integrative treatment of iatrogenic bile duct injuries. In a world where the best medical evidence defines the most effective therapeutic alternative, this book focuses on giving a solid and broad enough basis upon which medical teams can approach this disease.

Chapter 1 – This chapter, "Functional Anatomy of Biliary System (Clinical and Experimental Data)", represents the results of studies implemented since the late 1970s at the Department of Operational Surgery and Topographic Anatomy of Tbilisi State Medical University, under the leadership of Prof. Shalva Toidze, and was later conducted at the Alexandre Natishvili Institute of Morphology of Ivane Javakhisvhili Tbilisi State University. The complex design studies involve both clinical and experimental material, including the anatomical experimental data from autopsy liver material. The data from experiments, including up to 300 surgeries, 150 autopsies of the human liver and 200 biliary pathology modeling experiments implemented on stray dogs and Wistar rats, were all analyzed. Part of the human liver samples taken at autopsy from adult patients whose death was not related to the pathology of hepato-biliary-pancreatic zone were investigated through gradual maceration of parenchyma under spurts of water and separation of the portal tracts and hepatic veins.

The gross histo-topographic sequential slices from every segment of other parts of liver samples were studied to reveal the relationship (interactions) of the bile ducts and mucosal biliary glandswith other structures of the portal tract and hepatic vein tributaries as well. In the other part of the liver samples bile ducts and vessels were preliminarily injected with Indian ink-gelatin mixture for sharp visualization of the lumina of these structures.

The corrosion casts of both human and animal bile ducts were prepared by retrograde injection of the solidifying mass (latex and/or methylmetacrilate) into the common bile duct, which was followed by corrosion of liver tissue. The gross caliber structures were studied by binocular magnifier, and the small caliber structures – by a standard method of scanning electronic microscopy. The lumen relief of gross caliber bile ducts was studied by scanning the electronic microscope as well, after standard preliminary drying of preparations (at the critical point of transformation of liquid CO_2 into the gas, under the set of 100 Atm. pressure and 40°C). Both in dogs and rats the cholestasis was modeled via occlusion of the common bile duct, which was achieved by incision of the latter between two ligatures. The surgery was done through middle laparotomy under general anesthesia. (Sham operations were done in the control group, which implied the middle laparotomy and separation of common bile duct without its ligation or incision). The microscopic study of liver tissue was done by conventional methods of histology and immunohistochemistry. Regardless of the fact, that part of the studies was performed quite long time ago, they still don't have conclusions and their discussion is still ongoing. The authors think that much of the presented data will evoke the interest of professionals.

The authors would like to dedicate this publication to the memory of our teacher, renowned scientist and lecturer, Professor Shalva Toidze. Regrettably, the society of hepatologists has not become widely familiar with the results of the studies on the surgical anatomy of the liver and bile ducts implemented by the and his students until now.

Chapter 2 – The chapter is a review of the literature concerning anatomical variations of the extrahepatic biliary tract and its arterial blood supply, including the literature regarding arterial vascularization of all segments of the extrahepatic biliary system and aspects that are most important and essential for a surgeon. Different variations of formation, number and position of the gallbladder, hepatic ducts and common bile duct are reported in 1,6 to 47,2% of cases. The arterial blood supply of the extrahepatic biliary tract is different in particular parts. The gallbladder and cystic duct are supplied by a cystic artery. The blood supply to the right and left hepatic ducts and the upper portion of the common hepatic duct is from the cystic artery and the right and left hepatic arteries. The supraduodenal common bile duct is supplied by arterial branches from the right hepatic, cystic, posterior superior pancreaticoduodenal and retroduodenal arteries. The blood supply to the retroduodenal and intrapancreatic common bile duct is from the posterior superior pancreaticoduodenal and retroduodenal arteries. The proximal (hilar) part of the extrahepatic biliary tract has a very rich arterial blood supply. The arterial vascularization of the supraduodenal common bile duct is poor, in most cases as axial distribution (3- and 9- o'clock arteries), or less frequently - ladder distribution. It is a critical segment, in which most postoperative complications, such as biliary duct strictures, occur.

A surgeon should remember about the variability of the extrahepatic bile ducts and biliary tract arterial vascularization, in their particular parts, during surgical procedures, particularly such as cholecystectomy, biliary and biliary-alimentary anastomoses, pancreatoduodenectomy, liver transplantation and other procedures performed within the hepatoduodenal ligament. This knowledge will help avoid many serious postoperative complications.

Chapter 3 – Various imaging modalities, invasive and noninvasive, are useful for the assessment of bile duct anatomy in pre-surgical evaluation. In this chapter, I present characteristics of each modality and the new technical developments in this field. Assessment of the functional anatomy of the bile duct is important in evaluation of the risk factors affecting bile duct cancer. I show that MRI is the most appropriate modality for this purpose, because MRI facilitates analysis of bile and pancreatic juice flow, which may have associations with carcinogenesis in bile duct tumors. Although flow analysis of the bile duct with MRI has focused on continuous MRCP examination after secretin injection, a new method (time-SLIP imaging) is available for easier and faster flow analysis. I present various cases and clinical management approaches based on this new technique (time-SLIP imaging).

I present how various radiological modalities can be used to help differentiate between benignity and malignancy, stage tumors, select surgical candidates, and guide surgical planning when biliary disease is suspected. I also discuss how recent developments in imaging modalities contribute to the diagnosis of bile duct disease.

Chapter 4 – In general, complete circumferential sections of the biliary tract, with or without tissue loss, are classified in the literature as complex lesions. It is important to point out that the initial injury class is upgraded to a higher one as suggested by Bismuth, because the ischemic and/or inflammatory component leads to necrosis of the duct and may even compromise the confluence. Likewise, injury of the middle third of the hepatic duct may subsequently be upgraded due to the ischemic component. Many classifications have been created before and after the laparoscopic era. Before the introduction of this technique, the Bismuth-Corlette classification was, and perhaps still is, the most popular one. This classification only includes the complete section of the duct and the length of the stump of the proximal biliary tract.

Chapter 5 – The Strasberg's classification of iatrogenic biliary injury includes all variables and possible injuries, and thus it is a comprehensive basis to determine which therapeutic approach is chosen depending on the type of injury. In the case of type A injury, an endoscopic approach is preferred. Type B injuries, which require a right biliary tract anatomical variant, are generally managed symptomatically until the hepatic subsector becomes atrophic as a result of secondary biliary cirrhosis. Type C, in which a biliary fistula is presented, appropriate subhepatic drainage will prevent the formation of collections, and the duct may spontaneously occlude, leading to secondary biliary cirrhosis of the sector. Type D injuries are basically exclusive of laparoscopic cholecystectomy, in which the treatment depends on the severity of the damage; suture with placement of a T tube, endoscopic approach and biliodigestive derivation are feasable. The different type E injuries are usually managed through a Roux-en-Y hepaticojejunal anastomosis. Partial resection of segments of IV and V may be necessary to allow duct identification and execution of the anastomosis. The Strasberg's classification includes most variables and possible iatrogenic biliary injuries, thus we chose it as the basis for the design of potential treatment options.

Chapter 6 – When biliary tract injury is detected during surgery, conversion is necessary. Adequate exposure and dissection is critical. In patients with previous surgery, various kinds of anastomosis may be found. After obtaining a defunctionalized loop and mapping the biliary tract through thin dilators, the loop is anastomosed in a non-tense fashion to ensure a high quality derivation. The suture material used is important. The hepaticoduodenal anastomosis, from their point of view, has the disadvantage of exposing the anastomosis to acidic content and food residues that hinder its function. Hepatocholedochal anastomosis and choledo-choledocal anastomosis, even though they are comfortable procedures, have high failure rates. Stents can be placed during surgery or transendoscopically, and they are used by our group in complex cases. Neoformation of gallstones after biliodigestive derivation or prosthesis placement is due to the presence of inadequate biliary drainage and/or bile colonization.

Chapter 7 – *Introduction*: This survey analyzes the correlation between perioperative complications in patients who underwent hepatojejunostomy after a primary surgery (hepatoduodenostomy or choledoco-choledocal anastomosis), and those whom the first intervention was hepatojejunostomy. *Methods*: A quantitative and retrospective analysis was done, including patients in which hepatojejunostomy was performed at the "National Institute of Medical Sciences and Nutrition" from 1990 to 2010. The confidence interval was set at 95% and the statistical analysis was performed using Chi-squared test. *Results:* 116 patients were included; group 1 (*n=39*) was constituted by patients with previous repairs and group 2 *(n=77)* with patients without previous repair. Preoperative complications were found in *76% (30)* in group 1, whereas in the group 2 these complications were present in *54% (42)* (*p<.005*). Laparoscopic cholecystectomy was the most frequent type of surgery from the total number of patients, *66% (26)* in the group 1 and *44% (34)* in the group 2. Cholangitis was the most frequent complication found preoperatively; *66% (26)* in group 1 and *44% (34)* in group 2 (p=.04). The authors compared the proportion of postoperative complications in both groups, along with segment IV resection, and whether the confluence was preserved or not. In this regard, *30% (12)* of patients assigned to group 1 suffered this type of complications, while the group 2, *23% (29)*. *Conclusion*: In this study, patients with primary repairs had more preoperative complications than patients with no previous repairs prior to hepatojejunostomy.

Chapter 8 – Introduction: This study evaluates the postoperative outcome of patients who had hepaticojejunostomy as treatment for iatrogenic bile duct injuries, with previous use of endoprosthesis. *Methods:* A retrospective study was performed from 2005 to 2010. Patients who had endoscopic biliary stenting (minimum 6 months with 2 exchanges) previous to surgical reconstruction were included. Group 1 consisted of 25 patients repaired with endoscopic biliary endoprosthesis before surgical intervention and group 2 consisted of 75 patients who required surgical treatment as first approach. *Results:* Preoperative sepsis (p=0.012), number of preoperative episodes of cholangitis (p<0.001), postoperative stenosis (p<0.0001) and radiological intervention (p= 0.017) had a statistically significant difference between the two groups. A subanalysis of patients with criteria for endoscopic treatment failure (endoscopic treatment for minimum 1 year with 4 stent exchanges) was performed. Furthermore, the differences in the variables measured were statistically significant, and the stented group presented more complications. Conclusion: Management of bile duct injury must be multidisciplinary. When continuity of the bile duct is preserved, endoscopic biliary stenting is the treatment of choice. However, if the stenosis cannot be solved in a short period of time, it is necessary to promote early surgery to prevent postoperative long-term stenosis or radiological intervention. Early intervention would facilitate surgical reconstruction and improve long-term outcome.

Chapter 9 – *Background:* Hepatobiliary disease, especially issues concerning the gallbladder, is the most common indication for abdominal surgery in the elderly; therefore, cholecystectomies and bile duct injuries are expected to increase as the population ages. The aim of the study was to analyze the characteristics, management and outcome of bile duct injury repair in the elderly population through a 20-year period. *Methods:* A retrospective analysis of the institutional database identified all patients that underwent surgical repair of the biliary tract secondary to bile duct injury from July 1992 to July 2012. *Results:* A total of 486 patients were identified; 53 patients were identified as elderly population. They were allocated into two groups; Group 1 included 38 patients between 60 and 74 years of age and Group 2 included 15 patients with >75 years of age. The median age was 70 years. The authors found a direct correlation between the age of the patient and the amount of comorbidities associated; 64% of all patients had comorbidities, 58% in Group 1 and 80% in Group 2. Primary surgical repair was the most frequent procedure (51%) and the Hepp-Couinaud technique was performed in 70% of the cases. Postoperative complications were observed in 53% of the patients. Partial resection of segment IV-V was used in 51% of the patients and hepatectomy was necessary in 3 (5.6%) of the patients. Vasculobiliary injuries were found in 4 (7%) patients. Excellent outcome was achieved in 74% of the patients, successful outcome in 89% and poor outcome in 11% of the patients. Death occurred in 4 (7.5%) patients. *Conclusions:* The present study's outcomes confirm that bilioenteric anastomoses in the elderly is a safe procedure with acceptable morbidity and mortality, and that using different techniques in order to achieve an adequate anastomosis does not increase morbidity. Excellent outcomes are expected in specialized centers and poor results occur in older patients with co-existing morbidities.

Chapter 10 – *Introduction:* Injury of major vessels associated to bile duct injury in laparoscopic cholecystectomy has been reported with variable frequency. There is no consensus of what a surgeon has to do in this setting, although most of the reports show that there is no negative effect on long term results of reconstruction. *Methods:* The files of patients repaired at our hospital in the last three years in which hepatic arterial injury was specifically searched for at the operation were reviewed. In all cases an intrahepatic hepatojejunostomy was done. *Results:* A total of 195 cases were repaired, and the frequency of right arterial injury was 22% (43 cases). In 4 cases, the injury was identified at the index operation and in 25 cases within 36 hours. In the remaining 14 cases the repair was performed later. Postoperative cholangitis was found in 8% of the cases, with 4% requiring radiological and/or surgical reintervention to dilate the anastomosis. Of the patients that were repaired at the index operation or hours later, they observed that in 80% of the cases, retrograde flow of the injured hepatic artery was present. *Conclusion:* Almost one third of complex bile duct injuries have some type of arterial involvement. They are produced mainly laparoscopically. Moreover, most of the injured arteries have retrograde flow and do not need reconstruction.

Chapter 11 – Iatrogenic injury through operative trauma is the main cause of bile duct injury (BDI), accounting for 96% of all BDIs. The incidence of BDI has dramatically increased with the adoption of laparoscopy as the method of choice for gallbladder removal. Recent data suggests that incidence resulting from laparoscopic cholecystectomy is 0.3-0.7%, compared to 0.16-0.2% for the traditional open approach. Morbidity and mortality is reported to be as high as 47% and 9%, respectively. It is necessary to encourage surgeons to constantly avoid situations that increase the chance of causing a BDI. An example of such a circumstance is a patient who presents with a severely inflamed gallbladder, in which case the surgeon is advised to consider a two-stage treatment. The first stage would be to "cool down" the gallbladder with antibiotics and/or percutaneous or operative drainage. Thereafter, in the second stage, an elective cholecystectomy can be performed 4-6 weeks later. There are different diagnostic methods used to determine the presence of a BDI. In case a BDI is suspected during cholecystectomy, intraoperative cholangiography can be used to determine the type of injury. An unsuspected BDI may manifest with complications in the immediate post-operative period, or months to year later with symptoms secondary to cholestasis. The Strasberg Classification categorizes BDI from A through E. In type A through D, the defining characteristic is the intact communication between the intrahepatic ducts and the duodenum; in contrast, with Type E injuries this communication is lost. The goals of biliary reconstruction are: to provide definitive internal biliary drainage, to ensure long term anastomotic patency with low chance of stricture, and to avoid major post-operative complications such as bile leak, sepsis, organ failure and death.

Chapter 12 – The ampulla of Vater is a complex region adjoined by three distinct anatomic structures: common bile duct, pancreatic duct and duodenum. This region is lined by mixed intestinal, foveolar and pancreaticobiliary-type epithelium. Adenomas and adenocarcinomas are the predominant primary ampullary tumors. Neuroendocrine tumors, comprised of low grade neuroendocrine tumors (carcinoids) and high grade neuroendocrine carcinomas, are rare. Benign tumor-like lesions constitute a heterogeneous group of entities that includes primary sclerosing cholangitis, recurrent pyogenic cholangitis, inflammatory myofibroblastic tumor, and recently recognized autoimmune pancreatitis and IgG4-related sclerosing cholangitis. Stricture and obstructive jaundice are the most common presentations in ampullary tumors and tumor-like lesions. Despite the advances in imaging techniques, discriminating ampullary carcinoma from benign tumors and tumor-like conditions is still challenging. Differentiating IgG4-related sclerosing cholangitis from primary sclerosing cholangitis and cholangiocarcinoma is particularly important, as IgG4-related sclerosing cholangitis is often responsive to steroid treatment. Immunohistochemical stains can be helpful for histological diagnosis and staging, but they have limitations. The current classification system for ampullary carcinoma has limited value for predicting prognosis. Recent studies have suggested that histological differentiation (intestinal type vs pancreaticobiliary type) and sub-location (intra-AMP, AMP-ductal, peri-AMP-duodenal and AC-not otherwise specified) of ampullary carcinoma have prognostic significance. The treatment for benign tumors and tumor-like lesions is mainly endoscopic local resection. Pancreaticoduodenectomy is the most appropriate resectional procedure for large adenomas and early stage ampullary carcinomas, whereas stent or surgical palliation may be offered for late stage, unresectable cancers. In this review, the authors describe ampullary tumors and tumor-like lesions, and summarize different histological classification systems for ampullary carcinoma. They also address the challenges in discriminating malignant and benign ampullary lesions, and introduce the potential biomarkers for early diagnosis and predicting prognosis. In the meantime, the classical and emerging surgical treatment approaches will be illustrated.

In: Bile Duct
Editor: Miguel Ángel Mercado

ISBN: 978-1-63321-771-3

Chapter 1

Functional Anatomy of Intrahepatic Biliary System (Clinical and Experimental Data)

Dimitri Kordzaia, MD, PhD [1,*]***, Ilia Chanukvadze, MD, PhD*** [2,†]
and Mikheil Jangavadze, MD, PhD [3,‡]
[1]Ivane Javakhisvhili Tbilisi State University (TSU), Tbilisi, Georgia
Al. Natishvili Institute of Morphology, TSU, Tbilisi, Georgia
[2]Department of General Surgery, Tbilisi State Medical University (TSMU), Tbilisi, Georgia
[3]Department of Clinical Anatomy and Operative Surgery, TSU, Tbilisi, Georgia

Abstract

This chapter, "Functional Anatomy of Biliary System (Clinical and Experimental Data)", represents the results of studies implemented since the late 1970s at the Department of Operational Surgery and Topographic Anatomy of Tbilisi State Medical University, under the leadership of Prof. Shalva Toidze, and was later conducted at the Alexandre Natishvili Institute of Morphology of Ivane Javakhisvhili Tbilisi State University. The complex design studies involve both clinical and experimental material, including the anatomical experimental data from autopsy liver material.

The data from experiments, including up to 300 surgeries, 150 autopsies of the human liver and 200 biliary pathology modeling experiments implemented on stray dogs and Wistar rats, were all analyzed. Part of the human liver samples taken at autopsy from

*Dimitri Kordzaia, Professor, MD, PhD, Head of Department of Clinical Anatomy and Operative Surgery, Ivane Javakhisvhili Tbilisi State University /TSU/, Chief researcher of Al. Natishvili Institute of Morphology, TSU, Tbilisi, Georgia.

† Ilia Chanukvadze, Professor, MD, PhD, Department of General Surgery, Tbilisi State Medical University /TSMU/, Tbilisi, Georgia.

‡ Mikheil Jangavadze, Asistant Professor, MD, PhD, Department of Clinical Anatomy and Operative Surgery, TSU, Tbilisi, Georgia.

adult patients whose death was not related to the pathology of hepato-biliary-pancreatic zone were investigated through gradual maceration of parenchyma under spurts of water and separation of the portal tracts and hepatic veins.

The gross histo-topographic sequential slices from every segment of other parts of liver samples were studied to reveal the relationship (interactions) of the bile ducts and mucosal biliary glandswith other structures of the portal tract and hepatic vein tributaries as well. In the other part of the liver samples bile ducts and vessels were preliminarily injected with Indian ink-gelatin mixture for sharp visualization of the lumina of these structures. The corrosion casts of both human and animal bile ducts were prepared by retrograde injection of the solidifying mass (latex and/or methylmetacrilate) into the common bile duct, which was followed by corrosion of liver tissue. The gross caliber structures were studied by binocular magnifier, and the small caliber structures – by a standard method of scanning electronic microscopy.

The lumen relief of gross caliber bile ducts was studied by scanning the electronic microscope as well, after standard preliminary drying of preparations (at the critical point of transformation of liquid CO_2 into the gas, under the set of 100 Atm. pressure and 40°C). Both in dogs and rats the cholestasis was modeled via occlusion of the common bile duct, which was achieved by incision of the latter between two ligatures. The surgery was done through middle laparotomy under general anesthesia. (Sham operations were done in the control group, which implied the middle laparotomy and separation of common bile duct without its ligation or incision). The microscopic study of liver tissue was done by conventional methods of histology and immunohistochemistry. Regardless of the fact, that part of the studies was performed quite long time ago, they still don't have conclusions and their discussion is still ongoing. We think that much of the presented data will evoke the interest of professionals.

We would like to dedicate this publication to the memory of our teacher, renowned scientist and lecturer, Professor Shalva Toidze. Regrettably, the society of hepatologists has not become widely familiar with the results of the studies on the surgical anatomy of the liver and bile ducts implemented by the and his students until now.

Introduction

Specificities of Biliary Tract Architectonics with the Age Related Features

The specificities of the form (size and shape) and branching of intrahepatic bile ducts were studied on corrosion casts of the biliary tree.

In 72%, the common hepatic duct was created by the confluence of two – left and right hepatic ducts. The right hepatic duct, in turn, was created by the confluence of the ducts draining VI-VII and V-VIII segments (right lateral, or inferior and paramedian, or superior ducts) of the liver (here and thereafter below the numeration of segments and sectors are given according to the Couinaud classification). The right paramedian duct was observed to be the most variable, specifically in 17.7% of cases the duct or its tributaries would immediately empty into the common hepatic duct (Figure 1), in 9.5% - into the area of confluence of the right and left hepatic ducts and in 9.4% - into the right hepatic.

The left hepatic duct was created by the junction of the left lateral (dorso-lateral) with the left paramedian (ventro-lateral) ducts draining correspondingly into the II and III-IV liver segments. The biliary duct draining IV segment was observed to be the most variable. In 22% of cases, it would emptydirectly into the common hepatic duct (Figure 2).

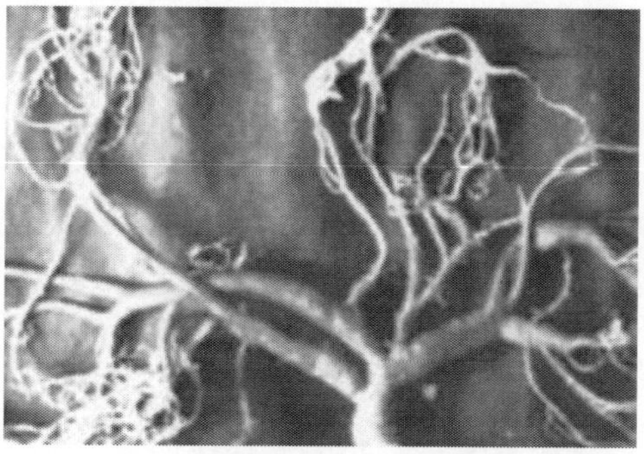

Figure 1. Right paramedian duct joining the common hepatic duct, corrosion specimen.

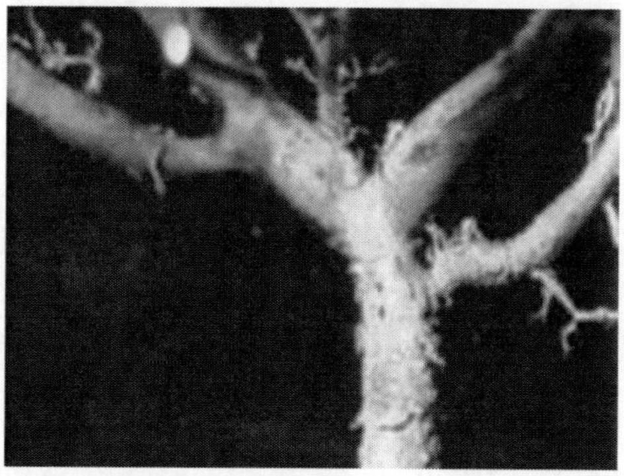

Figure 2. Bile duct of IV segment joining the common hepatic duct, corrosion specimen.

It is essential to consider the above mentioned and other similar variations of biliary duct topography during the surgery, especially in the case of reconstructive interventions on the biliary tract (Burke, McLean, 1989). For instance, in the case of stricture of the bifurcation area, when the duct draining the IV segment empties directly into the bifurcation site or superiorly to it but in very close proximity, formation of biliary-digestive anastomosis with the left hepatic duct will not restore bile drainage from the ventro-medial part of the left hepatic lobe (Couinaud, 1989). A similar situation is expected when the right paramedian duct directly empties into the bifurcation site or in close proximity (Pereira-Lima, 1992).

Therefore, the assessment of confluence patterns of hepatic ducts in the hepatic hilum, only by "manual and visual control", is related to high risks and requires the use of specific means of intraoperative investigation, which will allow both diagnosing of ductular pathologies as well as identification of their topography. But if the intraoperative investigation of the biliary tract is combined with debitometry, it additionally allows the evaluation of the functional status of major duodenal papilla (Niderle et al., 1981; Galperin, Volkova, 1988; Korolev, Pikovsky, 1990). The time spent on these investigations is fully compensated by resuming such "findings" as non-palpable stones, expansion area of structuring cicatrization, anatomical variations and anomalies of the biliary tree, etc., which, if left beyond consideration, involve high risk of complications. There is evidence that 23% of intraoperative damages of bile ducts in site of the confluence of segmental and lobar ducts, in addition to the large portion of 44% of damages occurring at the site of cystic and common hepatic duct junction, are directly conditioned by the underestimation of individual anatomy of the biliary tree (Nechay, Novikov, 1991).

The advancement of reconstructive surgery on biliary ducts, the development of radio-endobiliary and endovascular interventions and liver transplantations added practical significance to the topography investigation of the interaction of intrahepatic portions of vascular and biliary trees in liver segments.

Our data provided below relies upon the study of corrosion casts of biliary and vascular systems, as well as histo-topographic investigations of portal tracts.

It appeared that every branch of the intraorgan portion of the portal vein tree (segmental and smaller branches) might be accompanied by 1-4 bile ducts. When the number of ducts is more than one, one of them appears to be wider than the others. The right and left hepatic ducts, as well as the ducts from II, VI and VII segments are situated superior to the respective branch of the portal vein in more than 90% of cases. The duct from segment III is situated posteriorly while the duct from segment V is positioned medially to the branch of portal vein. The topography of the ducts from other segments and sectors with regard to the respective portal vein branches is relatively variable.

Considering the above-mentioned topography of intrahepatic bile ducts, we support the suggestion of Professor Z. Tskhakia that taking out the distal end of the transhepatic biliary drainage through the biliary duct of the V segment and the bed of the gallbladder is fully acceptable (Vinogradov, Tskhakaia, Pautkin, 1991) and safer, while the same action performed through the diaphragmatic surface of the liver is associated with increased risk of injury of hepatic vein branches crossing over the portal tracts (see below). With age, the biliary ducts become wider and they dislocate closer to the visceral surface of the liver; it is especially notable for the ducts of III and V segments. These circumstances make the method of transhepatic biliary drainage by Z. Tskhakaia more reasonable in elderly patients.

With the process of aging, the angle of confluence of ducts of III-IV segments into the respective collectors (dorso-lateral or left hepatic duct), as well as the left hepatic duct, confluence with the common hepatic duct approach 90° (Figure 3).

Such specificity of architectonics creates the favorable conditions for the development of bile congestion and infection in the left anatomical half of the liver, in contrast with right anatomical half, where the ducts flow into respective collectors through the dull angle. This fact is also evidenced by our clinical data, showing that 78% of cases of intrahepatic cholangiolithiasis were developed in the ducts of the left anatomical half of the liver. The ducts from the left lobe are more frequently injured by Caroli disease as well (Gordeev, Korneev, 1991), which may also be related to the biliary tree anatomy.

With the process of aging, the common hepatic duct and lobar ducts become markedly widened, while the range of their length between 0 – 6.3 cm (mean length 2.5 cm) and 0 – 5, 2 (mean length 1,9) does not seem to be related with age.

The diameter of the common hepatic and lobar ducts in old age exceed the same parameters in young subjects on average twice or more. With growing age, segmental and sub-segmental ducts tend to “shorten” and “widen”.

However, the total volume of the intrahepatic biliary tree is increased, which confirms the increased share of biliary ducts in common hepatic volume in elders.

The study of corrosion preparations of the biliary tree demonstrated that the casts of biliary ducts look like flattened cylinders (their cross sections resemble an ellipse rather than a circle).

In addition, the patterns of the separate ducts are not homogeneous.

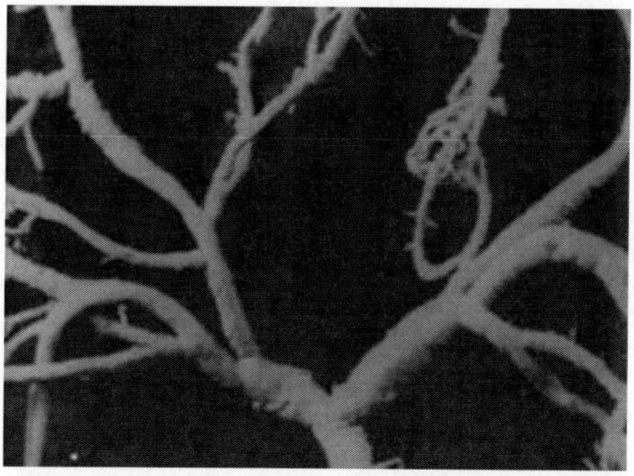

Figure 3. Confluence of left and right lobar bile ducts through 900 angle, male, 76 yr., corrosion specimen.

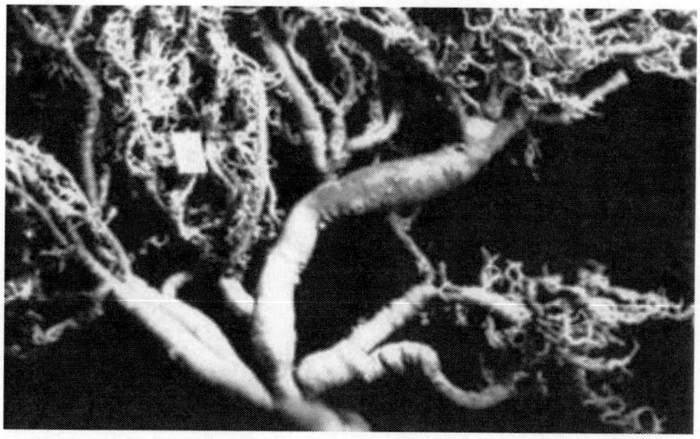

Figure 4. Local "narrowing" at the origin and confluence sites of biliary ducts, male, 65 yr., corrosion preparation.

Specifically, at the sites of duct origin and its confluence (beginning and end points) the casts are more narrowed; as general, the ducts' casts are narrower at the beginning point (Sh. Toidze et al., 1976).

The above-mentioned narrowing of the ducts is more typical for gross caliber ducts and is more markedly expressed in old age (Figure 4).

The quantitative assessment of the incidence of the biliary duct narrowing according to age and linear duct number was performed at the Department of Operative Surgery and Topographic Anatomy of Tbilisi State Medical University under the guidance of Prof. Sh. Toidze (results are presented in Table N1).

It is supposed that the comparable widening of ducts in their middle parts confirms that these sites are more sensitive toward biliary pressure.

Elias (1952, 1955) supposed that some smooth muscle fibers must be located at the sites of origin and confluence of bile duct segments, which may bear a sphincter-like function and participate in the regulation of bile flow. However, the recent investigations denied the presence of more or less expressed muscular layer, although they only confirmed the existence of separate muscular cells, which alone are unable to implement the sphincter function.

Table 1. Characterization of biliary duct lumens at the origin and confluence sites (given in %)

Intrahepatic bile ducts (according to linear order)	20 – 44 yr.			60 yr.		
	narrowed	moderate	widened	narrowed	moderate	widened
I line (lobar ducts)	55%	25%	20%	85%	7.5%	7.5%
II line (sectoral ducts)	45%	35%	20%	82%	10%	8%
III line (segmental ducts)	40%	50%	10%	75%	18%	7%
IV line (sub-segmental ducts)	25%	55%	20%	65%	20%	15%

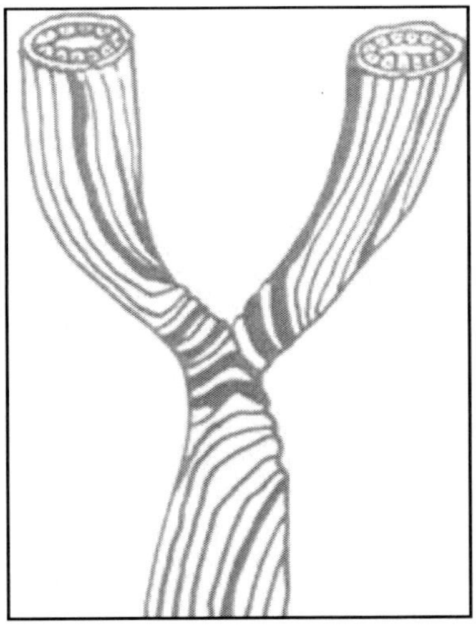

Figure 5. Direction of elastic and muscular (in black) fibers in the wall of bile ducts (scheme).

To clarify the reason of narrowing at the beginning and end points of bile ducts of the I-IV lines, we studied histological slices of sequential sections of bile ducts following their reconstruction. According to our data the walls of the I-IV line bile ducts show elastic and rarely, intermittent muscular fibers situated longitudinally along the axis of the ducts. However, at the sites of origin and confluence of the ducts these longitudinal fibers sharply change direction and localize circularly. These circular fibers are less compliant with the influence of biliary pressure compared with the longitudinal ones (Figure 5).

The Mucosal Glands of Bile Ducts

The description of the biliary pathway is impossible without describing the architectonics of the mucosal biliary glands. They represent the secreting constructions located in the wall (intramural glands) or outside of bile ducts (extramural glands).

The mucosal glands of biliary ducts are referred to as "Glandulae mucosae biliosae" in Paris Anatomical Terminology of 1955 and in the international nomenclature revised by

Tokyo Anatomy Congress in 1975. The name "peribiliary glands" and "mucosal biliary glands" became popular and finally accepted in English-language literature during the last several decades.

Since the 19th century it was already known that biliary ducts in humans and animals are provided by morphologically similar glandular structures. Several authors have described their characteristics. It was established that mucosal biliary glands consist of secretory (glandular), intermediate (cervical) and excretory (ductular) parts.

The last opens into the lumen of bile ducts. The orifices of these gland ductuli can be revealed as a small, sometimes, microscopically small, for aminaon the internal layer of bile ducts (M. Lavdovsky, T. Ovsyanikov, 1888, Venediktov, 1946, Marinozzi, G., et al., Sh. Toidze, I. Chanukvadze, 1978, Yamamoto K. et al., 1985; D. Kordzaya, 1990, Terada, et al. 1987, 1990, 1994; Ishida, et al., 1989).

The interest towards mucosal glands of bile ducts was raised in the last period (Cardinale, et al., 2011; Carpino, G., et al., 2012; Cardinale, et al., 2012). This was reasoned on one hand by the supposition that these mucosal glands represent the hearth of stem cell formation for biliary ducts and thus a source of regeneration of the epithelial duct cover (it is accepted that stem cells located in Hering's ductuli give origin to hepatocytes and biliary epithelial cells of the ductuli; thus the regeneration of biliary tract originates from two sources: the regeneration of bile ducts is initiated from mucosal glands and that of hepatocytes and initial ductuli – from Hering's tubules, respectively). On the other hand, the interest of researchers was directed towards the topic, which considered these glands as the sites for the development of different biliary pathologies, including cholangiocarcinoma (NakanumaY., et al., 1994).

Iamada et al. (1970) demonstrated the significant distinction between the glands of the animals with or without gallbladder. Specifically, the glands of the common bile duct in rats (without gallbladder) show marked absorptive and weak secretive function, while the biliary duct glands of the mouse (with gallbladder) reveal high mucin-secretive activity. The author explained this as the capability of the organism to neutralize the aggressive effect of the concentrated bile ejected from the gallbladder on the epithelium of the common bile duct.

The mucosal glands are provided both by extrahepatic and intrahepatic ducts. They are classified into intramural and extramural glands.

The intramural glands are located within the walls of the bile ducts. They are dispersed throughout the whole perimeter of the duct. These glands are generally tubular, lined with cuboidal or cylindrical epitheliocytes with a basal nucleus and light cytoplasm.

The extramural glands are located in the connective tissue around the bile ducts. These glands may be branched in tubular-alveolar type and composed of lobules enveloped by fibrous tissue. Each of such lobules includes serous and/or mucosal acini. The cells of mucosal acini have a cuboidal or short cylindrical shape and contain the nuclei disposed in basal region. Their cytoplasm is filled with numerous mucosal inclusions. The cells of serous acini have centrally located nuclei and comparatively dark cytoplasm. The secretory lobules of neighboring glands may communicate with each other and create some nodular conglomerate, which opens (drains) into the biliary lumen via several ductuli (Nakanuma Y., et al., 1994; Kordzaya, 1994). Usually the ductular part of the glands is located intramurally.

It is confirmed that mucosal biliary glands are not related with hepatocytes.

The maximal amount of extrahepatic glands is concentrated in the cervix of gallbladder, and at the confluence of hepatic and cystic ducts. The number of glands decreases at the supraduodenal and pancreatic segments of the common bile duct and rises again in close proximity to duodenal (Fater's) papilla. Based on the results of the study of corrosion preparations of biliary trees and histotopograms of portal tracts, it was demonstrated that mucosal biliary glands confluence with common hepatic and lobar ducts circularly - equally from every side, while the glands of sectoral, segmental and sub-segmental ducts generally confluence with the ducts along their lateral surfaces - the small radius ends (poles) of ellipsoid lumina of bile ducts (the anterior and posterior surfaces refer to the opposite sides of bile ducts' ellipsoid lumina circled with greater radiuses. These surfaces address the portal vein branch - from one side, and liver parenchyma - from the other side). Furthermore, the glands of segmental, sub-segmental and finer ducts are disposed symmetrically along the two parallel lines hypothetically drawn across the duct lateral surfaces, while their confluence points are located with 1-2 mm intervals between them. In some cases, these glands communicate with each other via their side branches and create so-called anastomoses (Figures 6-9).

Based on the investigations of corrosion preparations the following types of mucosal biliary glands have been classified: a) Tubular - simple, coiled and branched (without branching of the ductular portion); b) Alveolar - simple and branched (without branching of the ductular portion); c) Compound Tubular and/or Alveolar (with branching of the ductular portion).

The glands related to the common hepatic and lobar ducts are mostly of simple construction (the glands of complex structure are encountered at the origin of the lobar ducts (sites of confluence of sectoral ducts) and also at the angle created by the confluence of lobar ducts at the beginning of the common hepatic duct (C. J. H. Andrews, W. H. H. Andrews, 1979; Ishida et al., 1989; Kordzaia, 1990).

There is evidence that the number of biliary mucosal glands gradually increase in the postnatal period, achieving its maximum at the end of the 1st year (Spitz, Petropoulos, 1978).We have described some age-related peculiarities of these glands, which, in some aspects, account for the age-related specificities of the entire biliary bed.

According to the results of the corrosion specimen studies in the age groups of 20-44 years and 45-59 years, the number of casts of mucosal glands appeared to be identical. Namely, up to 20 patterns of mucosal glands, on average, are observed per each cm of common hepatic, lobar, sectoral and segmental ducts.

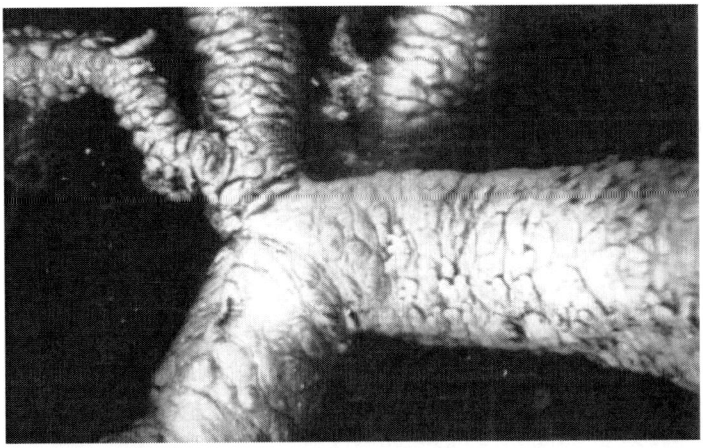

Figure 6. Mucosal biliary glands of common hepatic duct and its tributaries, corrosion specimen.

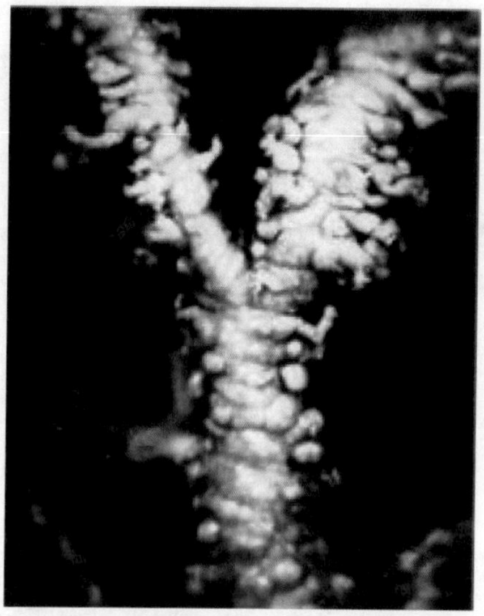

Figure 7. Mucosal biliary glands of segmental duct and its tributaries, corrosion specimen.

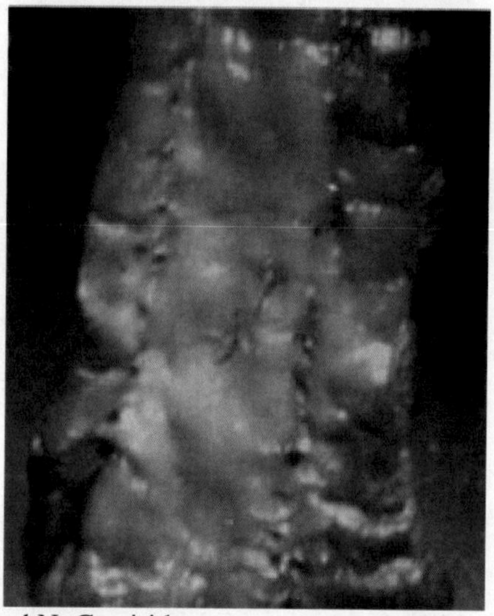

Specimen by Prof. Sh. Toidze and N. Gotsiridze.

Figure 8. Internal relief of segmental duct.

Sectoral and segmental duct glands reveal higher polymorphism compared with the glands of greater caliber (gross) ducts, in some cases their lengths achieve 20-30 mm (Figures 10-13).

It is noteworthy that when the right paramedian duct flows directly into the common hepatic duct, the number of mucosal glands on the hepatic duct dramatically increases distally to the confluence point. This fact can be considered as evidence of the hypothesis by Iamada et al. (1970), according to which the secretions of mucosal glands supposedly act to protect the duct walls from the irritation effect imposed by bile. In the mentioned case, the rise in the number of mucosal glands occurs simultaneously with bile "ejection" from the massive hepatic sector into the common hepatic duct (Figure 14).

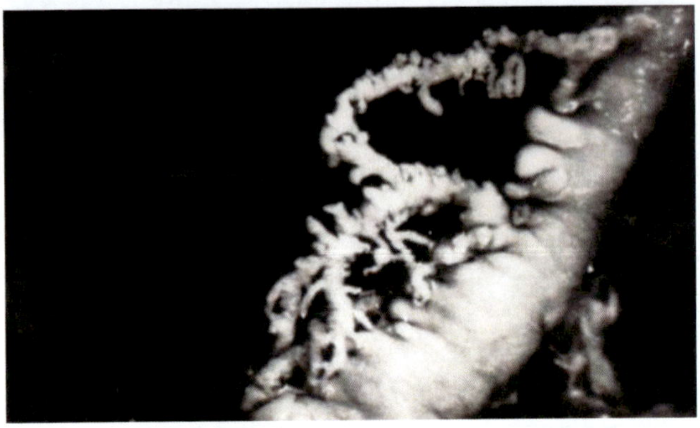

Figure 9. Anastomoses between glandular parts of extramural mucosal biliary glands, corrosion specimen.

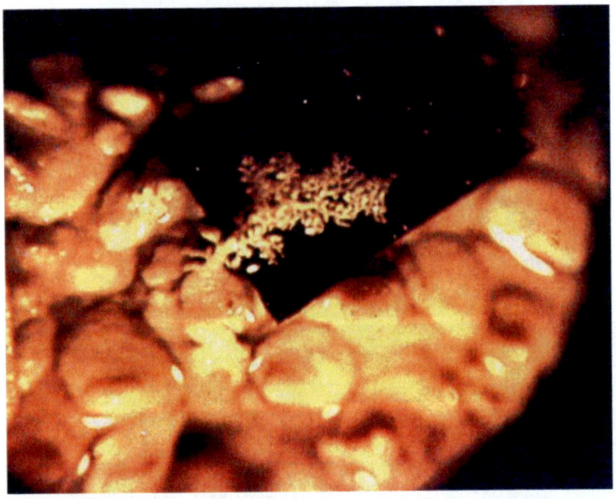

Corrosion specimen by Sh. Toidze.

Figure 10. Complex architectonic gland of common hepatic duct.

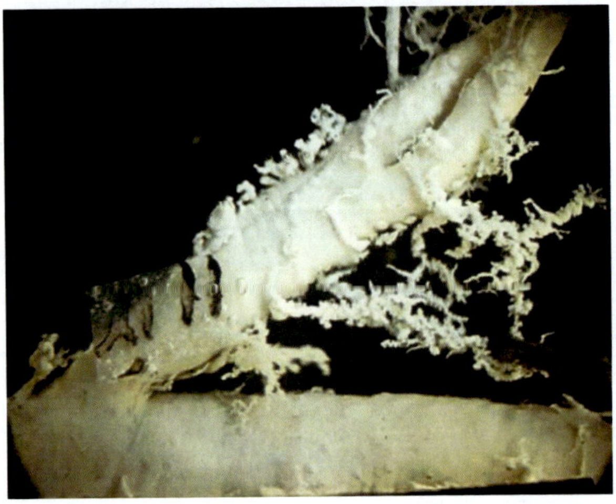

Figure 11. Anastomoses between glandular parts of extramural mucosal biliary glands, corrosion specimen.

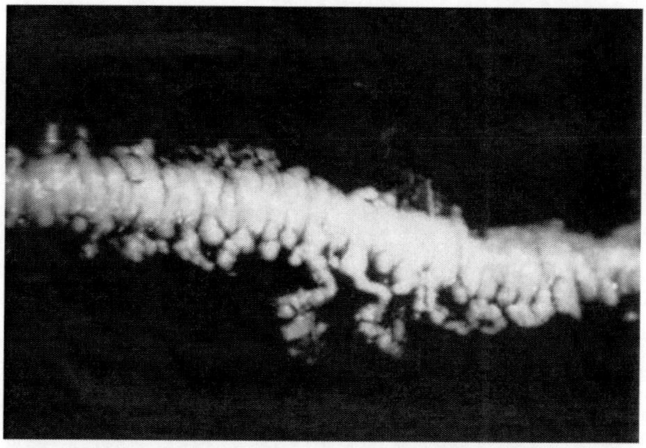

Figure 12. Mucosal biliary glands of segmental duct, corrosion specimen.

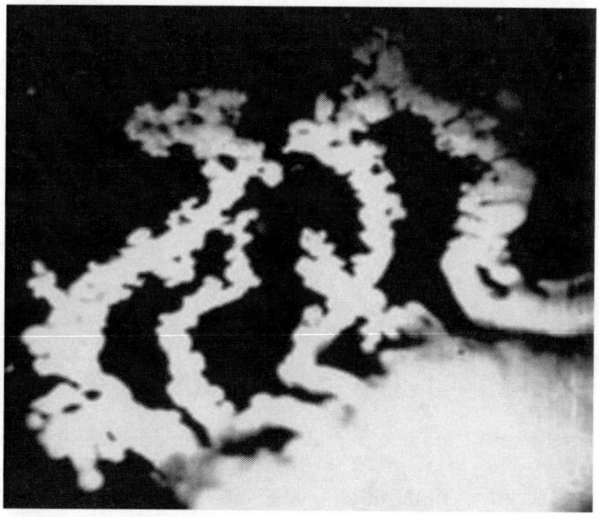

Figure 13. Mucosal biliary glands of segmental duct, corrosion specimen.

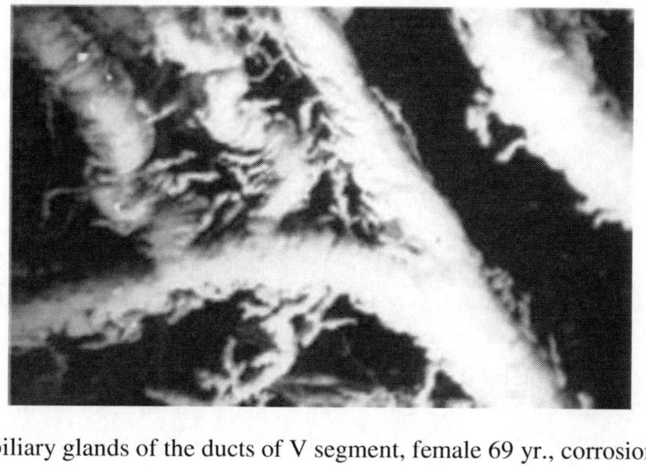

Figure 14. Mucosal biliary glands of the ducts of V segment, female 69 yr., corrosion specimen.

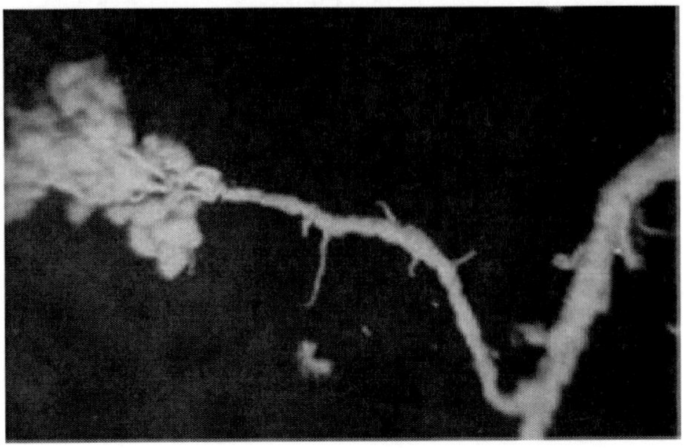

Figure 15. Sublobular and interlobular bile ducts with their networks of bile canaliculi, corrosion specimen.

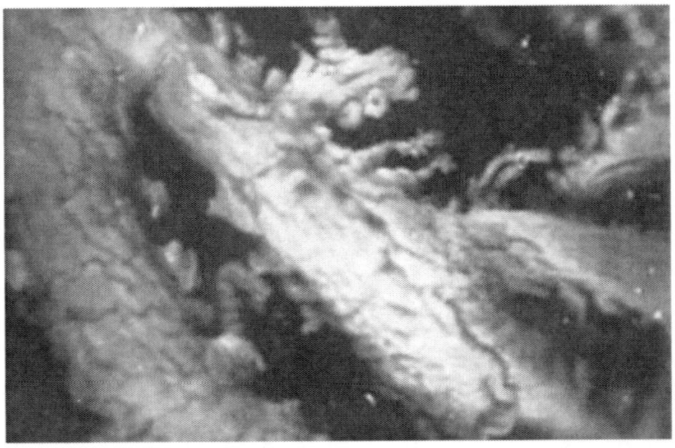

Figure 16. Mucosal biliary glands of segmental bile duct, female, 89 yr., corrosion specimen.

The histotopographic study of hepatic tissue revealed, that the extramural parts of the mucosal biliary glands supplying lobar and common hepatic ducts may be "penetrated" into portal plate in the hilar region; Furthermore, the extramural parts of glands of bile ducts, draining V segments, frequently achieve the cystic plate. Thus, their accidental injury during cholecystectomy must be taken into account; aside from the injury to aberrant ducts (see the sub-chapter "The aberrant Biliary Ducts"), the leakage of bile from the gallbladder bed following cholecystectomy can be considered as a result of the damage to these glands as well, moreover, it is well known that colecystectomy is followed by biliary hypertension.

Based upon these data, we categorically support the idea to leave thin tube (drainage) in the subhepatic space (near Vinslow's foramen) after cholecystectomy even if external draining of the common bile duct has been performed together with gallbladder excision.

The number of mucosal glands over interlobular ducts and their collectors (sub-lobular and septal ducts) is markedly decreased (Terada et al., 1987), (Figure 15).

This fact evidences the hypothesis that small caliber bile ducts mainly act to reabsorb the bile components from the bile collected from the bile canaliculi, in contrast with gross caliber ducts, which, as mentioned above, have a rich supply of glands and are characterized by highly active secretion. Above 60 years of age, the polymorphism of mucosal glands is less prominent. They become shortened, and the lumen of excreting ducts is widened (Figure 16, 17).The overall number of gland patterns also decreases.

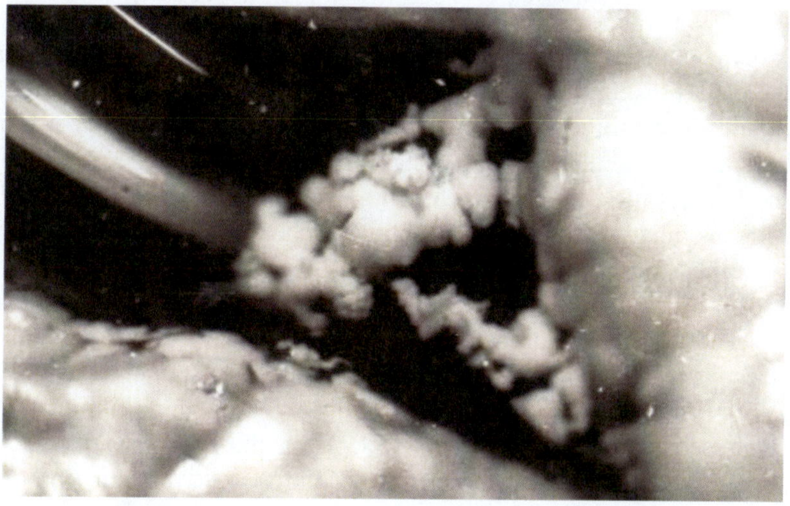

Figure 17. Mucosal biliary glands of segmental bile duct, female, 89 yr., corrosion specimen.

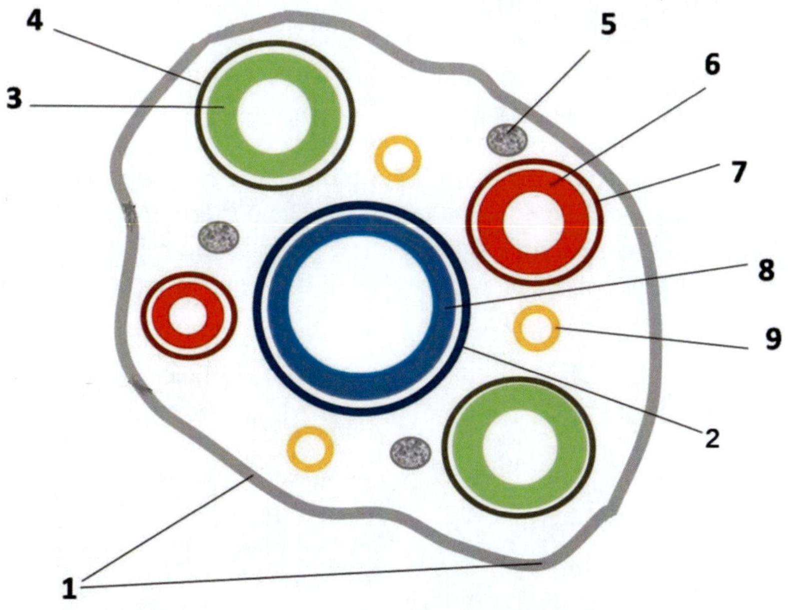

Figure 18. Standard portal tract: 1. perivascular fibrous sheath; 2. periportal tissue; 3. bile duct; 4. peribiliary tissue; 5. nerve; 6. artery; 7. periarterial tissue; 8. portal vein; 9. lymphatic vessel.

Regarding the Topography of Bile Ducts and Their Mucosal Glands Inside Portal Tracts

To reveal the spatial relationship between the biliary ducts and their mucosal glands with other structures of the portal tract, including the connective tissue layers and spaces, we studied the histograms/histotopograms of portal tracts after preliminary injection of the contrast medium (Indian ink and gelatin mixture) through the common bile duct.

The structure of the standard portal tract is presented inFigure18.

Analyzing the construction of connective-tissue framework of more than a thousand histograms/histotopograms of portal tracts, we have classified the fibro-vascular architecture of the portal complex as three consecutively arranged circular sheaths - fibrous-portal, fibrous-arterial and fibrous-biliary layers - enveloped within a fibrous sheath of the whole portal complex –a perivascular fibrous sheath (capsula fibrosa perivascularis - PNA), representing the intrahepatic derivate of Glisson's capsule (portal plate) rich with lymphatic network. The fibrous-biliary layer is located most peripherally. It is represented by branched gross and small caliber ducts, intra- and extramural mucosal biliary glands and peribiliary/ periglandular connective tissue, which is immediately surrounded by firmly attached peri-vasular fibrous sheath. The peri-glandular connective tissue represents the lateral branches of peribiliary connective (fibrotic) tissue. Its recesses contain the extramural portions of mucosal biliary glands. The adhesion of the perivasular fibrous sheath with its fibrous-biliary layer is so firm that their separation is almost infeasible even during the preparation under the microscope: separate extramural glands penetrate within the perivascular fibrous sheath and unite the above-mentioned two layers in one compound complex. This brings the lymphatic network of perivascular fibrous capsule in extremely close contact with biliary structures (Chanukvadze I., 1979, 2003, 2009, 2010, 2011, 2012).

In the magistral portal complexes the blind glandular terminals of extramural mucosal glands, related to the lateral surfaces of adjacent bile ducts, may reach each other and occupy almost all of the space between them (Figures 19-22).

However, the anterior (internal) surface of the biliary duct facing the center of the portal tract is in close relationship with the fibrous-arterial layer and is subjected to constant "trauma" - due to pulsation of liver arterial branches. The posterior (external) surface of the biliary duct is facing the parenchyma. Both of these surfaces are free from mucosal biliary glands or the glands situated on these areas are small and don't occupy the space inside the portal tracts (intramural glands).

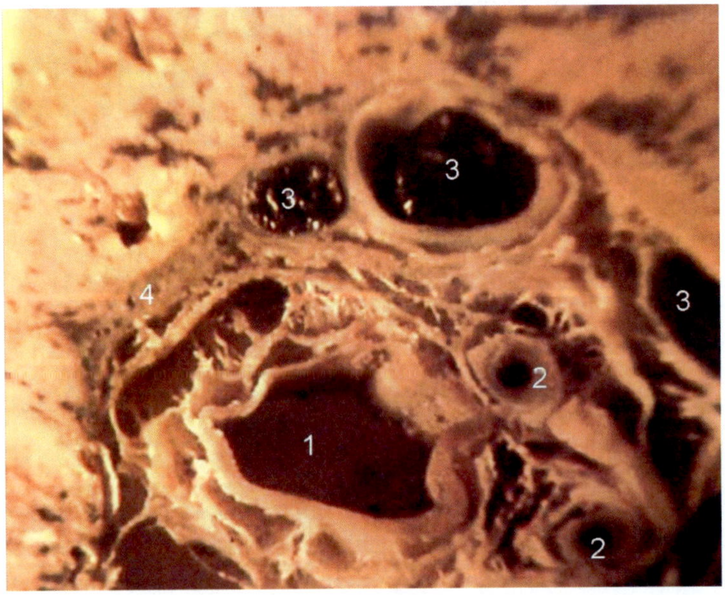

Figure 19. Lobar portal tract; 1. portal vein; 2. artery; 3. bile ducts are filld with ink-gelatine mixture; 4. mucosal biliary duct.

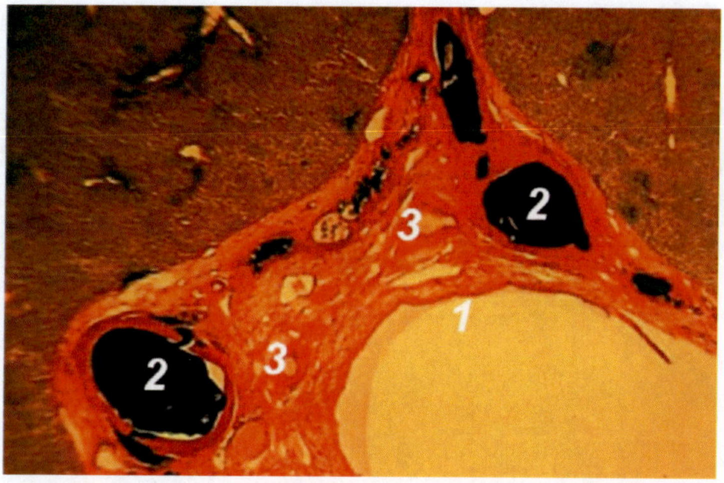

Figure 20. Gross histotopogram from the left hepatic lobe (32 year old male; magnification 1 X 8). 1.Major portal complex; 2.Hepatic vein; 3.Parenchyma; 4.Bile duct; 5.Portal vein; 6. Hepatic artery.

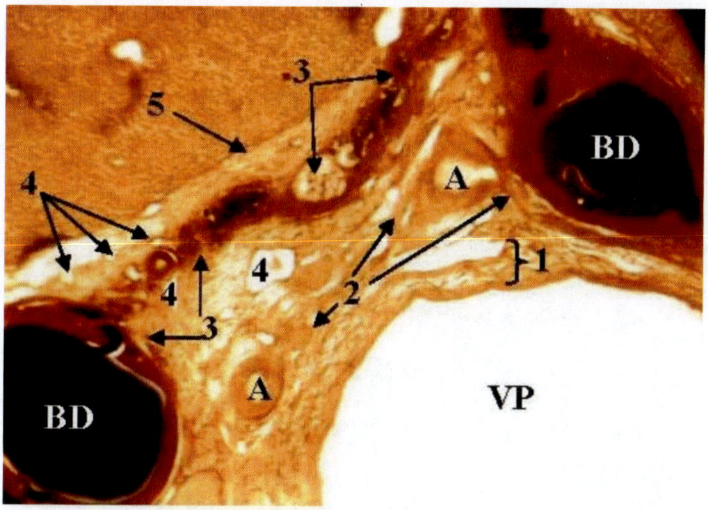

Figure 21. Fragment of portal tract; VP – portal vein; A – artery; BD – bile ducts (filled with ink-gelatine mixture); 1. portal fibrous layer; 2. arterial fibrous layer;3. extramural mucosal gland; 4. biliary fibrous layer; 5. perivascular fibrous sheath.

On the basis of all above, we have presented the structure of the portal complex not by traditional portal triad, but with all elements of the portal complex including the fibrous framework creating the soft skeleton of the portal tract – "skeleton mole" (Figure 23).

Aberrant Bile Ducts - Ducts of Lushka

In part of our liver specimens, we have described the ducts with unusual locations; they do not accompany the other elements of the portal complex and are frequently located beyond the liver parenchyma (e.g. within hepatic ligaments, portal plate and gallbladder bed) however they flow into the intrahepatic ducts.

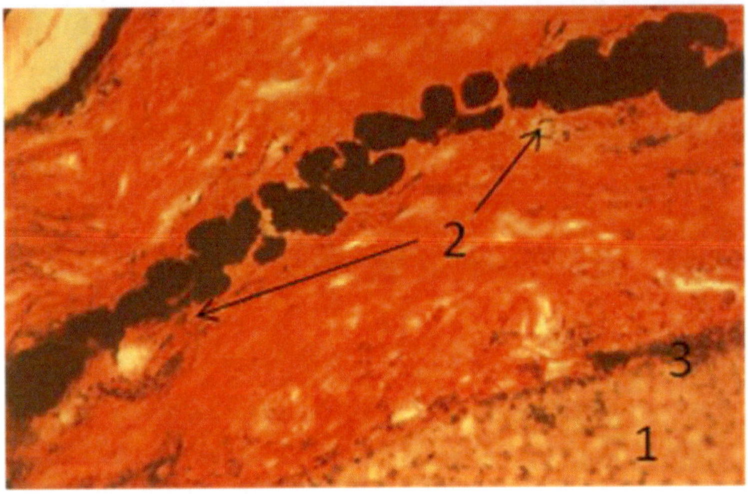

Figure 22. Fragment of portal tract; 1. parenchema; 2. extramural mucosal biliary gland (filled with ink-gelatine mixture); 3. perivascular fibrous sheath.

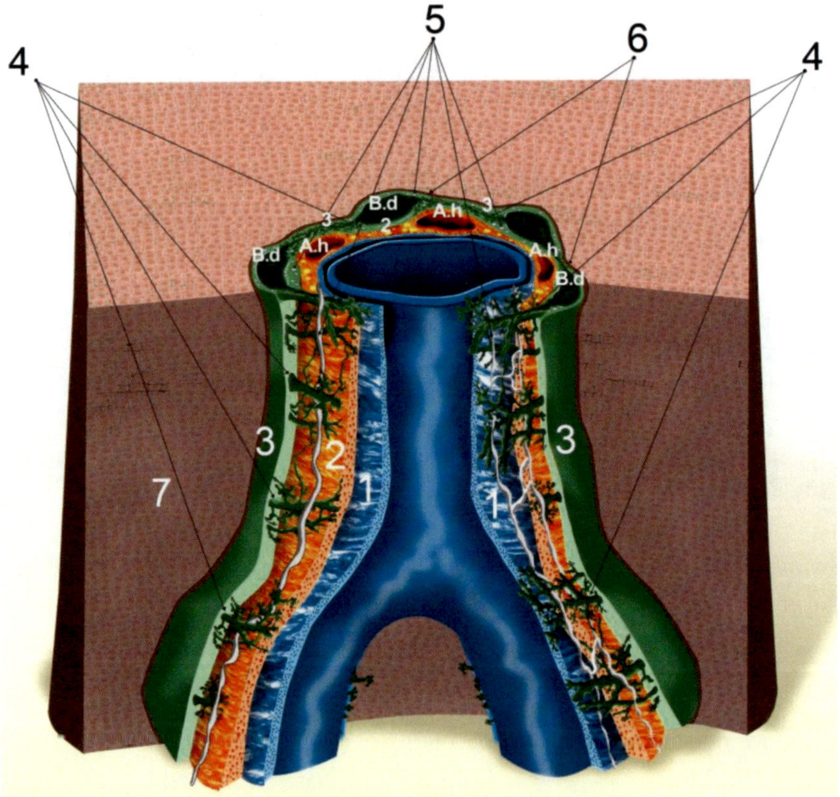

Figure 23. Vasculo-fibrous architecture of the major portal tract (per I. Chanukvadze) V.P. Portal vein; B.D. Bile ducts; A. Hepatic arteries. 1. Fibrous sheath of the portal vein; 2.Fibrous interarterial sheath; 3.Parabiliary connective tissue and perivascular fibrous capsule (6) forming an extensive outer fibrous sheath around the elements of the portal complex; 4.Mucous biliary glands; 5. Lymph ducts; 7. Hepatic tissue.

The aberrant ducts have become a subject of significant interest among the biliary tree abnormalities, due to the high risk of their injury during different surgical interventions with consequent complications. For instance, the intraoperative damage to the gross aberrant ducts due to the section of the left triangular ligament has been described, which occurred during left hepatic lobe mobilization performed in gastric resection surgery. This injury to aberrant ducts resulted in the development of biliary peritonitis (Niderle et al., 1982).

In our specimens, the aberrant ducts were found in falciform, left triangular and posterior coronary ligaments of liver, also in the connective tissue bridge situated on the posterior part diaphragmatic surface of the liver and bordered the channel for inferior vena cava. In addition, they have been found in Glisson's sheath, especially in the portal and bladder plates.

The aberrant bile ducts are named as "ducts of Lushka" after German morphologist Herbert von Lushka, who described them in 1863 (Ko K., et al., 2006). Generally, the duct of Lushka represents a short rudimentary biliary tube of approximately 1-2 mm diameter, located within the gallbladder bed (McQuillan T., et al., 1989). It carries bile from the duct(s) of the lateral hepatic sector to the common hepatic (McQuillan T., et al., 1989; Jenkins M., et al., 1994) or cystic duct (Jahanl M., et al., 2009). A Duct of Lushka may penetrate from gallbladder bed (cystic plate) into its adventitia but it does not empty into the bladder cavity. Thus, it may be considered as a subvesicular duct (McQuillan T., et al., 1989;JenkinsM., et al., 1994).

However, in two cases of colecystectomy we found the bile ducts coming out from the liver parenchyma and immediately flowing into the gallbladder. Taking into consideration that they are "sole" ducts – not accompanied by respective branches of the portal vein and hepatic artery - we consider referring them to the group of aberrant ducts as well. Possible topography of such aberrant ducts must be kept in account during cholecystectomy.

In most cases, they can be simply ligated (see chapter XXX). Non-ligated Lushka ducts at cholecystectomy may become a reason for bile extravasation and the development of biliary peritonitis afterwards. The inflammatory pathologies of gall bladder may be accompanied with marked proliferation of Lushka ducts, which microscopically resembles the image of adenocarcinoma (Healey J., Schroy P., 1953; Jahanl M., et al., 2009). The rare cases of intraductular and invasive adenocarcinoma of Lushka ducts have been also described (Healey J., Schroy P., 1953; Jahanl M., et al., 2009, Mori S., Kasahara M., 2001).Interestingly, recent histological studies show that in frequent cases, a duct of Lushka is not represented by a solid tube, but rather a network of small-sized ducts (Jenkins M., et al., 1994).

According to autopsy material data, the sub-vesicular aberrant ducts are presented in approximately 1/3 of the total population. However, our observation shows that aberrant biliary ducts are better and more frequently visualized in older age. They can be clearly seen under Glisson's sheath after injecting the biliary tract with latex (for the preparation of biliary corrosion casts) or different contrast masses (e.g. Indian ink). In several cases, we have discovered the cast of an originally shaped aberrant bile duct, which extended rather far from the respective collector. They were provided by the casts of mucosal glands disposed by keeping the "strict" order of paralleling, symmetry and intervals between them (Figure24).

In addition, since the aberrant ducts are not related to biliary capillary network, they cannot be bearing the function of bile drainage. They represent something like reservoirs, in which bile can be mobilized when biliary pressure increases. These ducts can also participate in the formation of the ultimate chemical composition of bile, as well (through the secretion of their numerous mucosal glands).

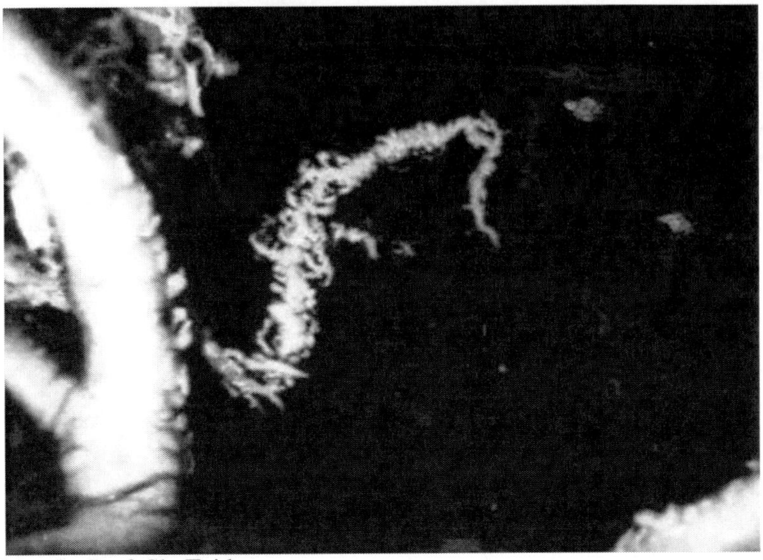

Corrosion specimen by Prof. Sh. Toidze.

Figure 24. "Aberrant duct"; male, 72 yr.

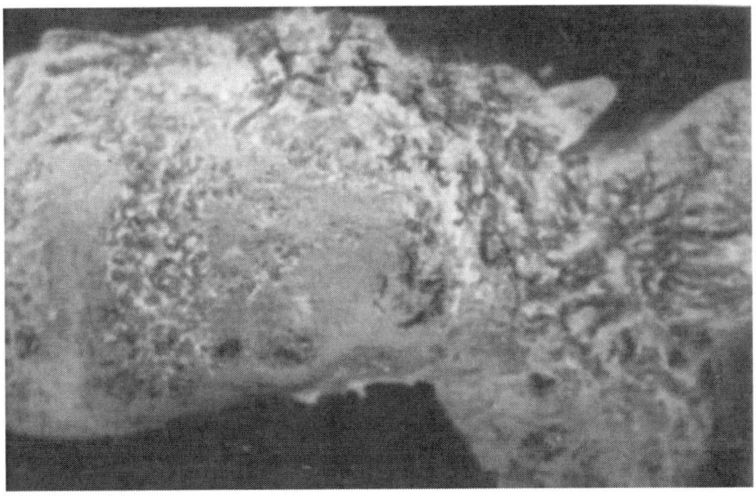

Specimen by Prof. Sh. Toidze.

Figure 25. "Vasa aberantia", female, 85 yr., superficial corrosion preparation of liver.

The fact that the aberrant bile ducts originate in the connective tissue structures, rich in the lymphatic network, like hepatic capsules and different ligaments, gives us the basis to suppose that they may be involved in establishing the biliary-lymphatic communication (interaction) in the setting of biliary congestion.

There is no uniform theory about the origin of aberrant ducts. Some researchers relate them to the anomalies of embryogenesis. Liver, intrahepatic bile ducts, gallbladder and extraheptaic bile ducts develop from hepatic diverticulum, which appears at the beginning of the 4th week of fetal development. The gallbladder is formed from the ventral part of the diverticulum, while the cranial part gives origin to primordial liver, which subsequently undergoes proliferation and generates hepatic cells and epithelium of intrahepatic bile ducts.

Proliferation of the last leads to the development of hepatic ducts, which originally have the shape of a plexus (ductal plate).Many of such ducts undergo involution in the 4th-5th weeks of embryogenesis and eventually create the familiar model of biliary tree architectonics. However, some of plates may be preserved. Thought, the aberrant ducts (ducts of Lushka) may result from such atypical involution of the fetal biliary plexi (ductal plates) (Champetier J., et al., 1991; Schneck C., 1994).

At the same time we also shared the opinion of Prof. Sh. Toidze, suggesting that the sharper appearance of aberrant ducts under the hepatic capsule in elders may be caused by the age-related involution of hepatic tissue, resulting in the depletion of small blood vessels and making the "sole" biliary ducts more visible (Figure 25).

Bile Ducts and Their Mucosal Glands in the Sites of the Porta-Caval Fibrous Connection – Less Known but Permanent Anatomical Structure

There are the less known anatomical details within the human liver formed through the confluence of fibrous sheathes of the portal canals and those of the hepatic veins in the areas where these structures come into contact and interdigitate (Figure 26).

Here the perivascular fibrous capsule (capsula fibrosa perivascularis – Paris Nomina Anatomica) enveloping the intrahepatic portion of the portal triad (the portal vein, the hepatic artery, and the bile duct) extends toward the hepatic vein and involves this vessel as the fourth element (Figure 27) (I. Chanukvadze, 1979, 1989, 2003, 2012).

We have implemented the term - "porta-caval fibrous connections" (PCFC) for the anatomical structure formed through the confluence of fibrous envelopes of the intrahepatic bile ducts and those of the hepatic veins (Chanukvadze, 1979, 1980, 2009).

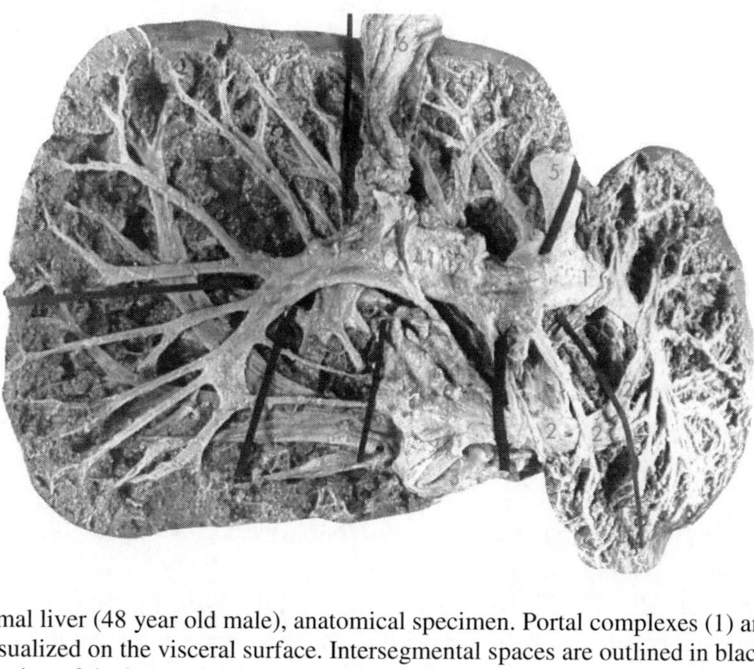

Figure 26. Normal liver (48 year old male), anatomical specimen. Portal complexes (1) and hepatic veins (2) are visualized on the visceral surface. Intersegmental spaces are outlined in black; 3. Inferior vena cava; 4.Portion of the hepatoduodenal ligament; 5.Round ligament.

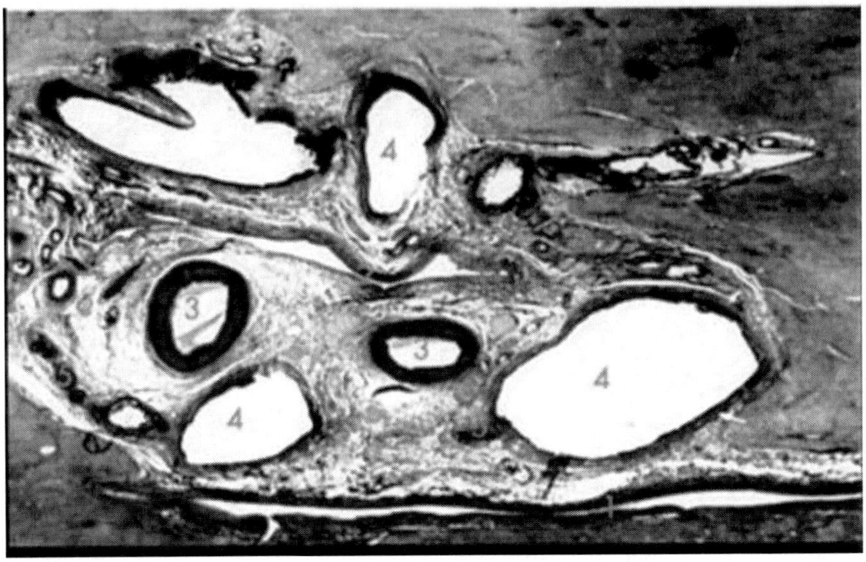

Figure 27. Sectoral portal complex and hepatic vein, histotopogram (68 year old male; magnification 1 X 8). 1.Hepatic vein; 2.Portal vein 3.Hepatic artery; 4.Bile duct; 5.Mucosal biliary gland (filled with an ink-gelatin mixture).

Classification of Intrahepatic Porta-Caval Fibrous Connections

The following forms of the intrahepatic porta-caval fibrous connections (IHPCFC) can be distinguished based on the area of fusion of fibrous sheathes of the portal tracts and the hepatic veins.

The complete fusion of fibrous sheathes of the portal tract and the hepatic vein with the surfaces facing each other (Figures 28, 29) was found in 72.5% of cases. This type of connection can principally be seen within II and III segments of the liver.

But despite the tight contact of the portal triads and hepatic veins in the areas PCFC, the narrow space between these structures, filled with loose connective tissue, can be always identified. This space is bordered by a portion of the perivascular fibrous capsule, which continues from the portal triad over the hepatic vein.

The above-mentioned space is traversed by small vessels (caliber up to 1.5 mm), branching-out from the hepatic artery branches and dislocating toward the hepatic veins, feeding their walls. These vessels can be observed through the injection of the hepatic artery system by an Indian ink-gelatin blend (Figure 30).

The number of vessels reaching the hepatic vein walls through the IHPCFC depends on the area of fused fibrous sheathes of portal tracts and hepatic vessels. Except for the arterial branches, the nerve fibers and lymphatic vessels are also found in the above-mentioned loose connective tissue space. The nerves extend from the portal complexes onto the hepatic vein walls and take part in their innervation. The lymphatic vessels create the communication among two direction-drained lymphatic plexi - accompanying portal tracts and the hepatic veins. These communicating lymphatic vessels should be taken into account in oncological practice as a potential path for metastases.

Partial fusion of IHPCFC occurs in sites where the perivascular fibrous capsule and the fibrous sheath of the hepatic vein, fusing with each other, leave the recess-like lateral spaces filled with hepatic tissue (Figure 31).

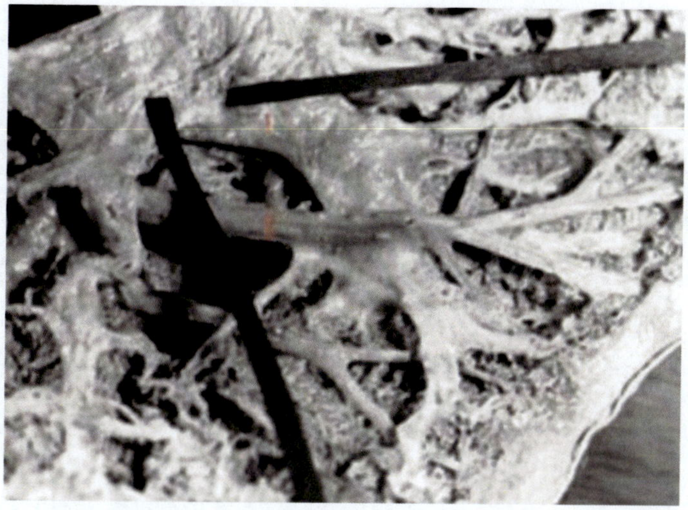

Figure 28. Hepatic segment III (42 years old male).Major portal complex (1) and left hepatic vein (2) form complete fusion of the IHPCFC.

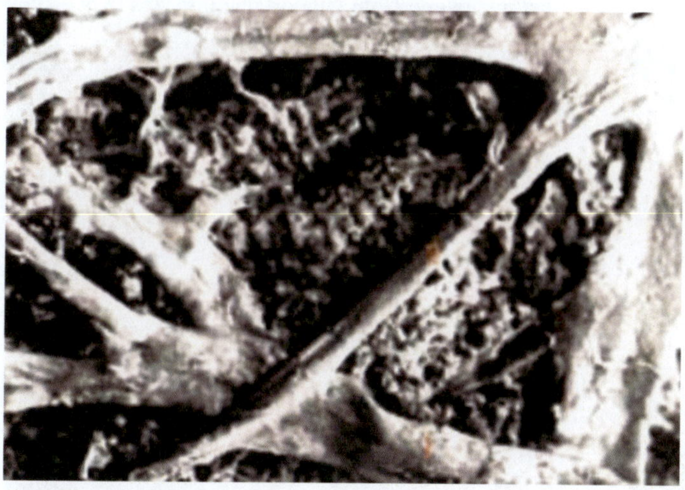

Figure 29. Hepatic segment II (56 year old male).Major portal complex (1) and left hepatic vein branch (2) form complete fusion of the IHPCFC.

Similar to complete fusion, these connections also contain arterial branches, the nerves and lymphatic vessels dislocating from portal complexes toward hepatic veins.

The separate form of IHPCFC is laminar connection.

It is formed through a fibrous lamina between the perivascular fibrous capsule and the hepatic vein sheath. They firmly attach portal tracts to hepatic veins.

These structures also contain small blood and lymphatic vessels (Figure 32).

Relationship of the portal tract structures with hepatic veins within IHPCFC is less variable: the hepatic vein in general is adjusted to the bile duct (78.2%). It is conditioned by an extremely peripheral location of the bile ducts within the portal tract.

Moreover, the bile ducts and their extramural mucosal glands are frequently the only structures of the portal area having contact with the hepatic vein (Figure 33).

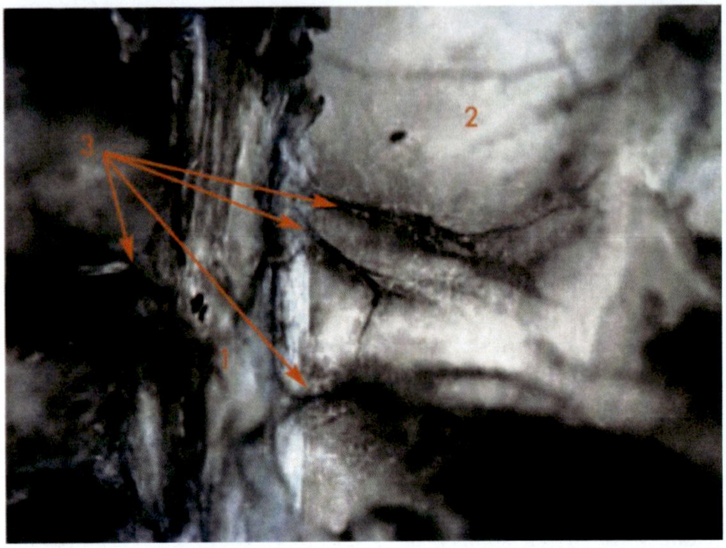

Figure 30. Gross sample from the liver of a 41-year-old male. 1. Portal complex; 2. Hepatic vein wall; 3.Small arteries injected with Indian ink extend from the portal complexes to hepatic vein wall.

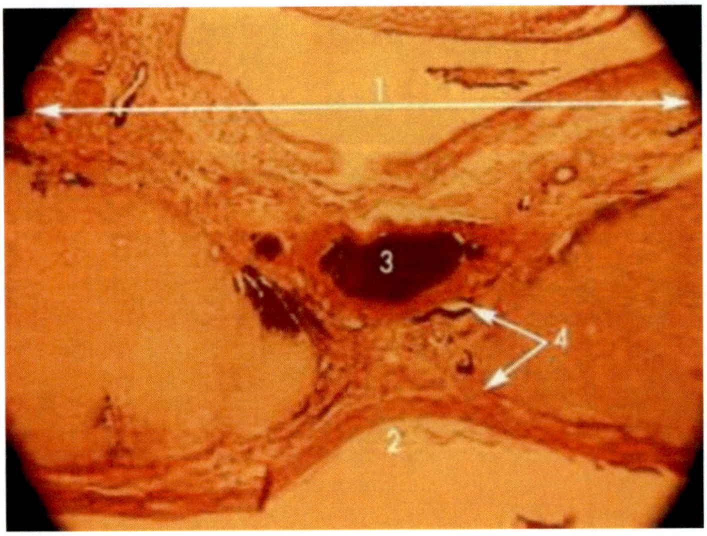

Figure 31. Hepatic segment II, histotopogram (62 years old male; X8). Major portal complex (1) and left hepatic vein wall (2) form the incomplete IHPCFC; 3. Bile duct (filled with ink-gelatin mixture); 4. Lymphatic vessels.

Therefore, the direct anatomical contact between the hepatic veins (from one side) and the bile duct and biliary mucosal glands (from the other) is a characteristic feature of IHPCFC. It appears that like arterial branches, lymphatic vessels and nerve fibers, the extramural biliary mucosal glands can also be dislocated from portal tracts toward hepatic veins and firmly attach to their wall. In 1975 we gave the pilot description of the extramural mucosal biliary glands (Chanukvadze I.) The location of these glands within IHPCFC creates an interesting situation: the branches (processes) of peribiliary connective tissue, containing the mucous glands, traverse free space within the IHPCFC and reach the wall of the hepatic vein (Figure 34).

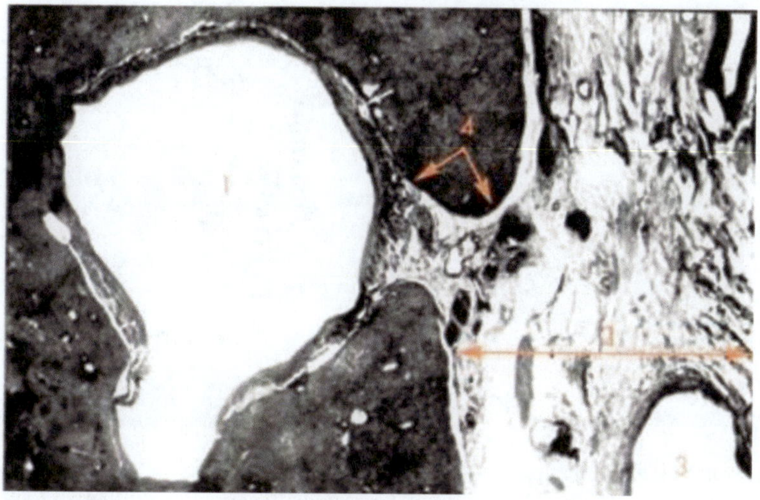

Figure 32. Hepatic segment IV; histotopogram (62 years old male; X8).Laminar IHPCFC. 1.Hepatic vein; 2. Portal field; 3.Bile duct; 4. Porta-caval fibrous connection contains lymphatic vessels.

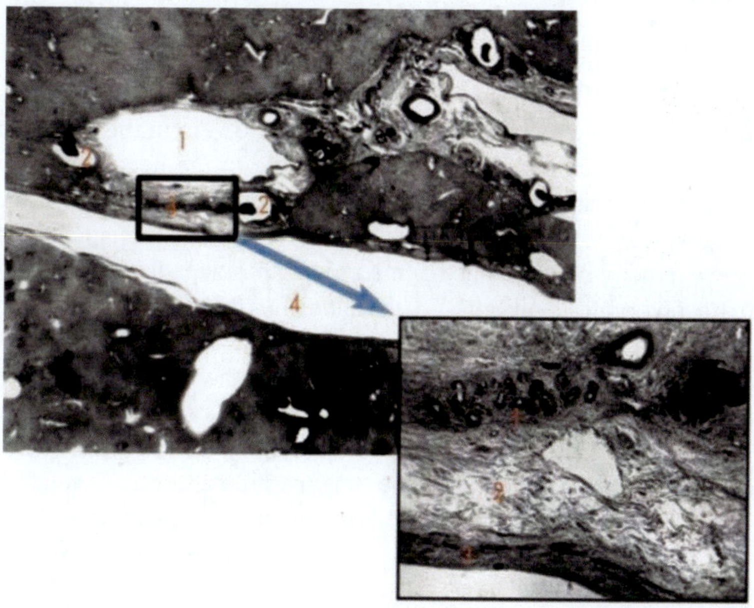

Figure 33. Porta-caval fibrous connection. 1. Parenchyma; 2. Glands of bile ducts from the portal complex zone; 3.Hepatic vein wall.

Specific importance should be given to the close relationship of extramural glands with hepatic veins in the area of the porto-caval fibrous connections.

We suppose that the immediate contact of hepatic veins with bile ducts and their extramural mucosal glands create actual conditions for the spread of pathological processes from the biliary tract (cholangitis and pericholangitis) to hepatic veins (Budd-chiary, Mellory syndromes) (Chanukvadze I., 1979, 1989; Toidze, Chanukvadze, 1978).In the setting of cholestasis, a dilated bile duct may compress the hepatic vein wall and thus significantly affect the draining function of this vein. This notion is supported by the results of the studies, which applied the filling of bile ducts with Indian ink-gelatin under high pressure.

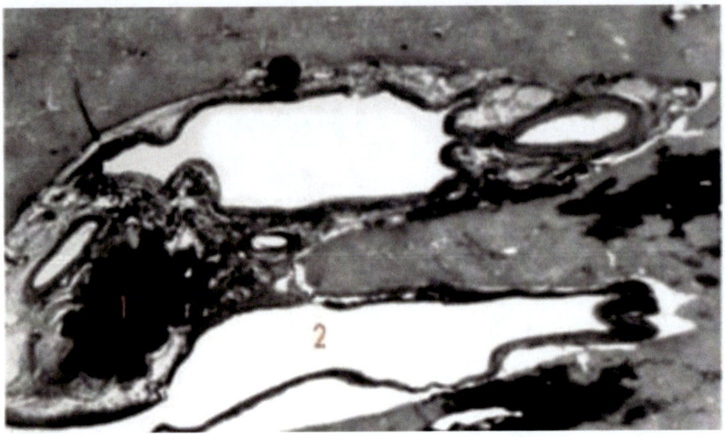

Figure 34. Portal complex and hepatic vein, histotopograph (83 year old male, magnification 1 X 8). 1. Dilated bile duct (injected with ink-gelatin mixture) obstructs the hepatic vein lumen (2) from the side of the portal complex.

Within the areas of porta-caval fibrous connections, injected ducts compressed hepatic veins, narrowing their lumens. Naturally, a complete or partial obstruction of the hepatic vein impairs its draining function and causes the congestion of caval blood within the liver.

In addition, age-related dilation of bile ducts may exert similar pressure on hepatic veins. Of the portal triad elements, the portal vein faces the hepatic vein in the region of IHPCFC in 15% of all cases. This configuration is most characteristic to the hepatic segment III, where the hepatic vein commonly margins the portal tract from beneath.

The close anatomical relationship between the portal and hepatic veins within the IHPCFC is of great practical importance for surgical intrahepatic portacaval shunting for which it provides a favorable condition. Of the elements of portal triad, the major hepatic artery borders the hepatic vein relatively rarely (4.4%).

The number of IHPCFC depends, to some degree, on the branching pattern of both the portal tract and the hepatic vein system. Thus, the number of IHPCFC per liver is much smaller when these vessels exhibit a "magistral" branching pattern (3-5 per liver) rather than a sparse pattern (up to 20 in total). However, the "magistral" pattern is characterized by more massive IHPCFC formed by a larger portal and caval branches (19-20 mm).

Internal Layer of Bile Ducts (Data of Scanning Electron Microscopy)

The application of scanning electronic microscopy (SEM) has provided the advantage of the study with magnification of surface reliefs by 10 – 100,000 times and higher, which facilitated the research, clarification and study of morphology of different cellular, tubular and connective-tissue structures of the liver.

Comparing the data retrieved by SEM of luminal surfaces of bile ducts with the date, received through the investigation of their corrosion casts, allowed us to describe precisely the peculiarities of the biliary pathway, including its age-related features (Kordzaia, 1990).

The SEM study of the reliefs of the common hepatic duct and the ducts of the I and II line ducts, obtained during the autopsies of adults (20-59 years), revealed the lumina of mucosal glands (10-12 patterns per 4 mm^2 area) with diameters ranging between 0.1-0.5 mm.

Large crypts (with diameters of up to 1 mm) were observed in the luminal surface of the common bile duct. They frequently appeared as crater-like grooves, with smaller lumina opening at their floor and walls (Figure 35). The corrosion casts of the mentioned construction may be presented in the shape of several trees (or bushes), which emerge on the small hill, following its radial direction (Figure 10).

In the 60-74 years age group, the general relief of bile ducts is more even. The above-mentioned perforated craters with smaller lumina are more prominent in the common bile duct; in addition, the diameter of the crater itself increases, while the depth decreases (Figures 36, 37).

In the 75-89 year age group, the relief of bile ducts shows widened and coarsened lumina of the ductuli of mucosal biliary glands, the diameters of which exceed 1 mm in some cases; In addition, the "craters" are flattened and deformed to such extent, that their walls cover the floor like a "cap". This creates the impression that the draining ducts of mucosal glands flow into the crater through their "lateral sides", under the umbrella of the "cap" (Figure 38).

However the epithelial cells lining the ducts are rarely and randomly observed while reviewing the micro-relief; the peculiarities described above actually depict the specificities of the sub-mucosal layer. The mentioned phenomenon represents one of the particular cases of the so-called embalmed cadaver changes. (The duct specimens were taken in autopsies performed in 6-32 hours after confirmation of death. It is proposed that to study mucosal relief by SEM, the specimens should be taken not later than 1.5-2 hours after death (Ravensky, 1977).

Considering this suggestion, to specify the age-related peculiarities of the luminar surface of the biliary tract, we studied the bile ducts of 10 adult dogs and 6 puppies of 2-3 months age immediately after their death. To conduct the comprehensive analysis we also studied the corrosion casts of the ducts.

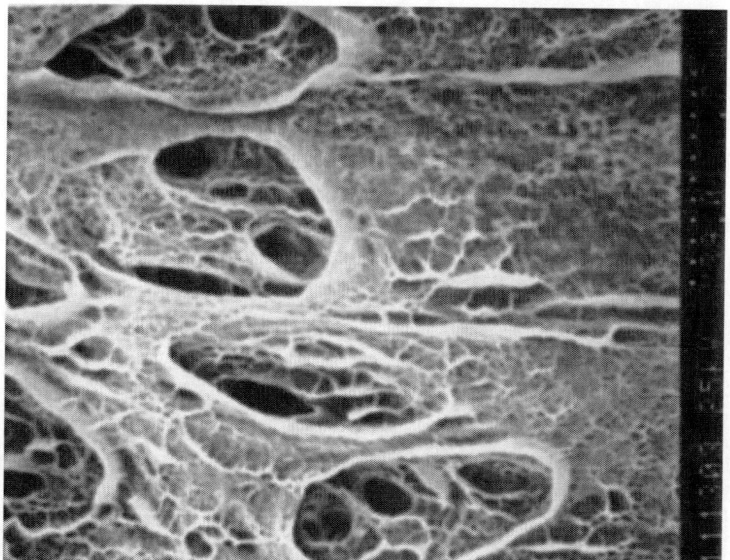

Figure 35. The scanogram of the lumen surface of common hepatic duct, male, 46 yr.

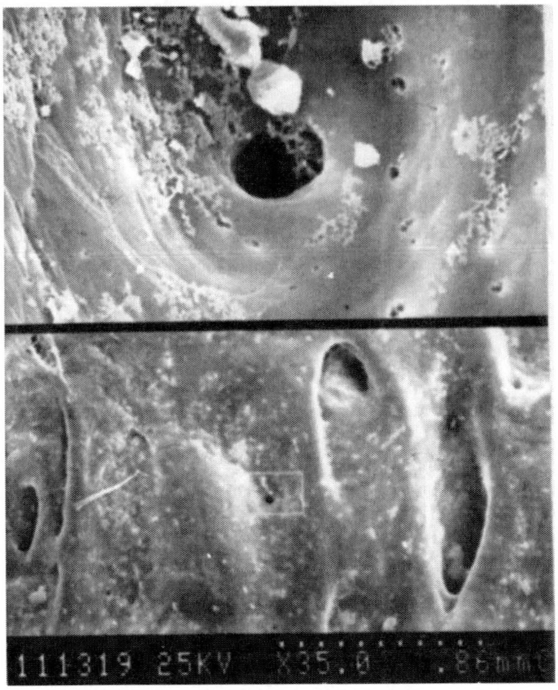

Figure 36. The scanograms of the lumen surface of common hepatic duct, female, 72 yr.

The corrosion preparations of I-IV line bile ducts of canines, like the human's duct patterns, are represented in the shape of slightly flattened cylinders, the diameter of which decreases insignificantly at the duct origin and confluence points. The surface of the casts is fine granular–rough. Slim, transversely disposed circular plicae (folds) are observed more clearly on the patterns of the I-II line, less clearly – of the III-IV line ducts, but again become more evident in patterns of smaller caliber. The casts of bile ducts are provided by casts of mucosal biliary glands, which sometimes are encountered as small hills or flat, leaf-like appendages (mostly on the I-II line bile ducts); in some cases they appear as branched appendages looking like a bush (mostly on the III-IV line ducts) but randomly as fine long tubular appendages with rare branching, extended significantly far from the respective duct (mostly seen on the IV-V line ducts).

In addition, it should be noted that in some cases the patterns of bile glands were not found at all on particular sections of the duct pattern. However, like the human biliary tract, the gland casts can always be found in the confluence sites of gross caliber bile ducts; the numerous lateral appendages of these glands may establish additional communication among the adjacent and/or joining ducts, thus creating the web-like structure.

The cast of mucosal glands of I line ducts are disposed evenly around the whole perimeter of the duct. On the II-IV line ducts, the glands tend to dispose at the two parallel lines drawn along the lateral surfaces of the ducts. But if such tendency is not observed and the glands are disposed around the duct more or less evenly, then the patterns of the glands associated with lateral surfaces of the ducts are longer and more polymorphic, compared with the patterns associated with the other two surfaces of the duct. The corrosion casts of mucosal biliary glands of small caliber ducts are mostly disposed in the same manner – along the lateral surfaces of the ducts. They are quite long, though less polymorphic.

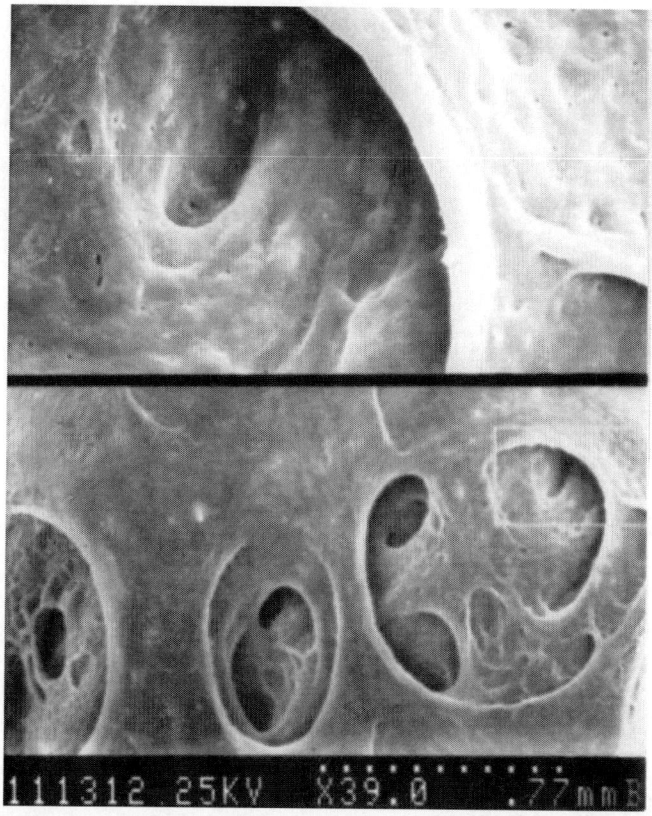

Figure 37. The scanograms of the lumen surface of common hepatic duct, female, 72 yr.

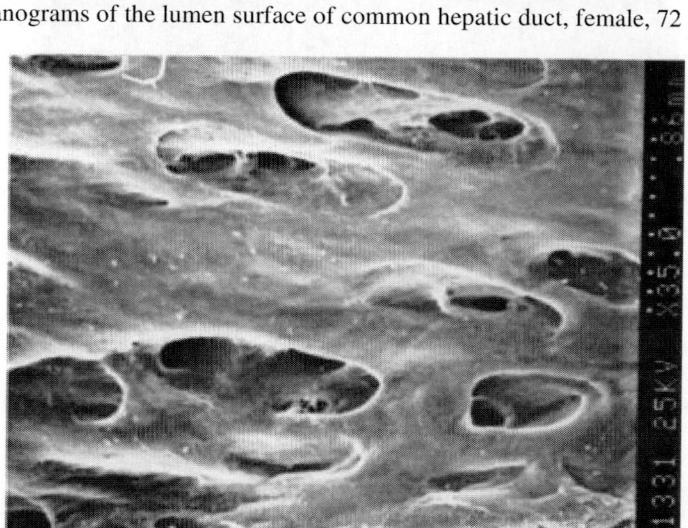

Figure 38. The scanogram of the lumen surface of common hepatic duct, male, 85 yr.

In addition, the remaining two surfaces of the same bile duct reveal "dwarf hills" shaped like semi-spheres or cones, which make the surface of the duct casts rough (granulated). Similar hills can be revealed as well at those sites of the casts of gross caliber ducts where typical glandular patterns are not observed (Figures 39-42).

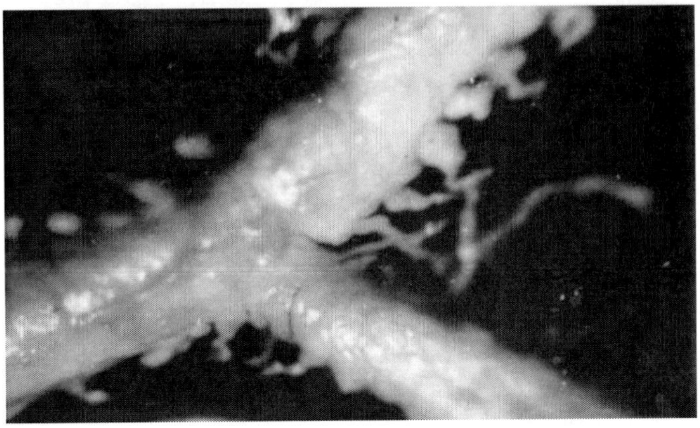

Figure 39. Segmental and subsegmental ducts and mucosal glands of canine liver, corrosion specimens.

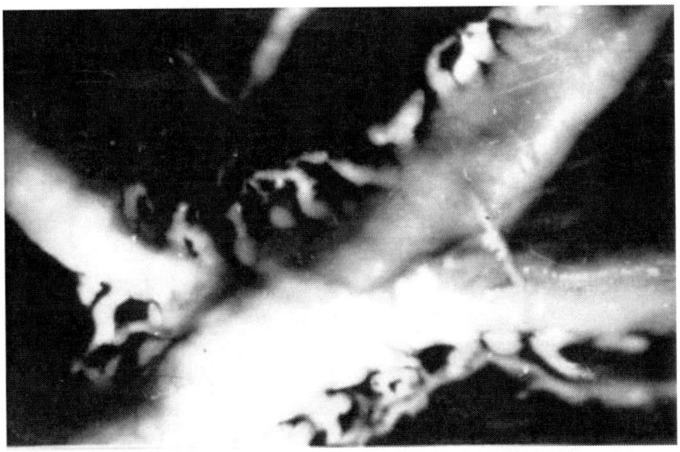

Figure 40. Segmental and subsegmental ducts and mucosal glands of canine liver, corrosion specimens.

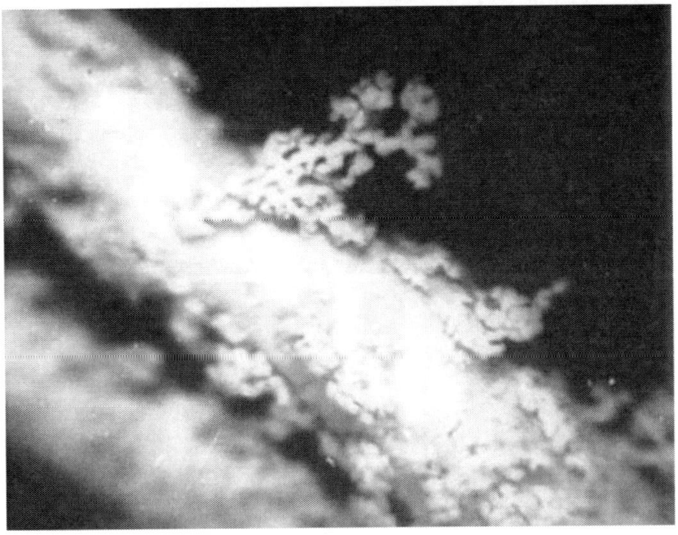

Figure 41. Segment and subsegmental bile ducts and mucosal glands of canine liver, corrosion specimens.

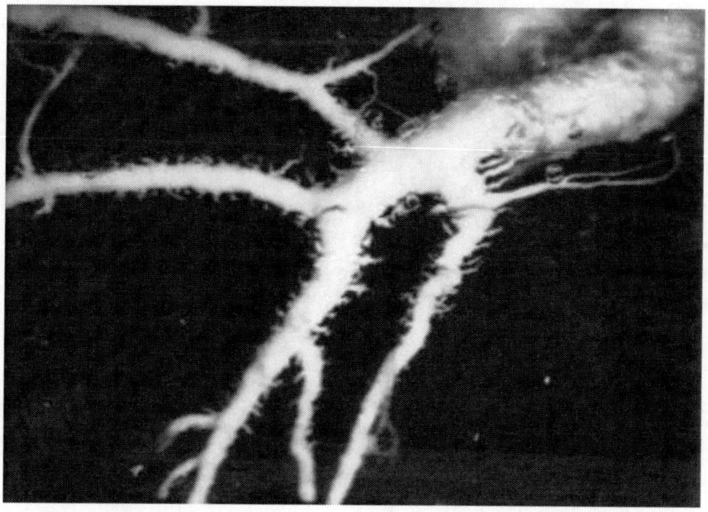

Figure 42. Segment and subsegmental bile ducts and mucosal glands of canine liver, corrosion specimens.

In puppies,the wrinkling of the relief of the biliary casts is less prominent, as well as the polymorphism of biliary mucosal gland patterns. In most cases, they are represented by small appendages with infrequent branching. The scanograms of internal relief of I, II and III line bile ducts of the canine liver show the wrinkling of the epithelial cover.

Furthermore the transverse folds appear to be deeper than the longitudinal ones. The mentioned wrinkles give a cellular appearance to the mucosal layer of bile ducts (Figure 43).

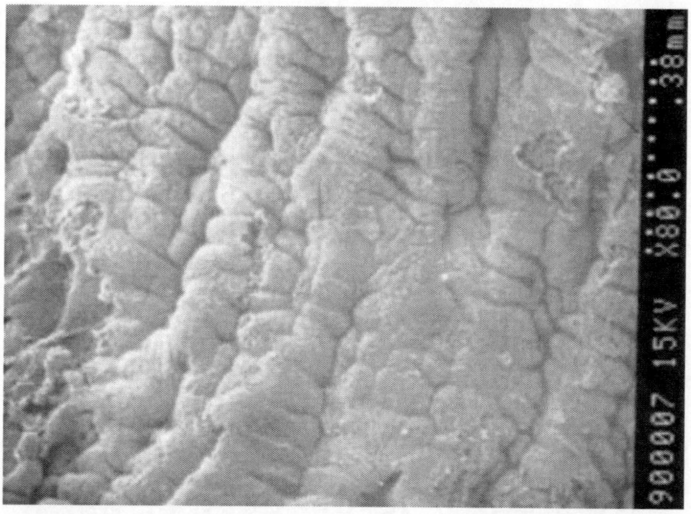

Figure 43. The scanogram of the lumen surface of lobar duct of canine liver.

SEM with higher magnification shows that the epithelial layer of I-III line bile ducts is composed of differently shaped cells. Part of the cells – with apical surface of 5 x 6 μm^2 – are abundantly covered by microvilli with the diameter of 0.1 μm and the length of 0.3-0.5 μm. The surface of these cells is polygonal and somewhat bulged. The margins between cells are well demarcated. This type of cell may co-exist with cells provided by small amounts of microvilli or with totally nude apical surfaces (Figures 44, 45).

On the apical surface of some cells, the microvilli are "replaced" by bead-like bumps, with diameters ranging between 0.5 μm – 4 μm, giving the impression that these beads should tear off from the cells (Figure 46).On the histological slices the content of such beads are mucin-negative (Gerlovin, 1982).

We consider the depicted images to illustrate the macro-apocrine-type secretion. The cells with microvilli, cells with nude apical surface and cells with "beads" over their apical surface may represent the cells of the same type at different stages of their functional activity: the villous epithelial cells in some cases begin to secrete the gross particles by the mechanism of apocrine secretion. The apical plasmalemma of these cells (usually creating micro-villi) evens out, expands and creates the envelope for mass excretion.

Finally, the corpuscles covered with plasmalemma detach from the cell and leave the "nude" apical surface, which gradually develops microvilli again (Figure 47).

Goblet cells with crater-like grooves on their apical surfaces covered by flake-like mass (mucus) are observed among the cells described above. The multiple invaginations observed on the scanograms of the mucosal layer of bile ducts represent the lumina of mucosal biliary glands lined by villous epithelial cells. These cells by their apical surfaces do not differ from similar cells lining the duct lumen (Figure 48). According to current investigations, the ductular compartment of mucosal biliary glands contain the stem cells providing regenerative capacity in case of injury of the mucosal layer in the biliary tree.

As mentioned above, both in humans and experimental animals, the mucosal biliary glands reveal the tendency to communicate with the ducts along their lateral surfaces. However, the study of internal reliefs of the III line ducts revealed that lumina of the gland ductuliare disposed almost evenly along the whole perimeter, but the lumina disposed at the "lateral" surfaces of the bile ducts are bigger in size.

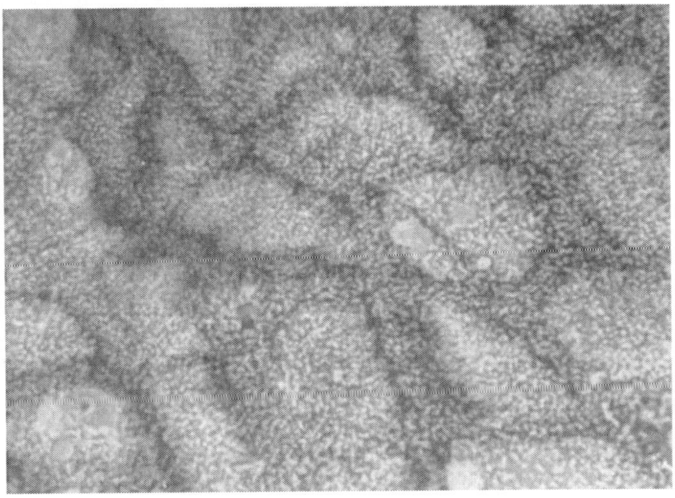

Figure 44. Scanogram of the lumen surfaces of epitheliocytes lining segmental intrahepatic bile ducts of canine liver.

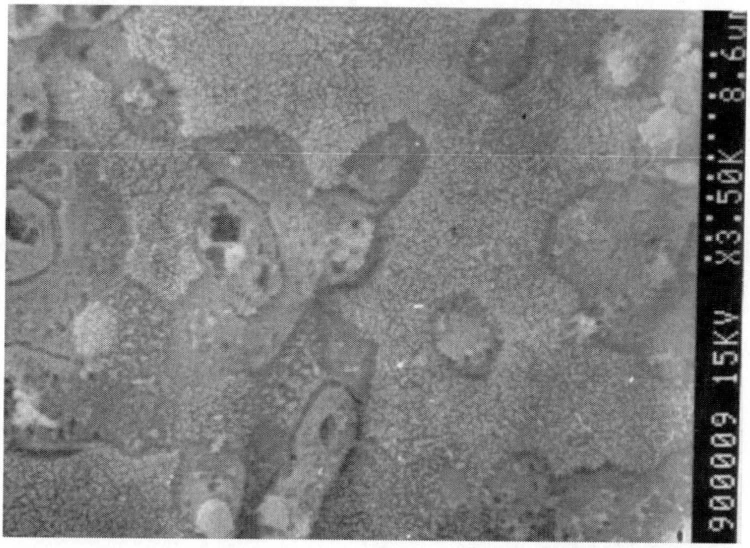

Figure 45. Scanogram of the lumen surfaces of epitheliocytes lining segmental intrahepatic bile ducts of canine liver.

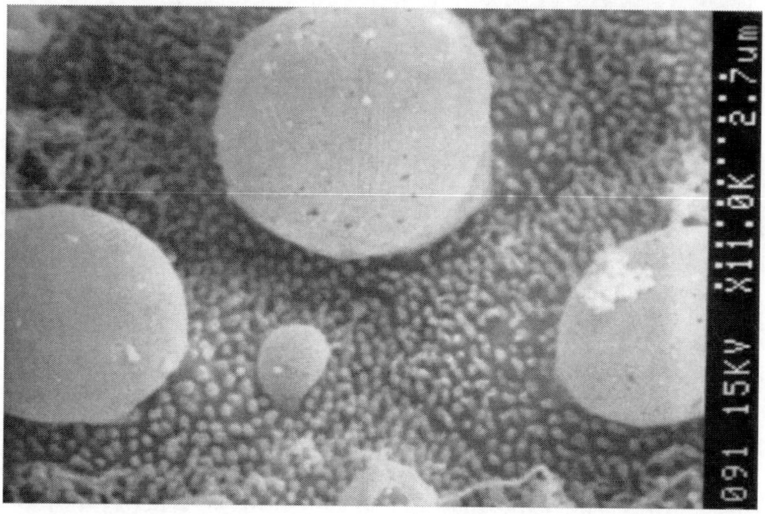

Figure 46. Scanogram of the lumen surfaces of epitheliocytes lining the II order bile duct in canine liver.

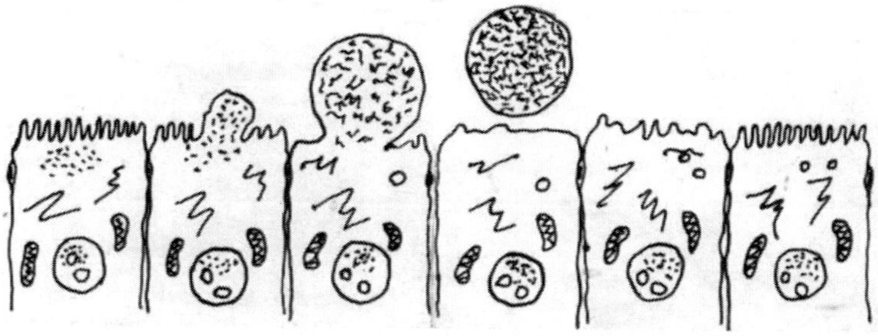

Figure 47. Changing dynamics occurring at the villous apical surfaces of the duct lining epitheliocytes (scheme).

It can be considered that biliary mucosal glands may flow into the bile duct from every side. However, the glands opening at the anterior and posterior surfaces are short (supposedly mostly intramural), because their extension is impeded by the fibrous-arterial layer or liver parenchyma (see above), or too twisted, which makes their "filling", by latex injected into the biliary bed through the common bile duct, impossible.

It must be mentioned that while studying the bile duct reliefs with an electronic scanning microscope, we found the higher number of lumina of mucosal biliary gland ductuli on each square millimeter, compared with the number of corrosion casts of the same glands. We may draw a hypothesis that not every glandular structure is filled when injecting biliary ducts with solidifying material; but if we suppose that not every gland is "filled", then we cannot assert that the pattern of every "filled" gland completely depicts its shape.

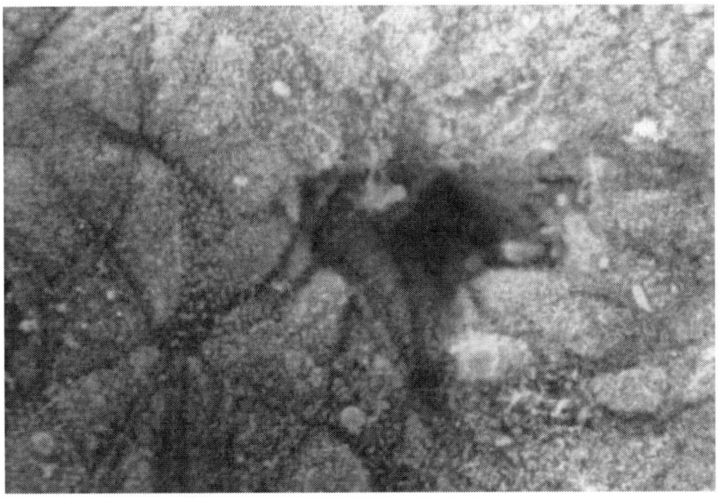

Figure 48. Lumen of ductule of mucosal biliary gland opened in the segmental bile duct of canine liver, scanogram.

Thus, we might have the casts of incompletely injected glands as well. We also consider that such incompletely "filled" glands correspond to the part of the small hills shaped like cones or semi-spheres giving rough form to the surfaces of the biliary casts. The above-mentioned allows us to consider the classification of forms of mucosal biliary glands on the basis of their corrosion specimen studies as suppositional.

Plasticity of Bile Ducts After Common Bile Duct Occlusion

Common bile duct ligation (CBDL) causes total dilation of the biliary tract. The degree (level) of dilation is directly related to the stage of bile congestion. The latex injected into the biliary pathway one week later after CBDL fills a significantly higher number of biliary branches, compared with normal conditions. Frequently latex even fills the interlobular ducts and terminal ductuli (Figures 49, 50).On 7-14th days following the CBDL the surfaces of corrosion cast of bile ducts are evened out compared with the cast patterns of normal bile ducts. The casts of mucosal glands are not observed on the gross caliber ducts. They are preserved only on finer ducts, although their shapes are more simplified. On 30-45th days of cholestasis, the latex injected into the biliary tree reaches the branches only to the V line, because the biliary corrosion casts appear as a "tree with cut off small branches" (Figures 51, 52). By the 30th day of the experiment, the number of mucosal glands grows even fewer, and on 45-60 days after CBDL they cannot be found, even on the thin bile branches. The abundant branching of the biliary tree with appearance of the casts of interlobular ducts and terminal ductuli at the early stage of experiment can be explained by overall dilatation of the biliary bed. However, at the subsequent terms of CBDL, the formation of "bile clots" within bile canaliculi and what's most important, in fine biliary (interlobular) ducts (Kartashova, Maksimova, 1979; Loginov, Aruin, 1985) blocks the distribution of injected mass toward biliary structures located proximally. Desquamation of epithelial cells also increases the severity of fine biliary path obstruction.

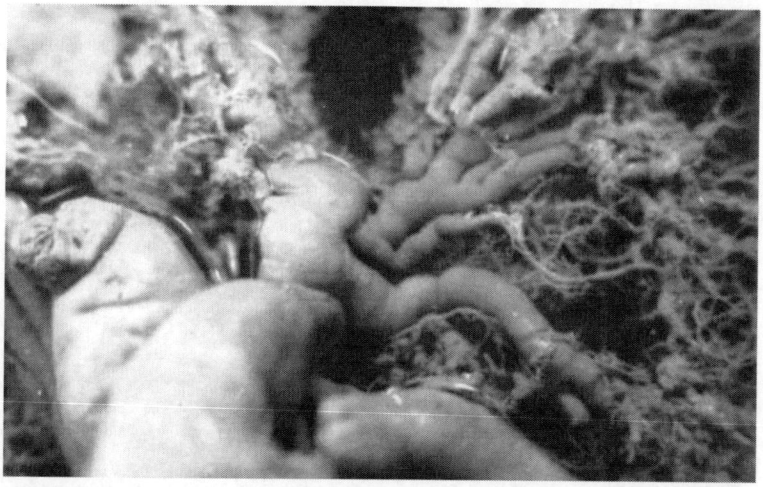

Figure 49. Intrahepatic bile ducts of canine liver, 7th day of cholestasis, corrosion specimen.

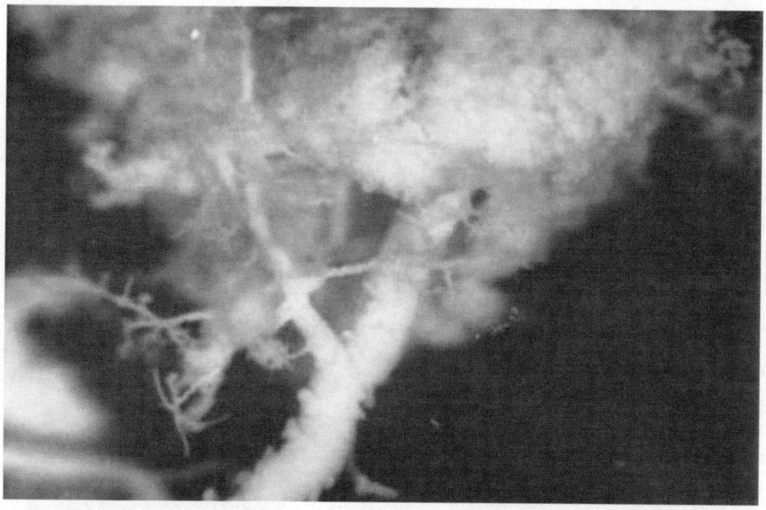

Figure 50. Septal, sublobular and interlobular bile ducts with network of bile canaliculi of canine liver, 7th day of cholestasis, corrosion specimen.

In the setting of biliary hypertension caused by CBDL, the gradual dilation of bile ducts supposedly results in the compression and cuddling of extramural parts of the mucosal biliary glands disposed within peribiliary connective tissue by surrounding fibrous-arterial and fibrous-biliary layers. This makes the “filling” of mucosal glands with injected medium impossible. But the glands of fine bile ducts are more densely “embedded” into peribiliary tissue and more reluctant to be subjected to dilation due to biliary hypertension. This explains why the patterns of mucosal glands over the casts of fine bile ducts account for longer preservation in a bile congestion setting.

The luminal relief of bile ducts in the setting of mechanical jaundice and biliary hypertension was studied by SEM and conventional histology.

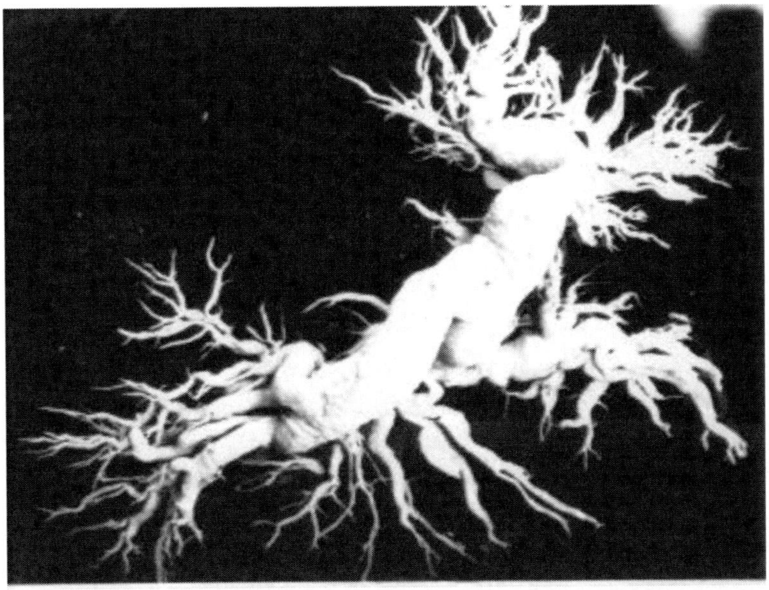

Figure 51. Bile ducts of canine liver at 30th day of cholestasis, corrosion specimen.

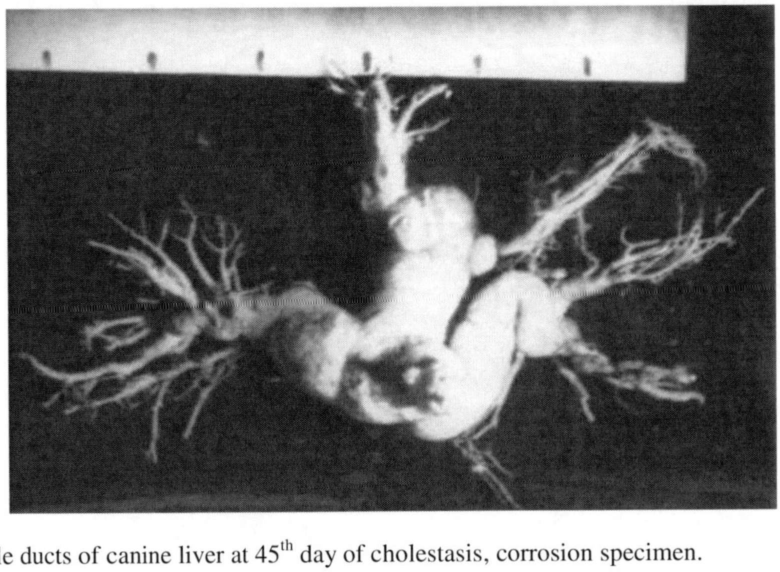

Figure 52. Bile ducts of canine liver at 45th day of cholestasis, corrosion specimen.

At the 7th day of bile congestion the level of wrinkling on the mucosal layer of common bile (magistral) duct, and I, II III line ducts was increased.

The apical surfaces of the cells located deep down in the crypts between neighboring folds are puffed out with their surface areas being smaller compared to the apical surfaces of the cells disposed over the "crest" of these folds (Figure 53). These cells are frequently cribrous (perforated). The cells with bulging surfaces develop swelling (mucoid dystrophy) while the cells with cribrous surfaces are in the stage of segmental-coagulation necrosis (denatured part of the cytoplasm has fallen out) (Figure 54).

The cribrous surfaced cells are frequently grouped, while the links between them are deranged.

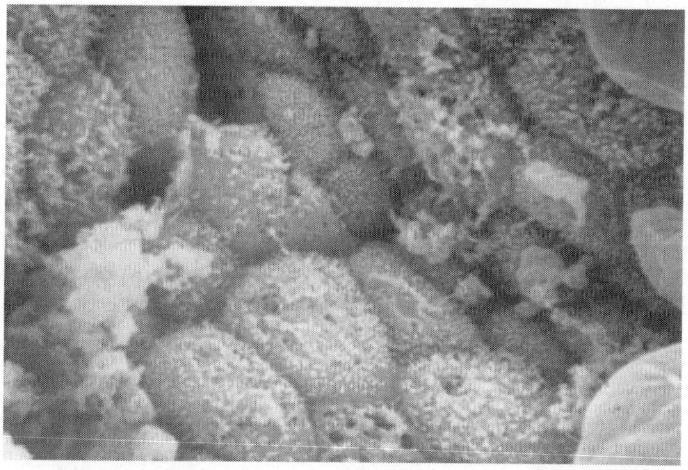

Figure 53. Scanograms of the luminal surface of epitheliocytes of segmental bile ducts of canine liver, 7th day of cholestasis.

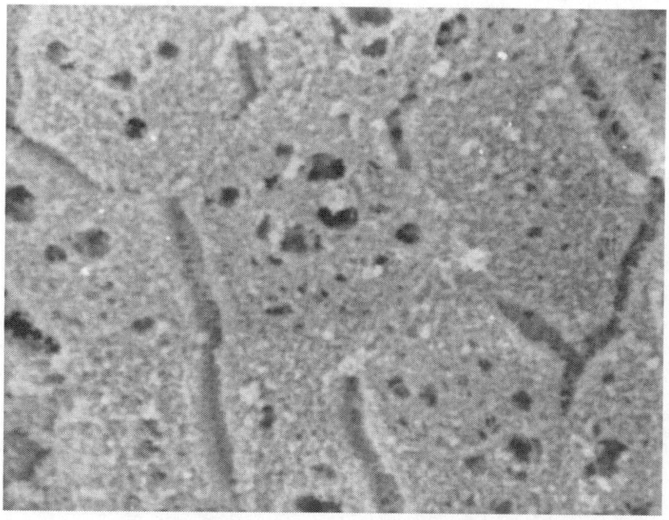

Figure 54.Scanograms of the luminal surface of epitheliocytes of segmental bile ducts of canine liver, 7th day of cholestasis.

According to some authors, such compromised bonds between the cells represent the open gates, through which the aggressive influence of bile is imposed on the duct wall (Zemskov et al., 1992). The number of “beaded” cells described in normal conditions is markedly increased at the 7th day of cholestasis. This data evidences the hypothesis by Yamada (1970), Alpini et al. (2010), etc., considering that the apocrine secretion in epitheliocytes lining biliary ducts is increased during the biliary pressure rise. The number of goblet cells is also increased. At the 14th day of cholestasis, the wrinkling of the mucosal layer is more evident. The severity of cells injury is also increased. The groups of cells, and sometimes the whole plasts with deranged bonds with surrounding cells can be observed, which seem to be “ready for desquamation” (Figure 55). The described lesions confirm that the longer the duration of cholestasis, the higher the risk of aggressive influence of bile on the structure of the duct wall.

On the 7th and 14th days from CBDL the lumina of ductuli of mucosal biliary glands are not visible. They are hidden among the enlarged folds of the epithelial layer of bile ducts.

It is well known that bile represents the chemotactic factor, which causes the activation of neutrophil granulocytes within the duct wall, their direction towards the lumen and intrusion into the biliary bed (Figure 56), (Fishzon-Ryss, Iu.I. and N. A. Postrelov, 1985). The bile leak into the mucosal defect in turn results in the degeneration of muscular and elastic fibers, the degree of which accounts directly for the restoration of normal geometric characteristics in bile ducts after relieving hypertension. By the 30th and 45th days of bile congestion the extensive plasts of biliary epithelium is desquamated (Figures 57, 58) and most of the remaining cells undergo severe dystrophic and necrotic changes (Figure 59). Multiple foramina are seen in the submucosal layer corresponding to the lumina of draining ducts of mucosal biliary glands (Figure 57). This fact proves that the invisibility of glandular lumina, in previous stages of cholestasis, resulted from their compression or blanketing by the wrinkles of the mucosal layer. The impeded discharge of gland secretions may, in turn, be causing the increased secretion of the duct epithelium itself. By the 30th day of bile congestion, the remnants of the epithelial cover of the ductular part of the mucosal biliary glands can be frequently seen inside the above-mentioned lumina, but by the 45th day it is almost impossible to see them.

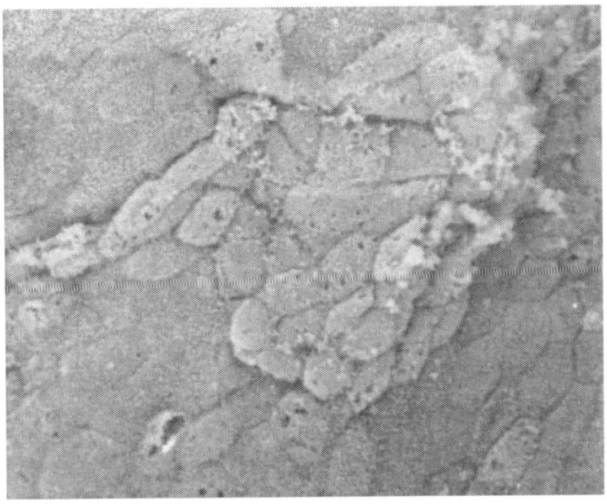

Figure 55. Scanogram of the luminal surface of lobar/segmental bile duct in canine liver, 14th day of cholestasis.

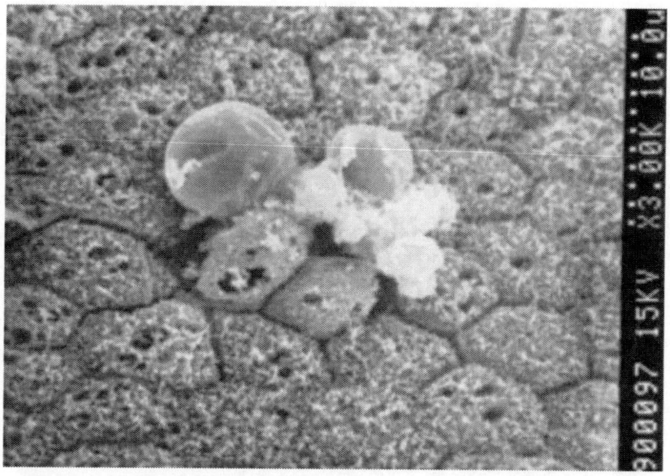

Figure 56. Scanogram of the luminal surface of lobar/segmental bile duct in canine liver, 14th day of cholestasis.

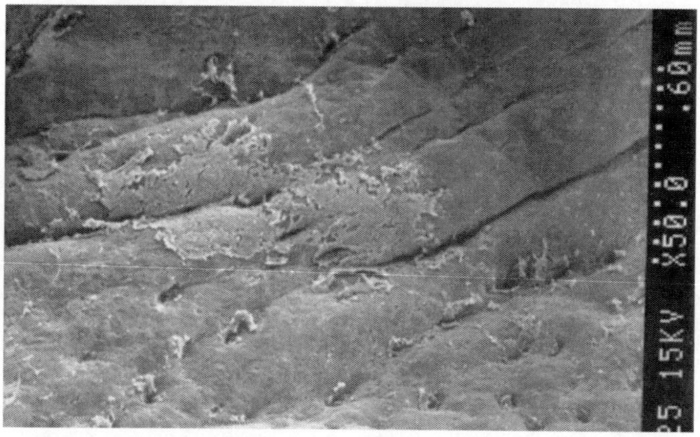

Figure 57. Scanograms of the luminal surface of lobar/segmental bile duct in canine liver, 30th day of cholestasis.

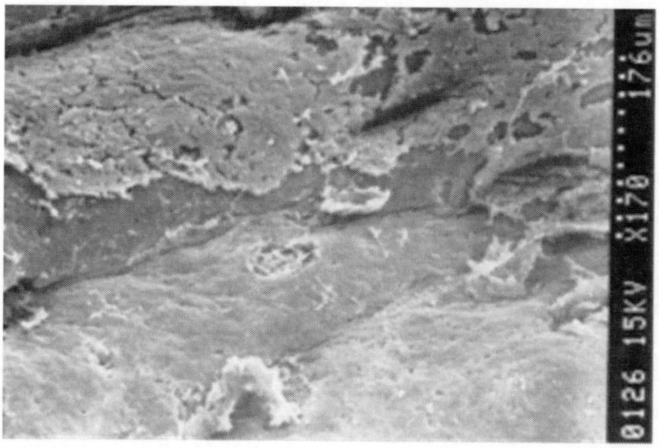

Figure 58. Scanograms of the luminal surface of lobar/segmental bile duct in canine liver, 30th day of cholestasis.

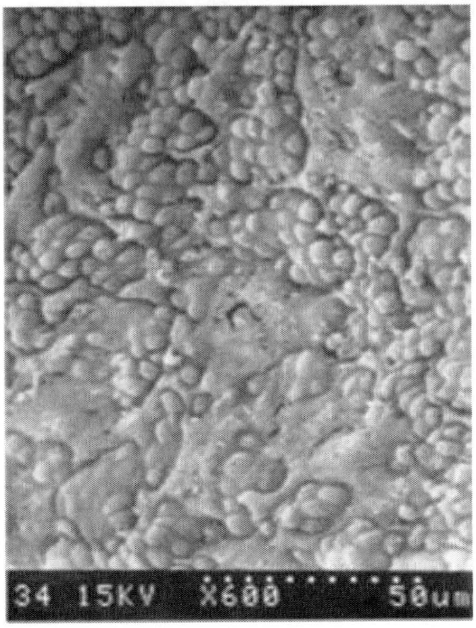

Figure 59. Scanograms of the luminal surface of lobar/segmental bile duct in canine liver, 30th day of cholestasis.

The histological study of the portal tract shows that viable epithelial cells are still preserved in the deeper secretive parts of mucosal glands, while the cells of the epithelial layer of bile ducts undergo the necrotic disorders. In case of relieving cholestasis, these viable glandular cells can function as a regeneration source for the ductular epithelium. According to current data, the cervical/ductular compartment of mucosal biliary glands indeed contain the stem cells, which can regenerate both damaged glandular and ductal epithelium as well.

Taking into consideration that interlobular ductuli of Hering are also a niche of hepatobiliary stem cells, it may be considered that the regeneration of impaired bile ducts can be accomplished via two sources: mucosal biliary glands and intralobullar ductuli.

By the 60th day of cholestasis, the wrinkles of the submucosal layer are moderately evened out. Epithelial cells are also more abundant, compared to the previous stage. At the background of dystrophic and altered cells are calyceal cells and the cells, covered abundantly with microvilli, can be observed. In addition, the apical layer of the latter is more protruded, compared to the normal type (Figure 60). The existence of the morphological-functional adaptation period of the liver with bile hypertensions and cholestasis is clearly proven (Galperin, 1976). The evidence for such adaptation is provided by the characteristics of the biliary duct relief in the setting of 60-day cholestasis described above.

We evaluate the cells covered with microvilli resembling normal cells as regenerates. However, protrusion of their apical surfaces indicates that dystrophic changes are already initiated within these cells and thus, such “improvement” is only temporary.

Regarding Bilio-Lymphatic Connections

The presence of specific linkage between the biliary tree and lymphatic systems within the liver has been a subject of research for a long time. The obvious evidence of such connections is provided by the fact that bile initially appears in lymphatic circulation and only afterwards reaches the blood, which is observed in the setting of common bile duct occlusion.

It is generally accepted that this linkage carries the compensative character and provides postponing of dramatic events resulted from cholestasis.

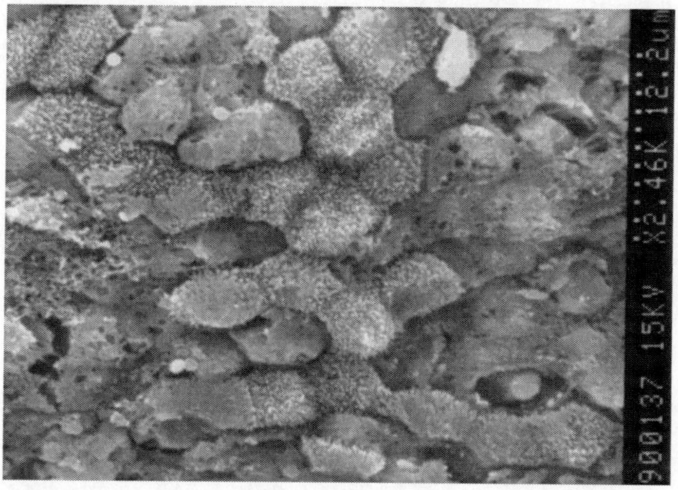

Figure 60. Scanograms of the luminal surface of epitheliocytes of segmental bile ducts of canine liver, 60th day of cholestasis.

There are no doubts that biliary-lymphatic connections exist at the level of hepatic profound structures (Briskin et al., 1986; Dumpe et al., 1983; Snegirevskaia et al., 1986; Bettezzati M., 1975). A causal relationship between increased biliary pressure in cholestasis and structural changes of intercellular connections is also undisputable (Virenkov et al., 1971) Biliary hypertension causes the change of direction of bile secretion by hepatocytes and bile transition into the lymphatic flow via the perisinusoidal spaces of Disse and periportal spaces of Mall (Toidze, Kordzaia, 1988; Kordzaia 1990).

The study of corrosion specimens of bile ducts of different calibers (from lobar ducts up to terminal ductuli) with binocular magnifier and/or SEM frequently reveals the trace of breached duct integrity, in the shape of solidified "extravasates" of injected medium (Figure 61). These "extravasates", in turn, frequently give origin to the casts of lymphatic vessels (Figure 62).

The study of corrosion specimens of white rat bile ducts with an electronic microscope at different stages of cholestasis and summarization of acquired results, with the level of pressure of injection of solidifying medium, demonstrated that the threshold of resistance of the bile ducts' wall falls in accordance with increasing terms of bile congestion. Thus, if by injecting a solidifying mass at the pressure of 100-120 mmHg in 1 month after CBDL the integrity of intact bile ducts can be breached, then the same result can already be achieved at the pressure of 30-40 mmHg. At this point, the bile duct casts are abundantly covered by solidified "extravasates" and casts of lymphatic vessels of different forms and sizes (Figures 63, 64).

However, it should be underlined, that in the above-mentioned cases, the pressures of 100-120 mmHg and/or 30-40 mmHg destroy the anatomical integrity of the biliary bed and promote the secondary filling of lymphatic vessels by the injected mass.

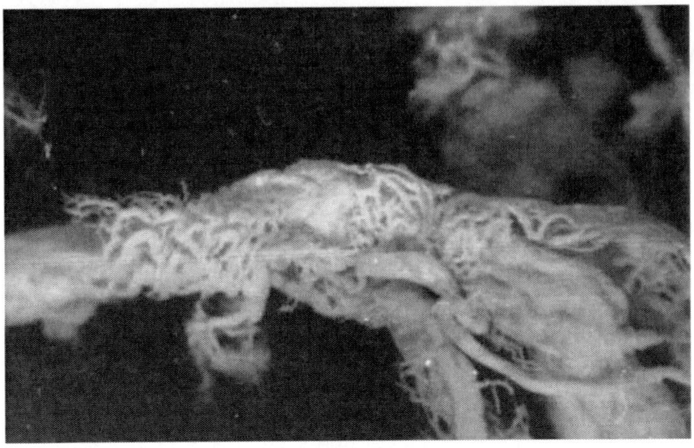

Figure 61. Bile ducts, "extravasates" and lymphatic vessels on 30th day of cholestasis, corrosion casts.

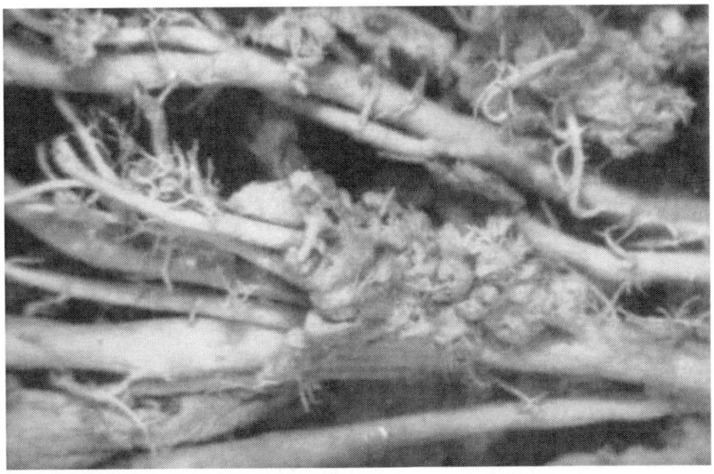

Figure 62. Bile ducts, "extravasates" and lymphatic vessels on 30th day of cholestasis, corrosion casts.

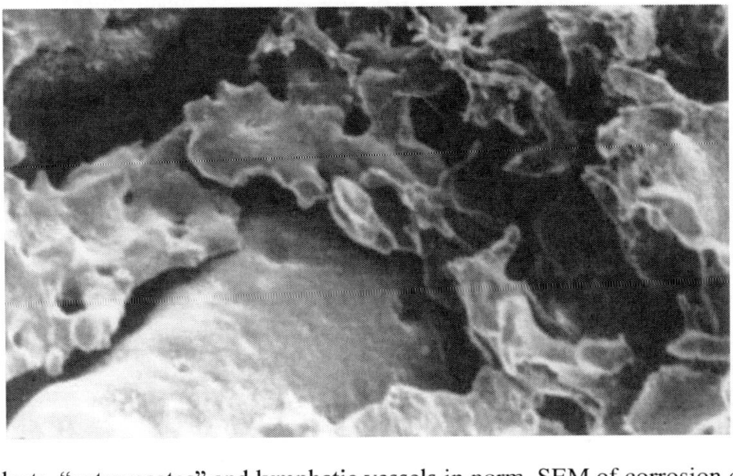

Figure 63. Bile ducts, "extravasates" and lymphatic vessels in norm, SEM of corrosion casts.

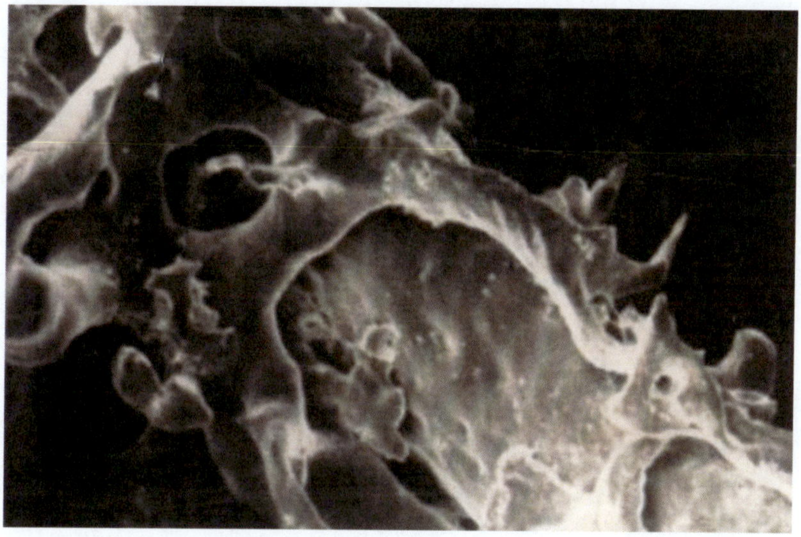

Figure 64. Bile ducts, "extravasates" and lymphatic vessels in norm, SEM of corrosion casts.

But in vivo, on the early terms of cholestasis, cholangio-lymphatic/cholangio-venous reflux can be developed already at the biliary pressure of 18-25 mmHg, by changing the direction of transcellular transport of bile miccelles (With, 1949; Mallet-Juy, 1963; Kinoshita et al. 1984, Kordzaia, 1990).

However, demonstrated below is the probability of another way of blocked bile transition into the lymphatic system, namely within the bounds of the intrahepatic portal tracts, which is realized by extramural biliary glands and lymphatic vessels.

Biliary-lymphatic connections are demonstrated in anatomical experiments as well: The mixed ink-gelatin mass injected through the common hepatic duct under pressure rapidly flows into the lymphatic ducts and visualizes both superficial (sub-peritoneal) lymphatic vessels as well as those in the hepatoduodenal ligament (Figures 65-67).

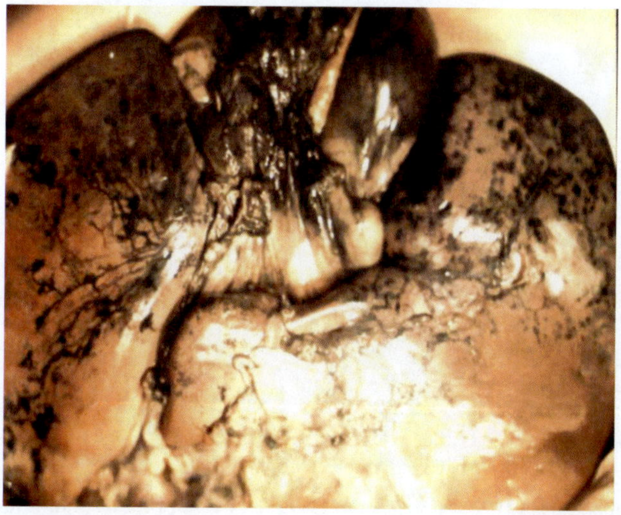

Figure 65. Lymphatic network on the visceral surface of liver after injection of ink-gelatin mixture through the common bile duct.

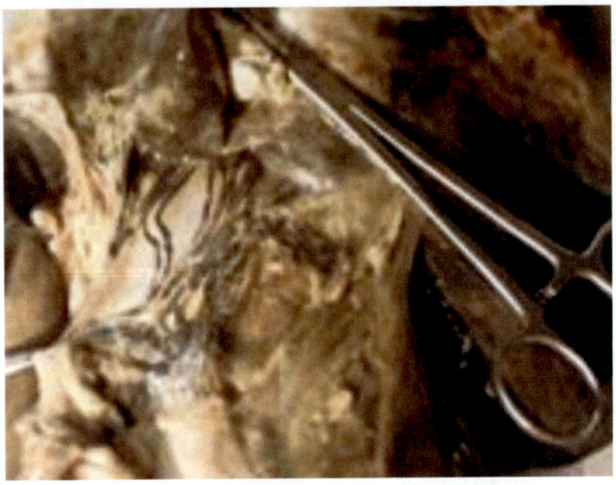

Figure 66. Lymph vessels revealed in hepato-duodenal ligament after injection of ink-gelatin mixture through the common bile duct.

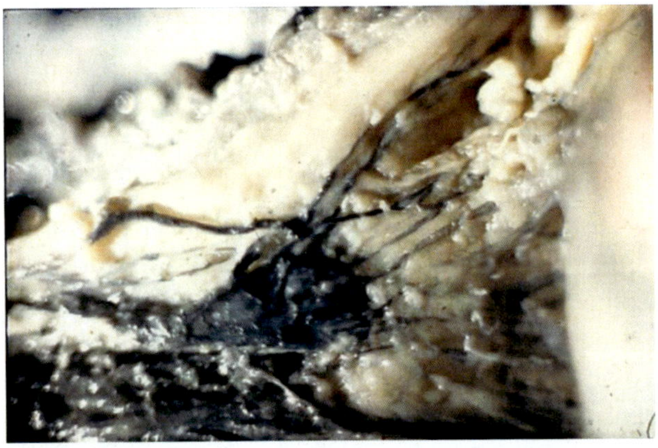

Figure 67. Lymph vessels revealed in hepato-duodenal ligament after injection of ink-gelatin mixture through the common bile duct.

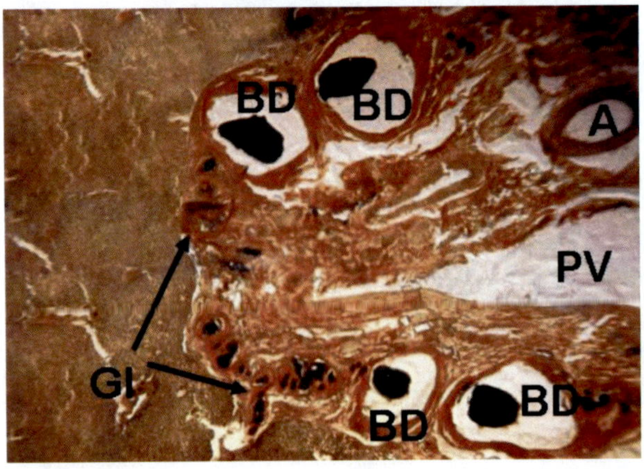

Figure 68. Segmental portal tract. PV – portal vein branch; A – artery; BD – bile duct (filled with ink-gelatin mixture); GL – extramural mucosal biliary glands (filled with ink-gelatin mixture) connecting two adjacent bile ducts; histotopogram.

As mentioned above, the extramural parts of bile duct mucosal glands are located within the fibrous-biliary layer or the most peripheral zone of the portal tract and occupy the areas between the bile ducts (inter-ductular space).Sometimes they even fuse (anastomose) with each other. This is well demonstrated both on histotopograms and corrosion casts (Figures 68, 69). Lymphatic vessels surround the compounded extramural mucosal biliary glands of lobar, sectoral and segmental magistral portal tracts. The close interconnections between these two structures are stably demonstrated on every specimen.

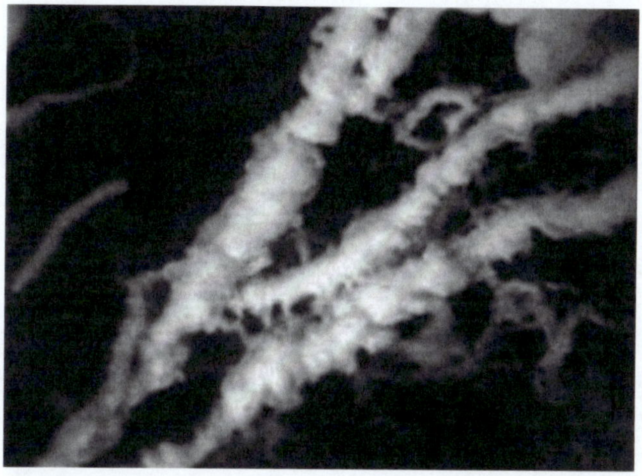

Figure 69. Intercommunication between segmental bile ducts by the glandular compartments of their mucosal glands; corrosion cast.

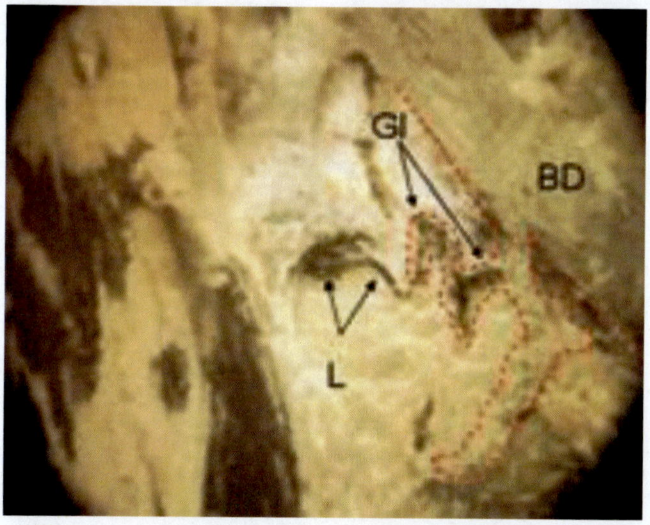

Figure 70. Portal region. BD – right hepatic duct; Gl – extramural mucosal biliary gland is filled by ink-gelatin mixture (through bile duct); L – lymphatic vessel is filled with ink-gelatin mixture through the mucosal gland; preparation under the magnifier; male 47 yr.

During the preparation under microscope, we have observed the flow of contrast mass (injected under high pressure through the common hepatic duct) from the glandular termini of mucosal glands into the parabiliary connective tissue spaces. From these spaces the ink-gelatine mixture transits into the lymphatic vessels (Figures70-72).

Supposedly the same happens in the setting of biliary hypertension. On the basis of these findings the intrahepatic portal tracts may be considered as one of the possible areas of the biliary-lymphatic connections where the congested bile (due to extraheptaic biliary occlusion) may leak into the lymphatic system (Chanukvadze I., et al., 2013).

Collaterals among the Intrahepatic Bile Ducts

The collaterals developed among the bile ducts of different line must be the subjects of a special discussion.

Studying the corrosion casts of the biliary tract at the 7th day of cholestasis small caliber collaterals (up to 1 mm in diameter) were observed between the adjacent segmental and subsegmental ducts (Figure 73).

At the 30th day of bile congestion, the collaterals are observed not only between adjacent, but also II-III line ducts of remote sites. In some cases several collaterals are arranged in parallel (Figures 74-77).

Development of collaterals clearly evidences the wide plastic capabilities of bile ducts. In addition to the development of new collaterals, new glandular structures pertinent to these collaterals are also formed.

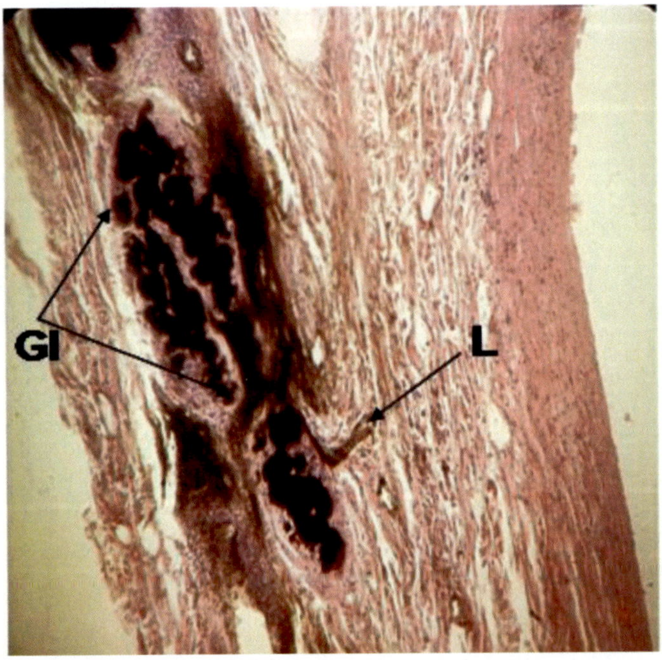

Figure 71. Fragment of histotopogram of portal tract, male 64 yr.; L – lymphatic vessel is filled by ink-gelatin mixture through the mucosal biliary gland (GL).

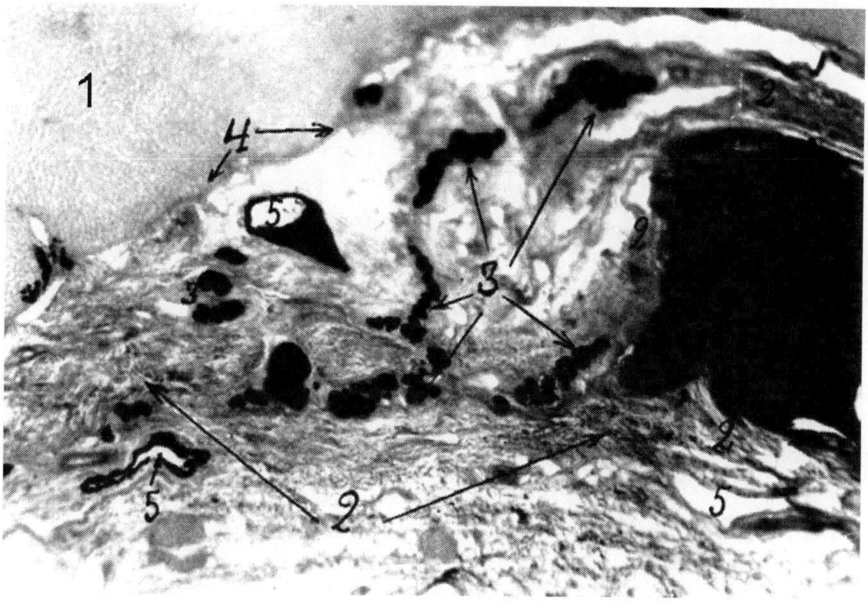

Figure 72. Fragment of histotopogram of portal tract, female 64 yrs; 1- liver parenchyma; 2- peribiliar connective tissue; 3 – bile duct and mucosal biliary ducts filled with ink-gelatin mixture; 4 – perivascular fibrous sheath; 5 – lymph vessel filled (partially) with ink-gelatin mixture.

This fact proves the relevance of the above-mentioned hypothesis that the number of mucosal biliary glands can increase further in the postnatal period (Spitz, Petropaulos, 1979).

It is established that there are no biliary collaterals under normal conditions (Hyortsio, 1947, Couinaud, 1954). Although the anastomoses created by interconnections of mucosal biliary glands of different bile ducts inside the portal tract or at the confluence sites of different bile ducts have been described (Figure 78). However, such bonds between the glands of adjacent ducts must not be considered as true collaterals.

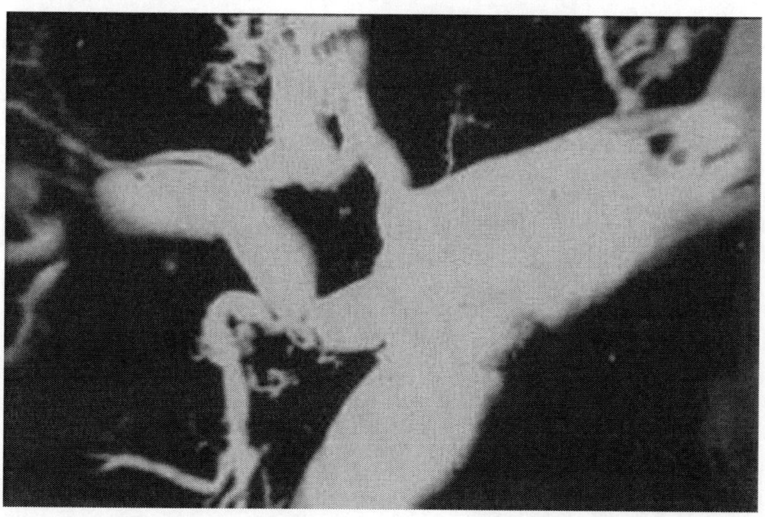

Figure 73. Collaterals between the segmental bile ducts of canine liver; 7th day of cholestasis; corrosion cast.

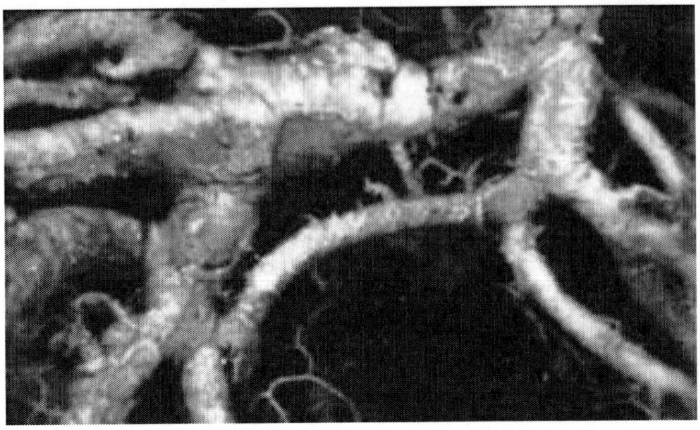

Figure 74. Collaterals between the canine bile ducts of different line; 30th day of cholestasis; corrosion cast.

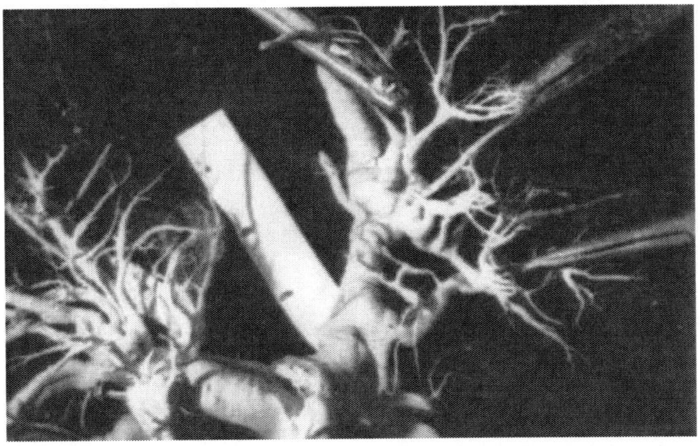

Figure 75. Collaterals between the canine bile ducts of different line; 30th day of cholestasis; corrosion cast.

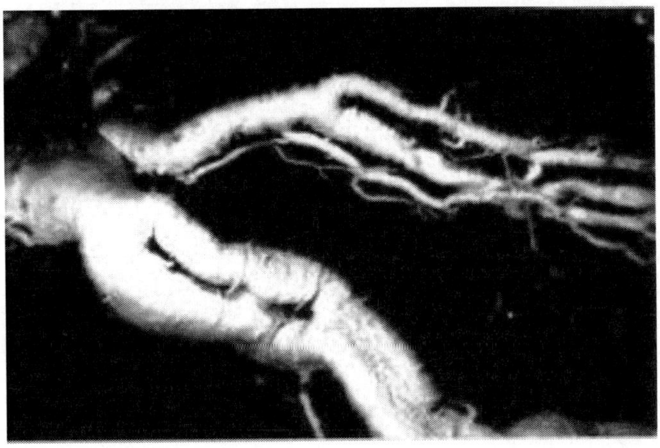

Figure 76. Collaterals between the canine bile ducts of different line; 14th and 30th day of cholestasis; corrosion cast.

The cause of the development of biliary collaterals must be sought in the phenomenon of bile ducts proliferation, which is so typical for extrahepatic cholestasis. Though the proliferation of biliary ducts is also described in other pathologies of the liver (Popper et al., 1962), in the CBDO setting it is more prominent, especially after 2-3 weeks of bile flow obstruction (Kartashova and Maximova, 1979).2 types of bile duct proliferation have been specified: the “sprouting” type and the “elongation” type. In respect to development of collaterals, great interest is evoked by the sprouting-type of proliferation occurring via “budding”, leading to the development of local saliences of the ducts, which act as additional reservoirs for congested bile. The saliences of different bile ducts may meet/conjoin with each other, which results in the creation of collaterals between these ducts. The fact that “collaterals” found on the corrosion casts of the biliary tract in the CBDO setting truly represents the anastomosing ducts and not artifacts, is evidenced by the following data: a) the surface pattern of collaterals does not differ from the patterns of intrahepatic bile duct surfaces; b) like duct patterns, the collateral patterns are also supplied by the casts of lateral branches and mucosal glands; c) histological study of hepatic tissue reveals the “sole” biliary ducts observed in particular zones at 30th, 45th and 60th days of CBDO.

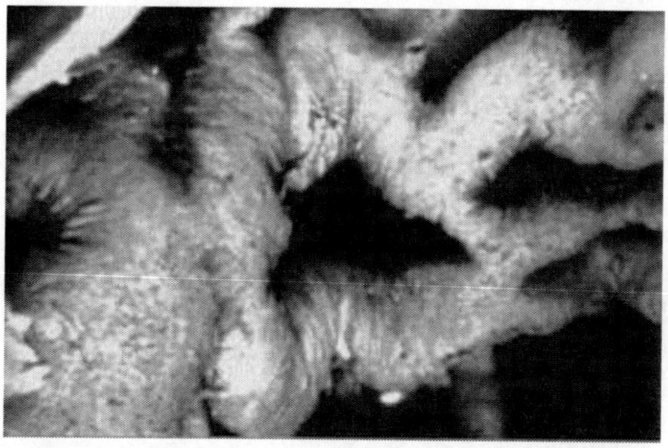

Figure 77. Collaterals between the canine bile ducts of different line; 14th and 30th day of cholestasis; corrosion cast.

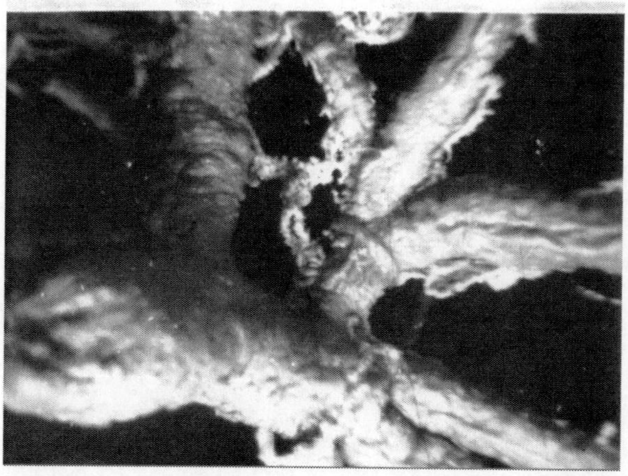

Figure 78. Anastomoses between the glandular compartments of canine extramural mucosal biliary glands drained into different collectors, corrosion cast.

They are not accompanied by respective branches of the portal vein and hepatic artery, but only by thin blood and lymphatic vessels (Figure 79, 80).

Considering the above-mentioned proliferation of bile ducts, with the development of collaterals among them; it might be considered a typical event for extraheptaic cholestasis.

Likewise in clinical practice, while performing percutaneous transhepatic cholangiography (with a Chiba needle), we have repeatedly observed the passage of contrast medium from the pool of the right hepatic to the left hepatic duct and then into the common bile duct – in the setting of distal occlusion of the right duct with tumor. The connection between right and left hepatic duct pools was created through the newly created collaterals of quite large caliber.

Based on the given data, the canine model of lobar (segmental) bile duct occlusion was developed (Kordzaia, 1990).It was already known that in the setting of ligation of the lobar branch of the canine portal vein, the lobe deprived of portal supply would adhere to adjacent intact lobes, with subsequent development of collaterals between the branches of intact and occluded portal vessels. This fact indicates that the autonomy of hepatic lobes (segments) does not represent the insuperable obstacle in terms of connection of ductular structures of remote sites (lobes, segments) (Figure 81).

On the 21st day after the ligation of canine lobar (segmental) bile ducts in an experimental setting, we demonstrated the development of biliary collateral conjoining the branches of the occluded bile duct with the bile ducts of the "intact" lobe (Figure 82). Emptying the bile from the "congested" lobe after development of anastomosis is achieved through the bypass route.

Considering this data, in the case of intra-operative traumatic injury to sectoral or segmental and specifically small ducts, the intervention may be limited by the ligation of these ducts. In one case of cholecystectomy, we ligated the atypically located duct, which flowed directly into the gallbladder from the liver parenchyma, and was accidentally cut while the gallbladder was being separated from its bed.

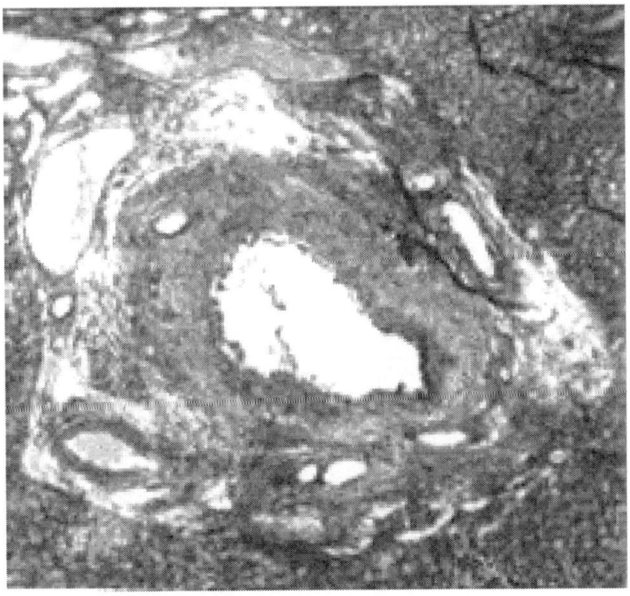

Figure 79. Sole bile ducts (accompanied only by thin blood and lymph vessels); 45th day of cholestasis; histotopogram of canine liver.

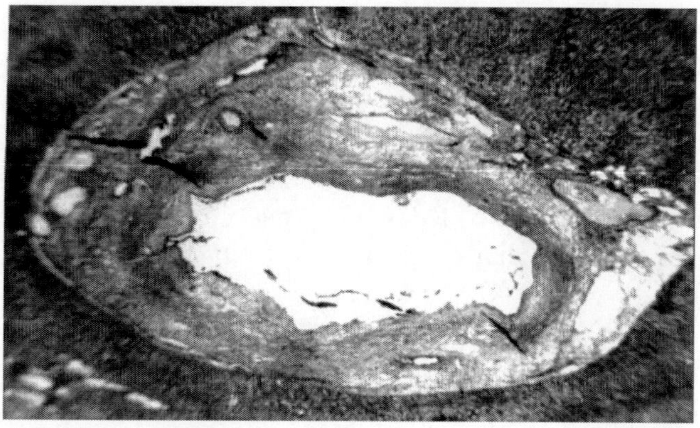

Figure 80. Sole bile ducts (accompanied only by thin blood and lymph vessels); 45th day of cholestasis; histotopogram of canine liver.

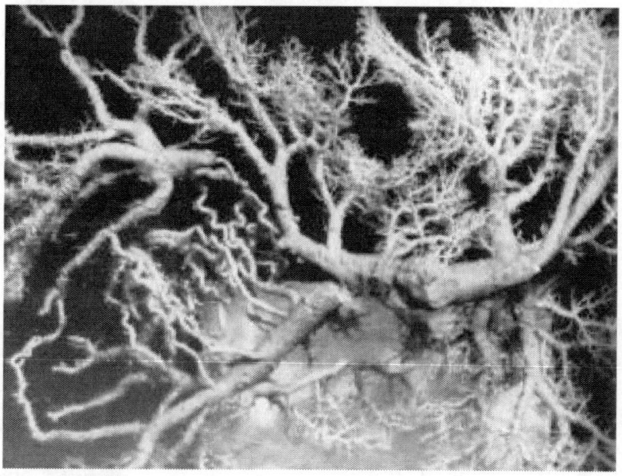

Specimen of Prof. Sh. Kevani Svili.

Figure 81. Anastomosis between two intrahepatic branches of portal vein developed after occlusion of one segmental branch situated among them; corrosion cast.

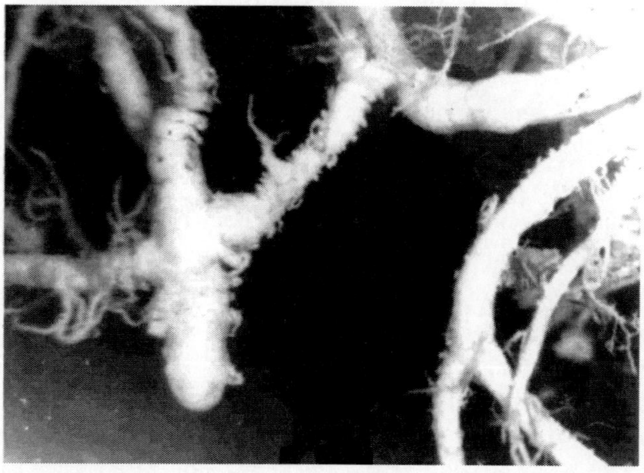

Figure 82. Anastomosis between intrahepatic bile ducts developed after occlusion of one segmental branch; corrosion cast.

Ligation of the mentioned duct did not lead to any complications postoperatively. Some authors, with the hope of developing anastomoses between bile ducts, suggest the creation of a biliary-enteric bypass at the segmental bile duct in cases of malignant tumors of portal site of the liver (Chei et al., 1988). Specifically, in the setting of tumor occluding bifurcation site of hepatic duct, creation of a biliary-enteric bypass at the biliary duct of different segments (most frequently, IV and V segments) led to emptying of both hepatic lobes in 12 cases from 22, which was achieved through the "communicative" biliary ducts.

Bile Ducts Transformation Following Cholecystectomy; Regarding "True Postcholecystectomy Syndrome"

The biliary tract of some animals without gallbladder is characterized by local ampoule-like widening (sacs), which represent the additional reservoirs of bile. However, the features of the biliary bed following cholecystectomy have not been studied profoundly. Furthermore, the necessity of clarification of the number of pathological processes developed in the postoperative period and summarized under the term "postcholecystectomy syndrome" requires a detailed investigation of the biliary system transformation after gallbladder removal (Mallet-Guy, Kestens, 1970). This syndrome separately discusses the "true postcholecystectomy syndrome", which implies the pain phenomenon developed after cholecystectomy. Moreover, this pain is not related to the technical pitfalls of surgery, nor the pathologies of other organs of biliary-pancreatic zone or of residual/relapsing cholangiolythiasis. It is conditioned by the "loss" of the gallbladder itself.

It has been observed that the intensity of pain gradually decreases 1 year after the operation and may totally disappear later on (Galperin, Volkova, 1988).

Analysis of our clinical data (154 patients) and comparison of these data with literature findings allowed us to confirm that the pressure in bile ducts usually increases and the gross caliber ducts dilate slightly following the surgery. In addition, this event occurs in patients from whom the "functioning" gallbladder was removed. It is accepted that biliary pressure increase is related to dysfunction of Odd sphincter, which in turn, is caused by "dys-adaptation" of sphincter-regulating mechanisms with a new regimen of bile excretion after excision of a "functioning" gallbladder (Purtokass, 1983). The rise of biliary pressure in the postoperative period following cholecystectomy was further evidenced by somewhat increased serum levels of alkaline phosphatase and bilirubin in 122 patients, which in 7 cases was accompanied by yellowing of sclera.

Above we have shown that biliary hypertension induces the proliferation of bile ducts and changes in their internal relief. To ascertain if biliary hypertension following the excision of a functioning gallbladder induces similar changes, we performed cholecystectomy in 22 canines. In 6 animals the gallbladder was removed on the second stage of the experiment. At the first stage these animals were subjected to "functional amputation" of the gallbladder, which was achieved by intracystic injection of a solidifying mass (latex), resulting in development of "rubber stones" filling/occupying the whole gallbladder volume.

The features of the biliary tract were studied after 3 months and at 1 year after cholecystectomy. At 3 months after cholecystectomy, the diameters of biliary casts were increased, relief appeared more wrinkled, and the patterns of mucosal glands were thickened and deformed with somewhat simplified architectonics (Figures 83, 84).

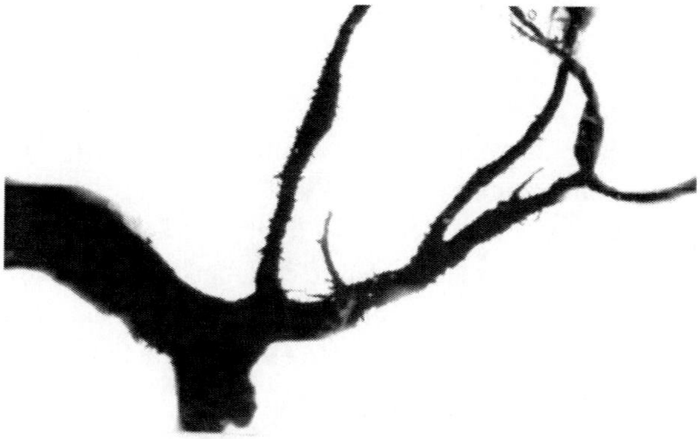

Figure 83. Intrahepatic bile ducts of canine (with small local dilatations). 3 months after colecystectomy; corrosion casts.

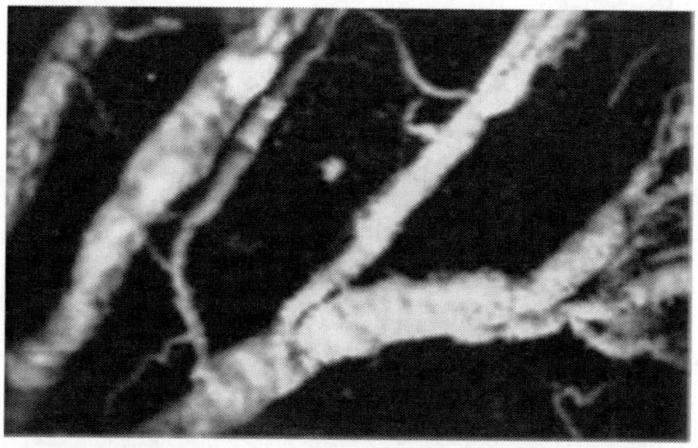

Figure 84. Intrahepatic bile ducts of canine (with small local dilatations). 3 months after colecystectomy; corrosion casts.

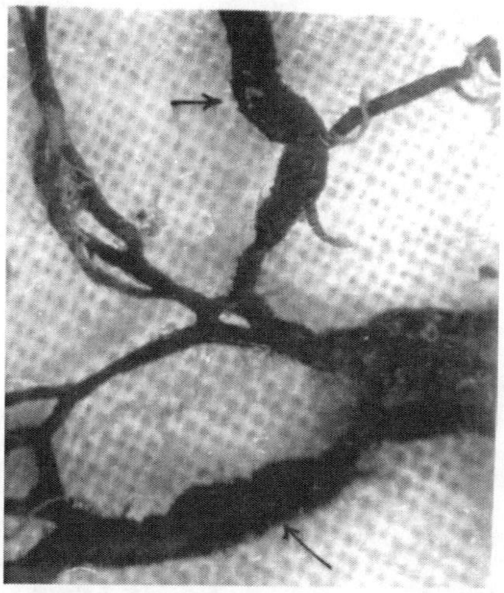

Figure 85. Intrahepatic bile ducts of canine (with small local dilatations and anastomoses);1year after colecystectomy; corrosion casts.

Collaterals were observed between II-V line ducts of adjacent zones (Figures 85-87). Spindle-like pouches (dilatations) disposed in line with each other were frequently seen. The study of corrosion specimens after 1 year of cholecystectomy revealed that collaterals and local dilatations were preserved. Histological investigation at 3 months following cholecystectomy demonstrated the increased area of portal tracts, their fibrosis and proliferation of bile ducts.

Development of circularly arranged muscle fibers was observed in the walls of gross caliber ducts, which, together with spindle-like dilations, can be considered as the development of "biliary micro-vesicles". SEM of duct relief revealed the image of intensified apocrine secretion at the background of increased number of plicae after 3 months following cholecystectomy. However, apocrine secretion was a rare finding at the 1st year after gallbladder removal, while the general image of relief somewhat resembled the relief of the gallbladder described by other authors (Mac Pherson et al., 1983) (Figure 88).The animals, in which the cholecystectomy was performed as a second stage trial, demonstrated the mentioned changes already after three months following the first surgery, whereas the cholecystectomy itself was not followed by any additional changes.

It may be concluded that removal of the functioning gallbladder resulted in transformation of the architectonics of the biliary tract demonstrated by dilatation of the ducts, development of spindle-like (ampule-like) local pouches, and proliferation of bile ducts with creation of collaterals among them.

Taking into account the data on biliary tract transformation during cholestasis, the changes following the cholecystectomy can supposedly be explained by the increase in biliary pressure. The dilatation of bile ducts, their proliferation and development of collaterals (which actually means to cut new passages within the liver) may be accompanied by the pain phenomenon, which clinically correlates with the "true postcholecystectomy syndrome" itself.

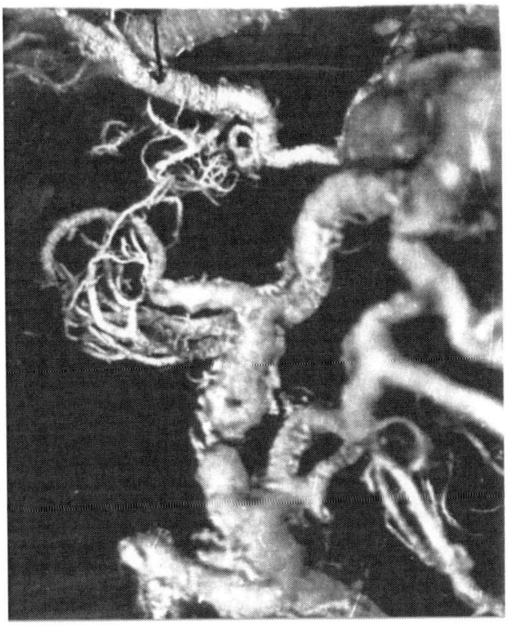

Figure 86. Intrahepatic bile ducts of canine (with small local dilatations and anastomoses);1year after colecystectomy; corrosion casts.

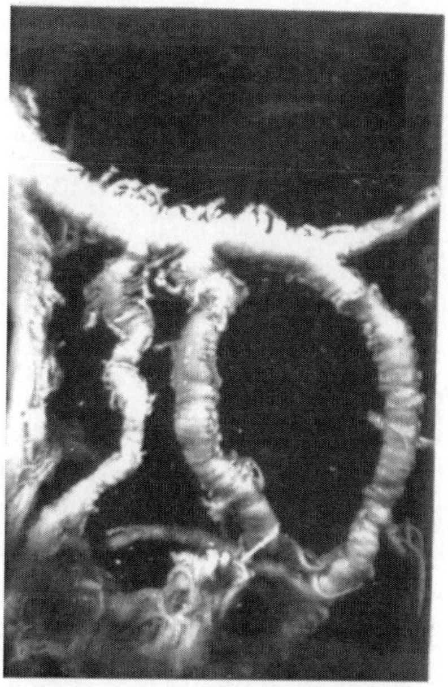

Figure 87. Intrahepatic bile ducts of canine (with small local dilatations and anastomoses);1year after colecystectomy; corrosion casts.

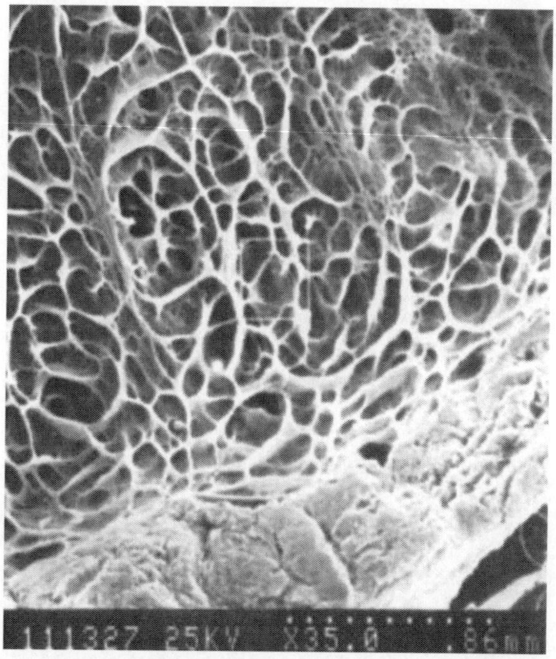

Figure 88. SEM of luminal surface of lobar bile duct of canine; 1 year after cholesistectomy.

Aside from the irritation of abundant sensitive nerve fibers located around the proliferating ducts, this pain can also result from contraction of "biliary micro-vesicles" representing the specific expression of adaptation to new conditions directed towards correction of the digestive function. The decline and further disappearance of clinical symptoms of the "true cholecystectomy syndrome", by about the 1st year following the cholecystectomy, should be related to the ending of transformation of the biliary bed after surgery.

Plasticity of Bile Ducts After Restoration of Congested Bile Drainage

The plastic ability of bile ducts may be observed not only in the bile congestion setting, but also after restoration of its drainage as well. For instance, the "narrowing" of the bile duct caliber down to its normal limits, evidenced after elimination of cholestasis, is widely described. However, the regeneration features of the biliary epithelial layer, also its adaptability with the digestive epithelium in the setting of biliary–digestive anastomosis (which represents an important practical issue), are rarely studied. The structural features of the bile pathway were studied at the 1st, 7th, 14th, 30th and 60th days following the correction of cholestasis of 14, 30 and 60 days duration. The biliary casts, prepared on the 1st and 7th days after correction of cholestasis, all mentioned durations similar to the patterns prepared in the setting of bile congestion. After 14 days of elimination of cholestasis of 14- and 30 days duration, the "amputated" ends of the biliary branch patterns are a little enlarged and supplied by the replicas of fine ductuli, which evidences the beginning of their recanalization and restoration of terminal ductular bile flow (Figures 89, 90).

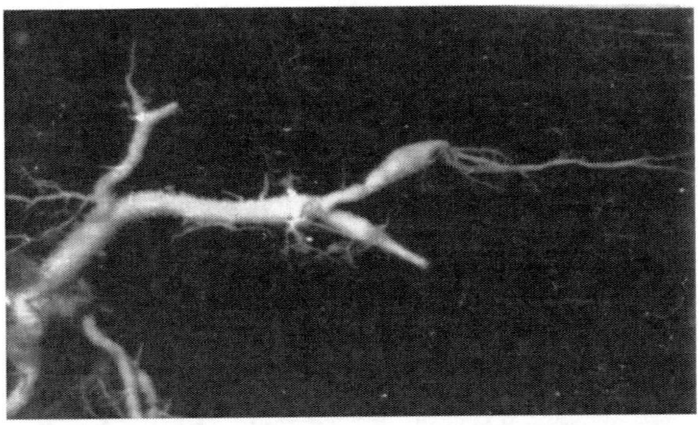

Figure 89. Intrahepatic bile ducts of canine after 14 days of elimination of cholestasis of 14- and 30 days duration; corrosion casts.

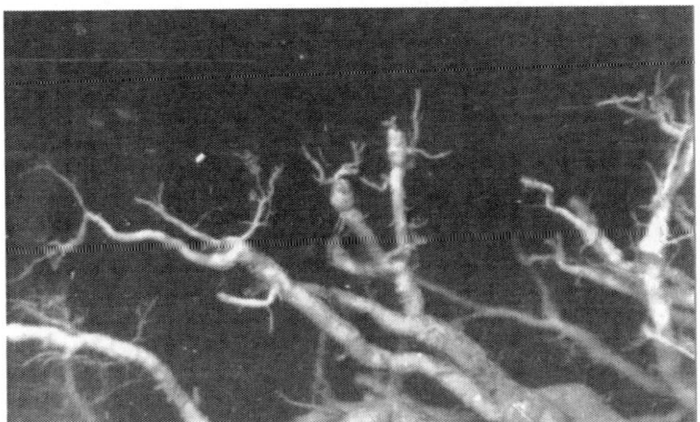

Figure 90. Intrahepatic bile ducts of canine after 14 days of elimination of cholestasis of 14- and 30 days duration; corrosion casts.

In addition, the casts of mucosal biliary glands, which have disappeared in the long-term cholestasis setting, emerge again on the casts of gross caliber bile ducts. Similarly the casts of fine biliary structures appear on the ends of corrosion specimens' branches by the 30th day of restoration of bile drainage following 60-day cholestasis (Figures 91, 92).

As mentioned previously, long-term CBDL is accompanied by blockage of fine biliary ductuli presumably by desquamated epithelium and bile clots. This block usually remains after liquidation of cholestasis; even the hepatocytes have regenerated their secretion toward bile canaliculi. This secretion pressure itself, before recanalization of terminal fine biliary ductuli, must be causing the local dilatation of these ductuli proximally to the "block" site. At the 60th day of elimination of cholestasis of 14- and 30-days duration, the corrosion specimens of bile ducts do not differ from normal variants by their general shape (Figures 93, 94). Whereas after 2 months of elimination of 60-days cholestasis the caliber of bile duct patterns still markedly exceed that of the normal pattern. In addition, at every stage, the casts of mucosal biliary glands are shorter and less branched compared with normal patterns (Figures 95, 96). The periductal and periglandular fibrosis associated with long-term cholestasis can be considered as the reason for the above-mentioned events.

The delayed recanalization of blocked fine biliary ductuli and restoration of canalicular-ductular bile flow after relief of long-term cholestasis are evidenced by clinical observations as well. The biochemical composition of bile starts to get back to normal limits after three or more days following the elimination of biliary obstruction.

We have registered a case, when after surgical correction of mechanical jaundice of 1-month duration (cholecystectomy, choledocholythotomy, external drainage of common bile duct) the biliary clots discharged into "white" bile of mucosal consistency at the 5th day following the surgery. A sudden darkening of excreting bile followed this discharge.

It must be noted that at every stage after deletion of biliary obstruction, the corrosion specimens of bile ducts remain in patterns of collaterals described in the cholestasis setting, which allows us to implicate that these biliary shunts preserve their functional activity after relieving the bile congestion and biliary hypertension.

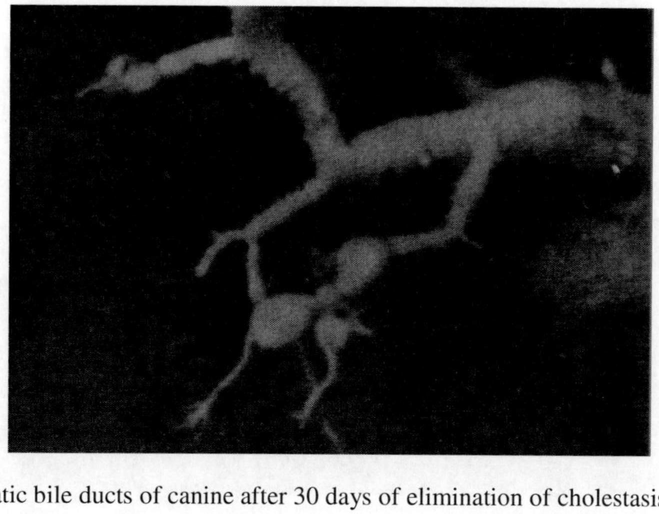

Figure 91. Intrahepatic bile ducts of canine after 30 days of elimination of cholestasis of 60 days duration; corrosion casts.

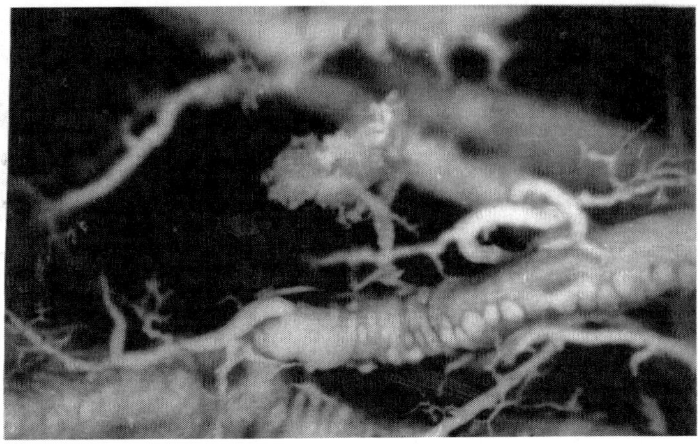

Figure 92. Intrahepatic bile ducts of canine after 30 days of elimination of cholestasis of 60 days duration; corrosion casts.

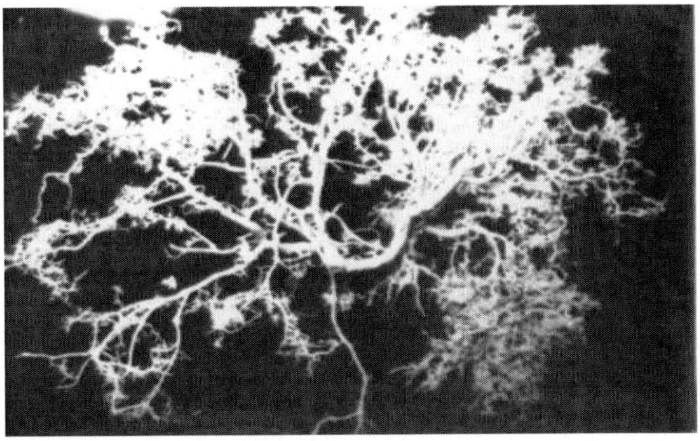

Figure 93. Intrahepatic biliary tree of canine after 60 days of elimination of cholestasis of 14- and 30 days duration; corrosion casts.

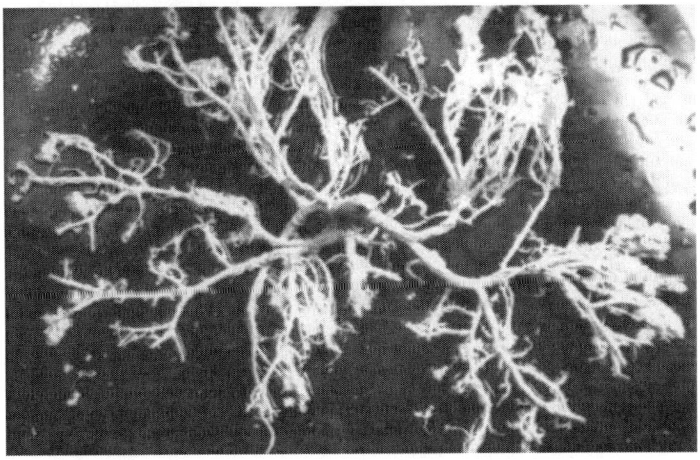

Figure 94. Intrahepatic biliary tree of canine after 60 days of elimination of cholestasis of 14- and 30-days duration; corrosion casts.

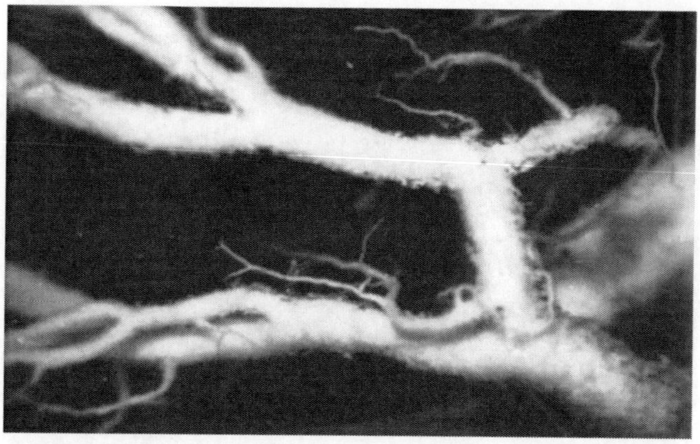

Figure 95. Intrahepatic biliary tree of canine after 60 days of elimination of cholestasis of 30 days duration; corrosion casts.

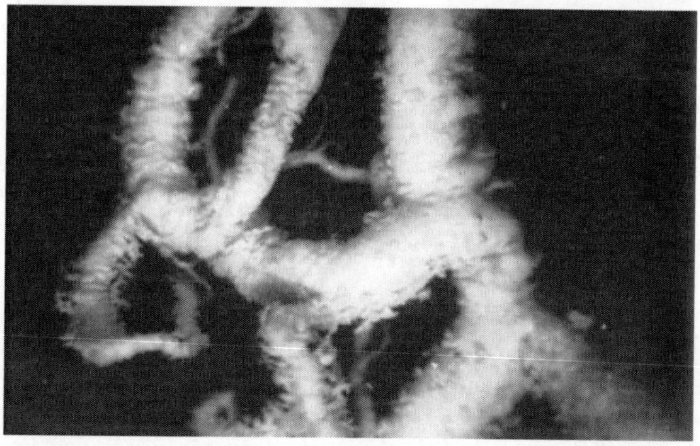

Figure 96. Intrahepatic biliary tree of canine after 60 days of elimination of cholestasis of 30 days duration; corrosion casts.

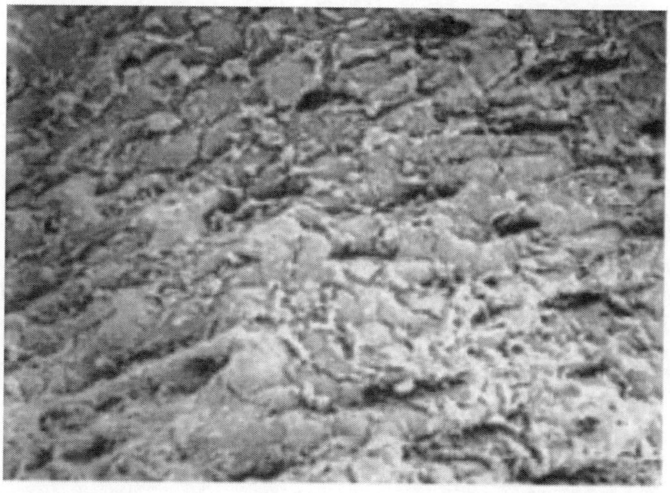

Figure 97. SEM of epithelial covering of canine lobar bile ducts in one month after elimination of cholestasis of 14 days duration.

The SEM of bile duct relief in 1 month following common bile duct external drainage after 14-days cholestasis showed that the epithelial cover of magistral, I, II and III line bile ducts is basically uninterrupted (Figure 97).

The apical surfaces of epitheliocytes are covered with microvilli, though compared to normal samples they are lower and thinner (Figure 98).

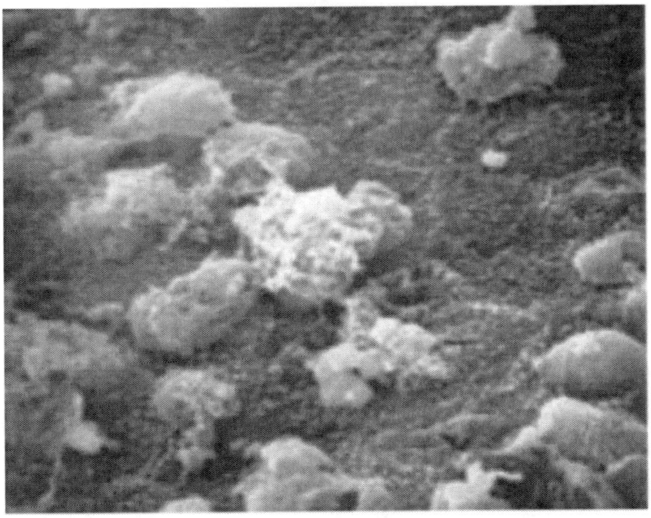

Figure 98. SEM of epithelial covering of canine lobar bile ducts in one month after elimination of cholestasis of 14 days duration.

Parts of the cells undergo dystrophic changes; their surfaces are protruded and sharply prominent in the general epithelial background. Compared with the respective stage of cholestasis, the number of dystrophic cells is markedly decreased. The goblet cells are fixed in stage of active secretion (Figure 99). After 2 months following the deletion of 2-weeks biliary obstruction, the epithelial cover of the bile ducts didn't differ from normal (Figure 100). However, the functional activity of both mucosal biliary glands and goblet cells is increased, which leads to increased production of mucus.

Due to the above, flake-like spots cover the relief of bile ducts at scanograms. This event can be explained by "splitting" information: In the setting of biliary congestion, "information of biliary hunger" leaks out from the digestive tract, which must be serving as a stimulus for increasing the secretion of the liver.

At the same time, the information about blockage impeding bile excretion is aired from bile ducts, which must be the result of the inhibition of the secretive activity of the liver.

The inter-regulation between the secretion stimulating and inhibiting mechanisms define the level of secretion by the hepatocytes, which account for biliary-lymphatic and biliary-venous reflux and the development of the mechanical jaundice syndrome. In case of external drainage of the biliary tract, the secretion-inhibiting information is cancelled, but the information on "biliary hunger" coming from the duodenum still remains, which becomes the reason for increased secretion of the liver. Though the latter becomes more and more difficult to achieve in the setting of external drainage the electrolytes, biliary acids, pigments and cholesterol are permanently lost. For this reason, the liver switches the secretive reserves of bile ducts in the shape of increased activity of mucosal glands and goblet cells, which results in the image manifested by SEM.

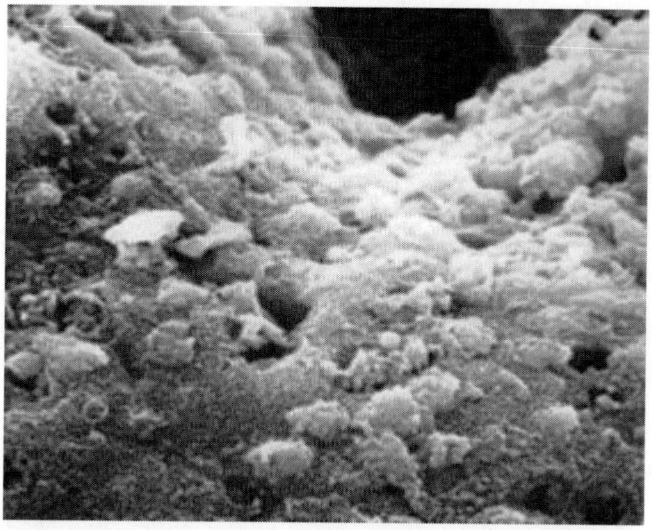

Figure 99.SEM of epithelial covering of canine lobar bile ducts in one month after elimination of cholestasis of 14 days duration.

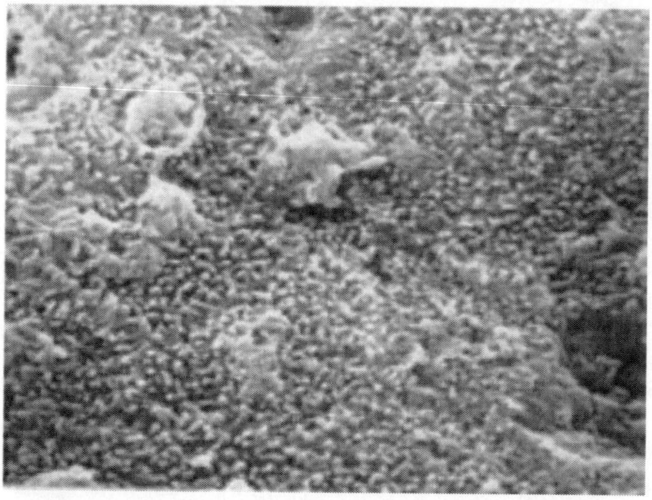

Figure 100. SEM of epithelial covering of canine lobar bile ducts in two months after elimination of cholestasis of 14 days duration.

After 1 week from the external biliary drainage, performed in the setting on the 30th day of cholestasis, the epithelial cover of bile ducts is represented fragmentally. In addition, it is evidenced that restoration of the epithelium is achieved via epitheliocytes lining the excretory ductuli of mucosal biliary glands (Figure 101).

One month later after deletion of cholestasis of 30-days duration, the epithelial cover is almost totally restored (Figure102).

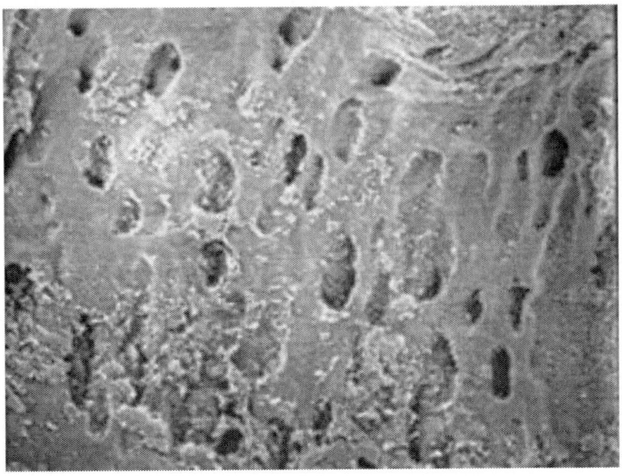

Figure 101. SEM of epithelial covering of canine lobar bile ducts in one week after elimination of cholestasis of 30 days duration.

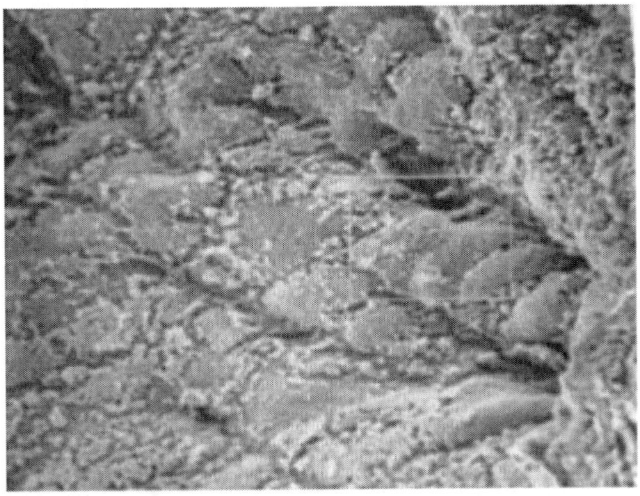

Figure 102. SEM of epithelial covering of canine lobar bile ducts in one month after elimination of cholestasis of 30 days duration.

Significant portions of epitheliocytes are covered with microvilli, which are shorter and blunter compared to normal samples. The goblet cells are frequently observed (Figure 103).

At 2 months following the external drainage of bile ducts, performed on the 30th day of cholestasis, most of the epitheliocytes lining the ducts undergo dystrophic changes, compared with the previous stage. Many of them are fixated within the state of apocrine secretion (Figure 104). The implemented investigations have shown that bile ducts can restore their caliber and epithelial cover quite rapidly after deletion of bile congestion through the external drainage. Such recovery depends on the terms of bile congestion, and it also depends on the time elapsed after restoration of bile drainage. Moreover, obtained data indicates that full restoration of morphological-functional status of the bile ducts is quite a long process. In addition, the external biliary drainage resulting in acholia itself represents a pathological condition, prolongation of which leads to severe changes not only of the bile ducts and liver, but the whole body as well.

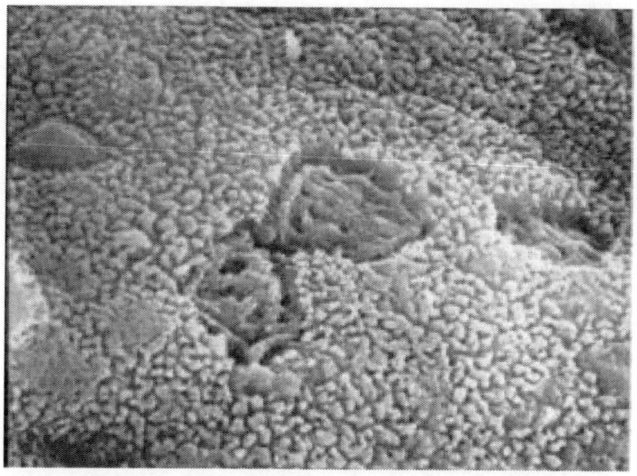

Figure 103. SEM of epithelial covering of canine lobar bile ducts in one month after elimination of cholestasis of 30 days duration.

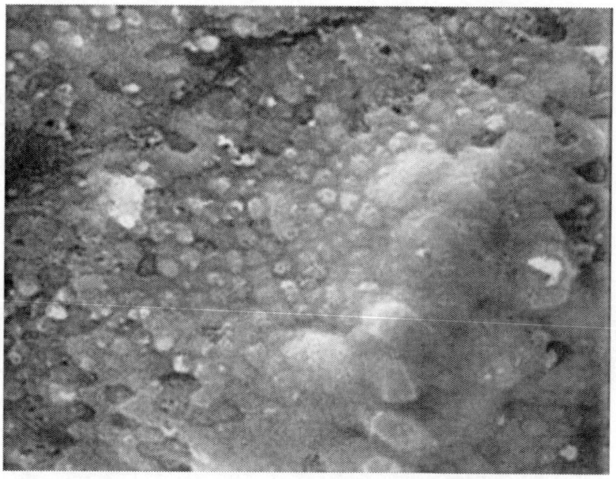

Figure 104. SEM of epithelial covering of canine lobar bile ducts attwo months after elimination of cholestasis of 30 days duration.

In one group of animals the bile congestion was relieved by formation of artificial bilio-digestive anastomosis. The choledocho-duodenal anastomoses were accomplished with #6.0 Prolen thread, using penetrating and precise sutures. While using the penetrating suture, we were turning the mucosal layer outside (with externally located ligatures). The distance between adjacent ligatures was 2.5-3 mm.

After 2 months following the creation of bilio-digestive fistula, on the 30th day of bile congestion, the study of bile duct relief by SEM reveals several specificities: the relief of magistral, I and II line bile ducts appear markedly wrinkled. The shape of the wrinkles, which is typical for the ducts epithelial cover, has disappeared and it resembles the relief of the duodenal mucosal layer of the same animal (Figures 105-107).

A significant amount of bacterial colonies is observed over the wrinkles, which are the result of compromised biliary tract autonomy (Figure 108). Each separate wrinkle resembles intestinal villus, both by shape and general overview of the surface (Figure 109). The epithelial cover of the bile ducts as well as the apical microvilli of epitheliocytes are restored.

In addition, the shape of apical surface of most of the cells somewhat differ from normal samples – they are shaped like spindles and covered with thin and short microvilli. The goblet cells also have the same spindle-like shape (Figure 110), which is somehow unusual for this type of cells.

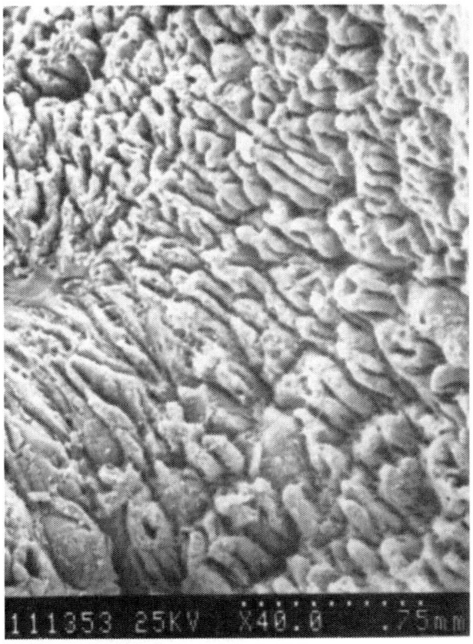

Figure 105. SEM of epithelial covering of canine lobar bile ducts after 2 months following the creation of bilio-digestive fistula on the 30th day of bile congestion.

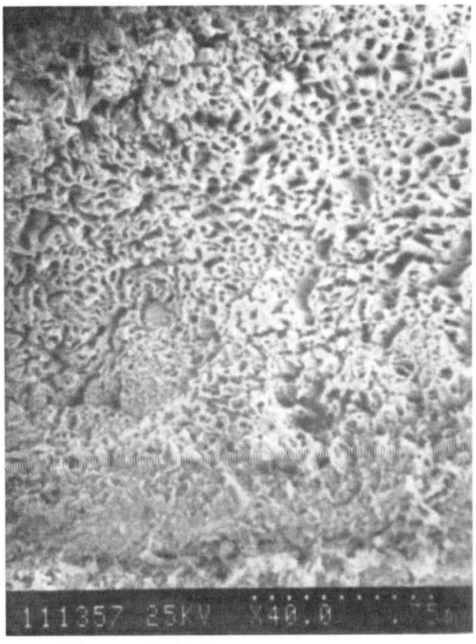

Figure 106. SEM of epithelial covering of canine lobar bile ducts after 2 months following the creation of bilio-digestive fistula on the 30th day of bile congestion.

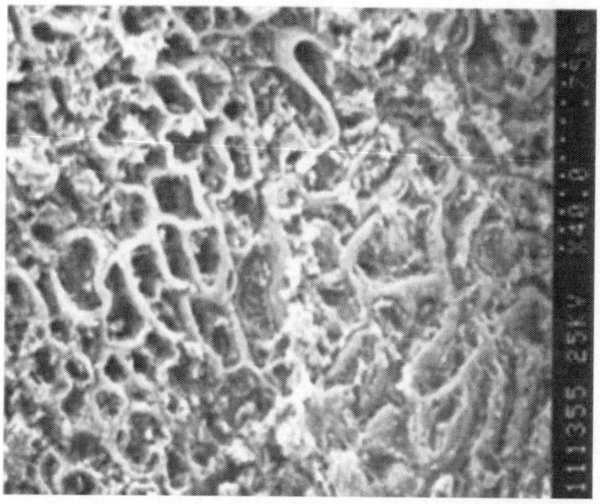

Figure 107. SEM of epithelial covering of canine lobar bile ducts after 2 months following the creation of bilio-digestive fistula on the 30th day of bile congestion.

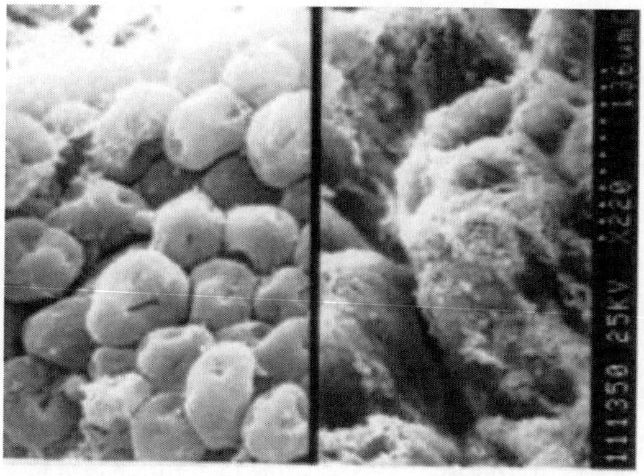

Figure 108. SEM of epithelial covering of canine lobar bile ducts after 2 months following the creation of bilio-digestive fistula on the 30th day of bile congestion; The significant amount of bacterial colonies is observed over the wrinkles (108).

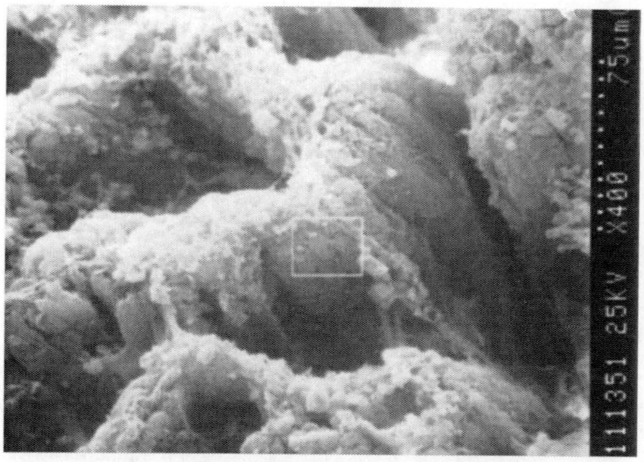

Figure 109. SEM of epithelial covering of canine lobar bile ducts after 2 months following the creation of bilio-digestive fistula on the 30th day of bile congestion; The significant amount of bacterial colonies is observed over the wrinkles (108).

The mutual transition of intestinal and biliary epithelium is quite simple. The projection line of the suture can differ on small magnification, but on large magnifications this landmark is gradually lost (Figure 111).

The confluence site of the epithelium of two organs demonstrate how the so-called transitional zone is created, construction and relief of which reveals close resemblance to the construction and relief of both intestinal and duct epithelium wrinkles (Figures 112, 113).

The secretive activity is increased to some extent, which is conditioned by the overproduction of both goblet cells and mucosal biliary glands. This can be explained by the irritation of these glands with duodenal content.

Increased secretion of mucus itself provides the prevention of ascending cholangitis, as it provides "self-cleaning" of the ducts while rinsing out from bile ducts the masses deposited there as a result of enteric-biliary reflux.

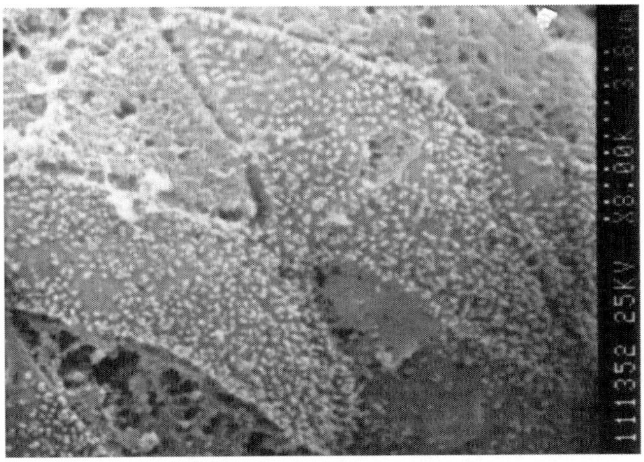

Figure 110. SEM of epithelial covering of canine lobar bile ducts after 2 months following the creation of bilio-digestive fistula on the 30th day of bile congestion; the cells shaped like spindles.

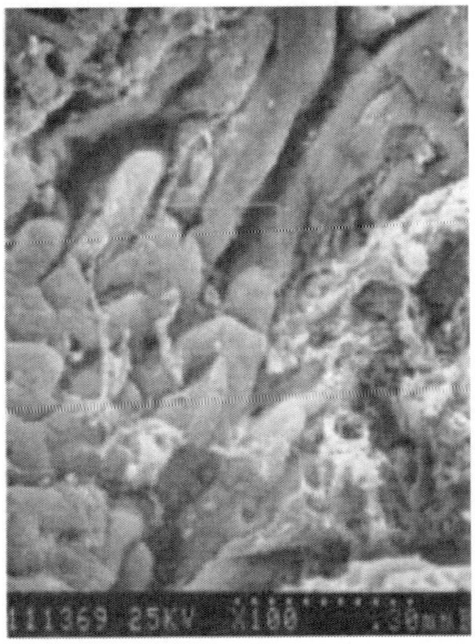

Figure 111. SEM of epithelial covering of the region of biliary-digestive anastomosis after 2 months following the creation of fistula on the 30th day of bile congestion.

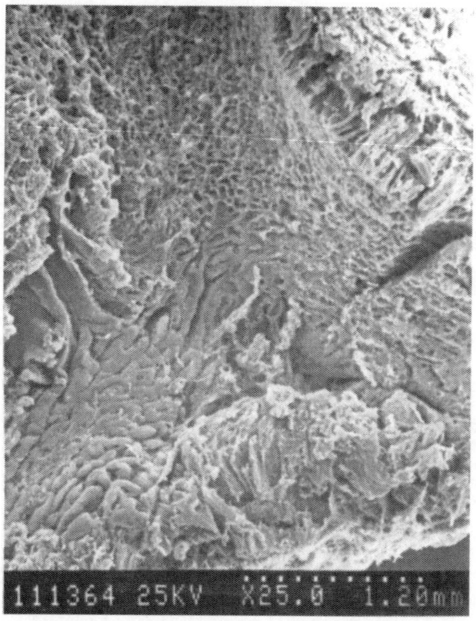

Figure 112. SEM of epithelial covering of the region of biliary-digestive anastomosis after 2 months following the creation of fistula on the 30th day of bile congestion.

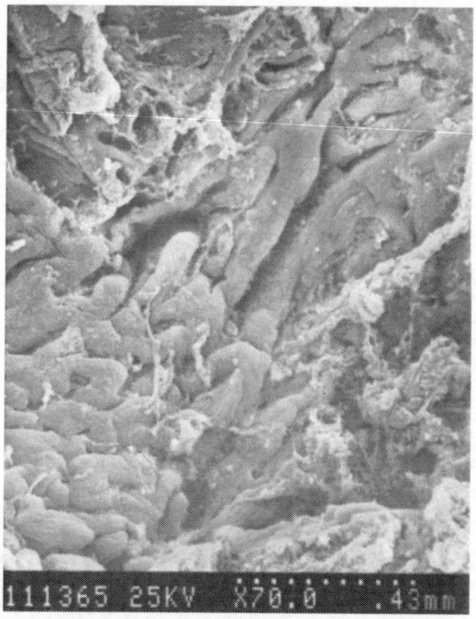

Figure 113. SEM of epithelial covering of the region of biliary-digestive anastomosis after 2 months following the creation of fistula on the 30th day of bile congestion.

Actually, this is one of the advantages of choledocho-duodenal anastomosis against cholecystic-duodenal anastomosis: the high absorptive capability of gallbladder (lacking of mucosal glands) creates perfect conditions for the development of ascending infection in bile ducts even in cases of the smallest stasis and entero-biliary reflux. However, it is confirmed that numerous mucosal glands supply the gallbladder cervix and the cystic duct. This fact provides the evidence for recommendation, that in case forming the choledocho-digestive anastomosis is impossible,, it is reasonable to create cystic-duodenal anastomosis, which should be free of above-mentioned complications as the secretions of mucosal glands may provide "self-cleaning" of the area of fistula and maintain the sterility of the bile (Vitebsky, 1988). At 2 months from creation of choledocho-duodenal anastomosis, on the 60th day of CBDL, the changes of the biliary duct relief is quite similar to the pattern described above but resembles the construction of the duodenal mucosal layer even more (Figure 114).

Summarizing the results of the studies on bile ducts after deletion of bile congestion and biliary hypertension, it can be concluded that restoration of the cannalicular-ductular passage of bile and regeneration of the epithelial cover of the bile duct as well as of the zone of biliary-digestive anastomosis depends on the terms of cholestasis on one hand, and on the duration of the period following the restoration of bile drainage, on the other.

Specifically, the shorter the first and the longer the other, the reparation and regeneration events seem to be more comprehensive. In the setting of bilio-digestive anastomoses, the relief of bile ducts is transformed into intestinal type, while in the zone of suture a so-called transitional epithelium is created, which demonstrates the resemblance of both the intestinal and duct epithelium as well.

Early Ductular Reaction Following Bile Duct Ligation

Common bile duct ligation (CBDL) represents a well-established in vivo model for the study of biliary proliferation including both - cholangiocyte and bile ductular proliferation. This proliferative response of biliary structures in bile retention is regulated by the complex interaction of several factors, including gastrointestinal and neuroendocrine hormones as well as autocrine or paracrine signalling mechanisms (Alpini G.,et al., 2002; Mancinelli R.,et al., 2009; Glaser S.S. et al., 2010). It is considered that biliary hypertension represents the proliferative trigger for biliary structures in the biliary occlusion setting, however, dynamics, as well as the mechanisms of this process require further comprehensive investigation.

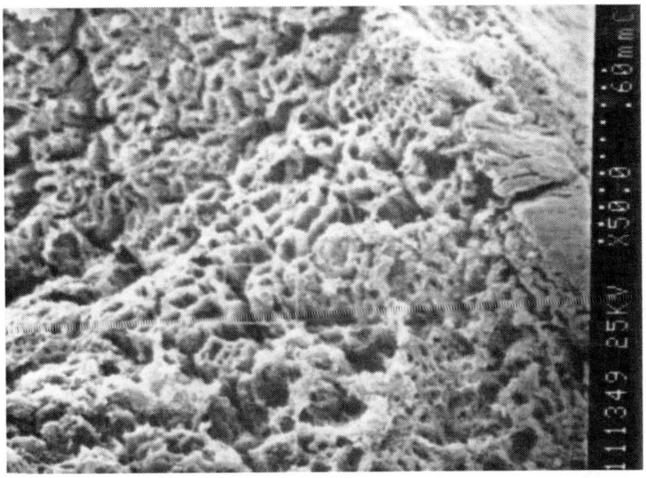

Figure 114. SEM of epithelial covering of canine lobar bile ducts after 2 months following the creation of bilio-digestive fistula on the 60th day of bile congestion.

According to several studies the appearance of new ductuli is evident on the second or third days after CBDL and is associated with increased mitotic activities of the biliary epithelia (Shibayama Y., 1990; Burt A.D., R. N. MacSween, 1993; Marucci L., 1993; Demetris A.J., 1999).

It has been demonstrated that "newductules" originated from proliferated biliary epithelial cells even in vitro. Initially, ductular proliferation appears in the periportal areas and then gradually advances intralobularly. It is considered to be more evident at one week after biliary obstruction (Glaser S.S.,1990).

However, we have previously demonstrated that amount of ductular profiles increases in the liver of CBDL rats already at several hours after biliary obstruction (Aslamazishvili T.,et al., 2007). The origin of "new" bile duct profiles and mechanisms, which can be involved in such early DR, is currently unknown, and needs to be elucidated. It is conceivable that early DR after BDL is not related to mitotic activity of existing biliary epithelia and proliferation of bile ductules.

To identify the origin of "new" ductular structures that appeared within 24 hours in response to biliary obstruction,36 inbred male Lewis rats weighting 250-300 g were subjected to common bile duct ligation (n=24) or sham operation (controls, n=12) under ethyl-ether narcosis. The animals were killed on 3, 6, 12 and 24 hours after CBDL (6 animals in each group); part of the dissected liver samples (median lobe) were frozen at -80ºC for immunohistochemistry and part fixed in 10% neutral buffered formalin, embedded in paraffin and used for a routine histological examination.

Liver sections of 5 μm thickness were stained with hematoxylin and eosin. Fixed in 10% neutral formalin and/or frozen liver sample with standard histological (Hematoxilin-eosin stained slides) and immunohistochemical investigations.

Frozen liver samples were sectioned on cryostate microtome (Leica 800 Cryostat Microtome CM1800) and immunostained for Ki67 (1:150) (ab16667, Abcam plc, Cambridge, UK), pan-Cytokeratin antibody [AE1+AE3](neat) (ab961, Abcam, plc, Cambridge, UK) and OV-6 (1:100)(MAB2020 RandD Systems, Inc.) using appropriate protocols provided by antibody suppliers. Sections were counterstained with haematoxilin.

Data for the average number of ductular profiles were analyzed by the one-way analysis of variances (one-way ANOVA). In ANOVA, for the average number of ductular profiles the factor was time. Planned comparisons between the average numbers of ductular profiles were made using *t*-tests. Statistical tests for the average number of ductular profiles were two tailed.

It appeared that CBDL was accompanied by a significant (2-4 folds) increase of ductular profiles while in sham operated animals statistical analysis revealed no significant effect of the time factor for the number of ductular profiles ($p<0.05$).

Biliary Epitheliocytes and "Reactive ductules' cells" were strongly positive for CK and OV-6 at all time points. "New" ductular profiles appeared around the portal tracts of all sizes: from large to the finest (Figure 115 a, b) also intralobullarly, sometimes several hundreds microns away from the portal tract (biliary ducts) (Figure 115 c).

These "neoductules" were located in the spaces of Disse (Figure d); the cells composing the neoductuli were small and uniform with light, oval, sometimes spindle-shaped nuclei and scant cytoplasm. They are Ki67-negative, but equally immunopositive for Pan-Cytokeratine and OV6. No Ki67 positive staining of any type of cells was observed.

These results demonstrate the appearance of "newductules" in 3-24 hours after CBDL.

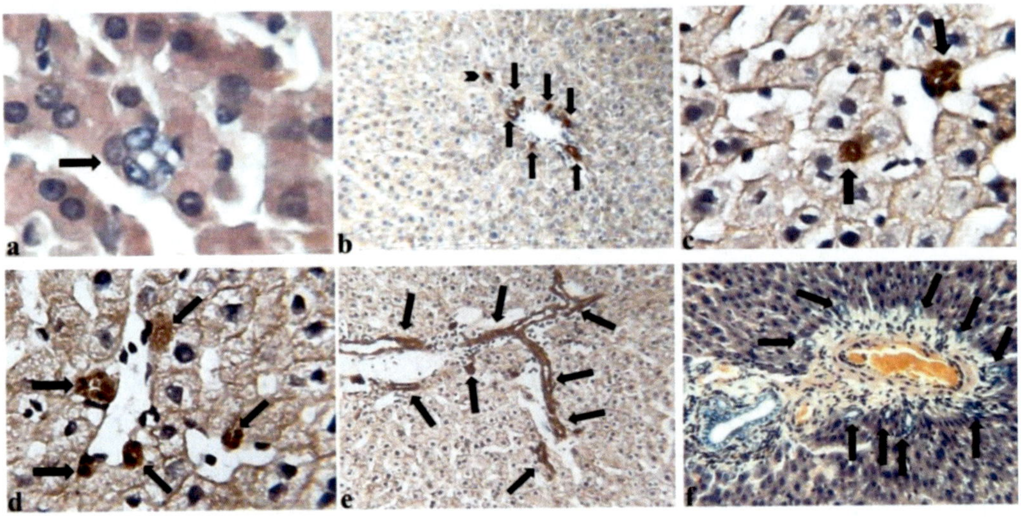

Figure 115. Histology and Immunohistochemistry of liver tissue after CBDL a) Intralobular bile ductuli (arrows), Hand E, 6 h after CBDL; b) Bile ductuli in the small portal area (arrows), intralobular bile ductuli (arrowhead), H and E, 6 h after CBDL; c) "Newductuli" surrounding widened sinusoids (arrows), CK, 12 h after CBDL; d) "Newductuli" surrounding widened sinusoids (arrows), OV6, 12 h after CBDL; e) Bile ductuli surrounding portal vein (arrows), CK24 h after CBDL; f) Bile ductuli surrounding portal vein (arrows), H and E24 h after BDL.

However, the negative reaction of cells covering the lumens of these newductules towards Ki67 antibodies indicates that this phenomenon cannot be associated with proliferation of existed bile epithelial or any other cells. These data are in correlation with the results of our previous investigation showing that the indexes of mitoses of cholagiocytes and hepatocytes are originated from the second day of CBDL (Azmaiparashvili, et al., 2009). They confirm that the increased number of ductular profiles at 3, 6 and 12 hours after CBDL is not associated with cell proliferation. It must be related with widening of existing lumenar structures covered by epitheliocyte (or epitheliocytes-like) cells.

One of the possible sources of increased ductular profiles can be the lumens of biliary mucosal glands, which are widened due to raised CBDL-induced biliary pressure (as it was described on autopsy liver specimens (Terada T., Y. Nakanuma, 1992) and in dogs after biliary obstruction (Kordzaia D., 1990). However, in rats, unlike dogs, cats and guinea pigs, the amount of mucosal biliary glands is much smaller and the majority of them are attached to the extrahepatic but not the intrahepatic bile ducts (Yamamoto K.,1985). The topography of the newly appeared ductuli (they position along the perimeter of portal vein lumen remotely but not adjacent to bile ducts, also intralobularly) excludes the possibility of their glandular origin.

Next epithelial-lined tubular structures located at the portal areas, which can be a source of DR is periportal biliary plexi described on biliary corrosion casts in rats (Murakami T., et al., 2001). In these plexi the bile ductules are anastomosing with each other, and forming a plexiform network around the portal vein branch or at the periphery of portal canal (Figure 116). This network of bile ductuli forms larger ductuli to drain into the intrahepatic bile ducts in the portal canal. We suggest that the periportal biliary plexus is the basis for numerous ductular profiles, which appear in the periportal area already in the few hours of bile congestion. But, according to our data, at 6 h after CBDL the ductular profiles also appear inside the lobules, far away from the portal tract.

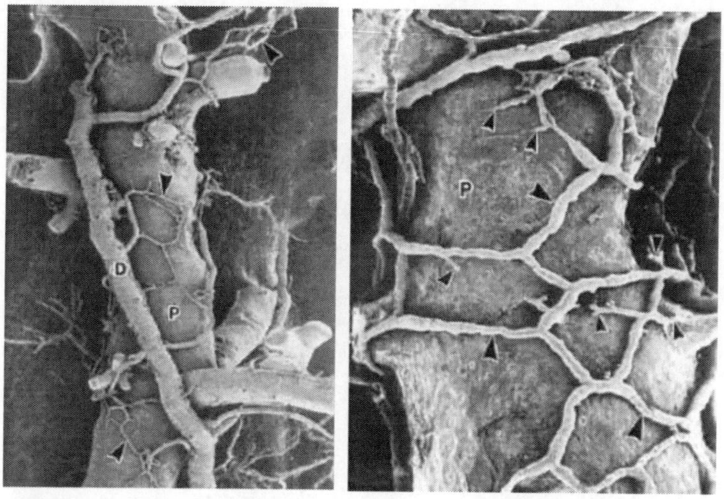

Figure 116. Periportal biliary ductular plexus (arrowheads). In this case, portal vein branches (p) were concomitantly replicated. D bile duct. X40.

The figures are provided by kind permission of Prof. T. Murakami.

Obviously, the periportal biliary plexus cannot be the source for these structures. They should be cross- and tangential sections of the finest bile ducts ramifications, bile ductules and Hering's ductules, which are established to pass the limiting plate and spread quite far inside the lobulli (Roskams T.A.,et al., 2004).These finest biliary structures, which lie within the lobule and not at the limiting plate, are not readily apparent on routine histological staining (Saxena R., N. Theise., 2004). But the increased biliary pressure due to BDL can be a sufficient factor for their dilatation and appearance on microscopical slices. Ductular profiles can represent the sections of the finest biliar-biliary anastomoses, which are evident on SEM of corrosion casts (Murakami T.,et al., 2001).

They can also be an intercalated portion of the biliary ductuli, creating the finest plexi at the bordering areas with limiting plates (Takahashi-Iwanaga H., T. Fujita., 1992).

Normally there is on average one Hering's ductile per 10 μm of bile duct length. (Saxena R., N. Theise, 2004). The comparative analysis of the results of Scanning Electron Microscopy of corrosion casts (SEMCC) of portal and biliary trees stipulates the conclusion that frequently the angles of ramifications of the sinusoids from the thinnest portal branches appear different with angles of ramification of biliary ductuli from the finest interlobular bile ducts (Motta P.M., et al., 1978; Yamamoto K., et al., 1985; Kordzaia D., 1990.;Murakami T.,et al., 2001;Yoshida K., et al., 2010).The above-mentioned peculiarities of the architecture of vascular and biliary structures are schematically presented on Figure 117. It can explain the suggested mechanism of appearance of ductular profiles inside the liver lobule caused by widening of biliary ductule lumens due to biliary hypertension. Localization of described "neoductuli" in the spaces of Disse confirms this suggestion, because perisinusoidal spaces are the only areas where the biliary ductules, Hering's ductuli and/or the finest biliary-biliary anastomoses can be placed.

In conclusion, our data indicates that the appearance of "new biliary ductuli" starts with in a few hours after CBDL and is mediated by widening the finest biliary ramifications, biliary ductules and periportal biliary plexi and is not associated with proliferation of existing bile ducts/ductuli and their epithelial cells.

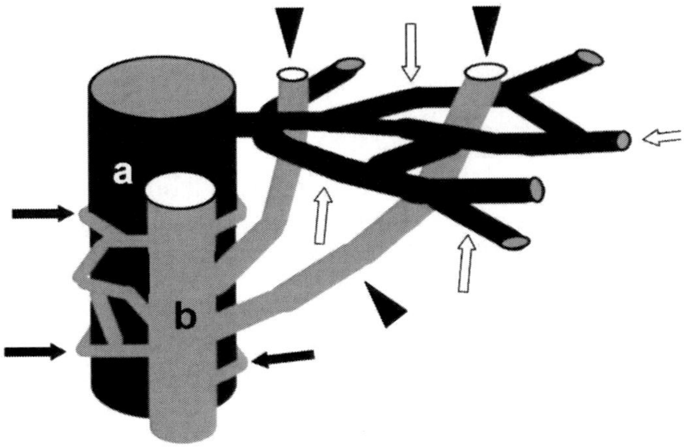

Figure 117. Architecture of the finest vascular and biliary structures: interlobular portal vein (a), interlobular bile duct (b), periportal biliary plexus (black arrow), Canals of Hering and intralobular ductules (arrowhead), sinusoids (white arrow).

Do Bile Ductuli Accompany the Tributaries of Hepatic Veins?

A significant number of papers dedicated to the architecture of hitherto unknown or less-studied tubular structures of the liver has been published in recent years, with clarification of their possible role and functional importance in the development of different pathological processes. These works particularly addressed the identification of reliable stereomorphology of the functional unit of the liver and the topography and architectonics of finest biliary branches – colangioles and Hering's ductuli (Saxena R., et al., 1999; Roskams at al., 2004; Teutsch H., 2005; Dezso K., et al., 2009).

This is hypothetically explained by the fact that conventionally accepted models of functional liver units, like "classic lobule", "secondary lobule", "acinus", etc., and their corresponding microcirculatory networks, cannot adequately interpret all manifestations of different clinical and experimental pathologies of the liver and biliary system. It is also considered, that a microcirculatory module of the liver, unlike the standard modules with three circulatory pools, additionally includes the fourth component - bile circulation (Saxena R., et al., 1999; Sulaberidze G., et al., 2006).

One of the pathological phenomena that triggered the investigation of the functional morphology of liver lobules in depth and especially the finest branches of biliary tract is the Ductular Reaction (DR). DR is a well-known phenomenon in many acute and chronic liver conditions in humans as well as in rodents, histologically expressed by the increased amount of ductular profiles (Desmet V., 2011; Roskams T., et al., 2003). The investigation of DR genesis led to a new stage in the research of the morphology of liver lobular structures with special accents on cellular structures composing the biliary bed. Three possible types of ductular reaction have been established: I. "typical" (caused by the proliferation of existing bile ductuli), II. "atypical" (caused by the transdifferentiation of hepatocytes toward biliary epiteliocytes) and III. caused by the proliferation of progenitor cells (oval cells) in the liver (Desmet V., et al., 1995; Roskams T., Van Eyken P., 1995; Priester S., et al., 2010).

Typical ductular reaction develops after acute biliary obstruction both in human as well as in rodent models. Appearance of new ductuli associated with increased mitotic activity in the biliary epithelium is evident from the second/third days after Common Bile Duct Ligation (CBDL) in periportal areas, which gradually advance to the intralobular compartment later on (Burt A., MacSween R., 1993; Demetris A., et al., 1999; Marucci L., et al., 1993; Shibayama Y., 1990).

It is considered that after CBDL, newly developed ductuli are originating from the preexisted biliary ductuli (Slott P., et al., 1990) and their amount is increasing in a time-depended manner after BDL (Dirlik M., 2009; Alpini G. et al., 1998; Gaudio E., et al., 2006; Franchitto A., et al., 2012; Alpini G., 1998; Gaudio E., 2006; Antonio F., 2012).

However, we have previously shown that DRin rats already develops within several hours after CBDL. Obviously, this early DR could not be a result of proliferation. We confirmed that it develops as a consequence of widening of less known periportal biliary plexi as well as intralobular bile ductulii (including Hering's ductuli) due to increased biliary pressure caused by CBDL, which provides their apparent visibility.

In addition, we showed that several intralobular ductulii are quite long and penetrate deep into the lobular parenchyma (Azmaiparashvili E., et al., 2012; Kordzaia D., et al., 2012).

These findings are consistent with the data provided by other researchers (Theise N., et al., 1999; Saxena R., et al., 1999; Roskams T., et al., 2004).

In the current study about DR specificities at early stages following CBDL in the rat liver we drew attention to the ductular profiles (DP) that are directly attached to the tributaries of hepatic veins of different caliber – from large to sub-lobular and central veins. The intentional search of the ductuli of the above-mentioned localization showed us that in rare cases they may also be found in normal conditions, but in the setting of biliary congestion they were seen more frequently with a clearer and sharper appearance.

The special review conducted in the PubMed database could not yield any data regarding the above-mentioned paravenous ductular profiles.

The profound target investigation of the of DPs, discovered immediately at the central and sublobular veins, showed that they are CK 19-, CK 7- and OV6-positive, which evidenced their biliary origin (Figures 118, 119).

The forms and sizes of DPs in the adventitia of the large tributaries of the hepatic veins are different and confirm that ductuli may be situated transversely, tangentially or longitudinally towards the vein branches. Sometimes DPs are accompanied by small vascular profiles.

On the histological specimens of rat livers from both - control and CBDL groups can be found the sites of crossing of different size portal tracts and hepatic vein tributaries. These sites are characterized by integration (fusion) of connective tissue sheaths of the above-mentioned structures.

The perivascular capsule - the derivate of the liver sheath - surrounding the portal triad extends to the hepatic vein and includes it as a fourth component. The part of DPs located at these sites has a traditional, periportal location, while the other part of DPs are dislocated (moved) towards the hepatic vein branch and situated within its connective tissue sheath (adventitia) (Figures 120, 121).

In several cases fine ramifications of portal tracts are communicating with the large branches of the hepatic vein.

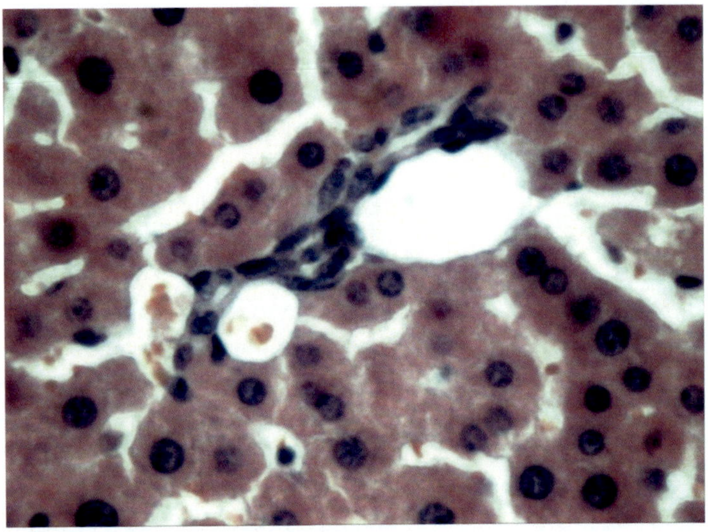

Figure 118. Central and sublobular veins with accompanying CK19-positive and OV6-positive ductular profiles, BDL-6; X200; 118) H and E; 119) CK19; 120) OV6.

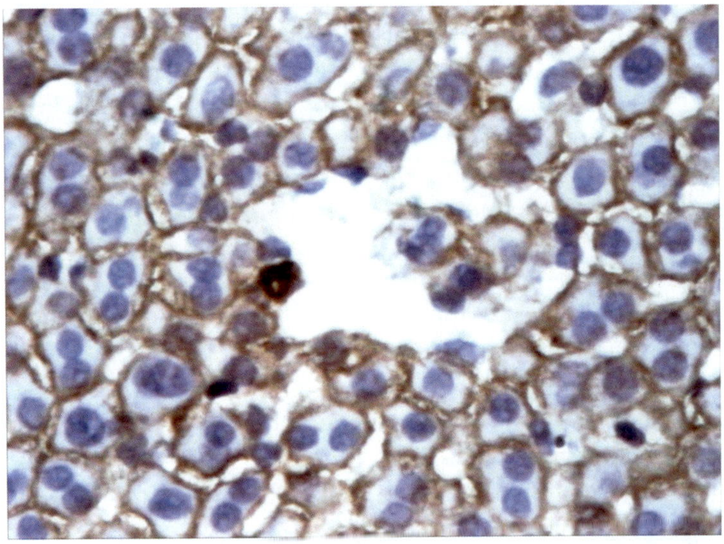

Figure 119. Central and sublobular veins with accompanying CK19-positive and OV6-positive ductular profiles, BDL-6; X200; 118) H and E; 119) CK19; 120) OV6.

In such cases bile ducts and blood and lymph vessels of the portal tract are directly "continued" into paravenous connective tissue (adventitia)making it bulge out in this area (Figure 122).In the specimens prepared after the injection of contrast medium into the biliary system via CBD, the injected ink is manifested in portal and perivenous DPs as well as in bile canaliculi (Figure123), which confirms the intercommunication and continuity of the lumina (beds) of the mentioned structures.

At the same time, the lumina of blood vessels and sinusoids are contrast medium-free.

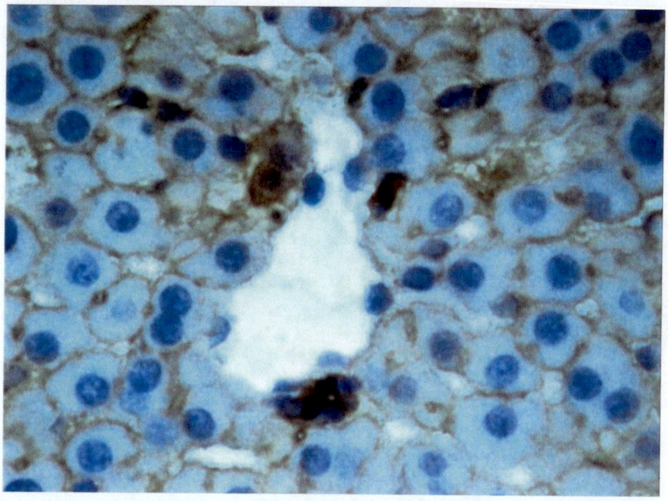

Figure 120. Central and sublobular veins with accompanying CK19-positive and OV6-positive ductular profiles, BDL-6; X200; 118) H and E; 119) CK19; 120) OV6.

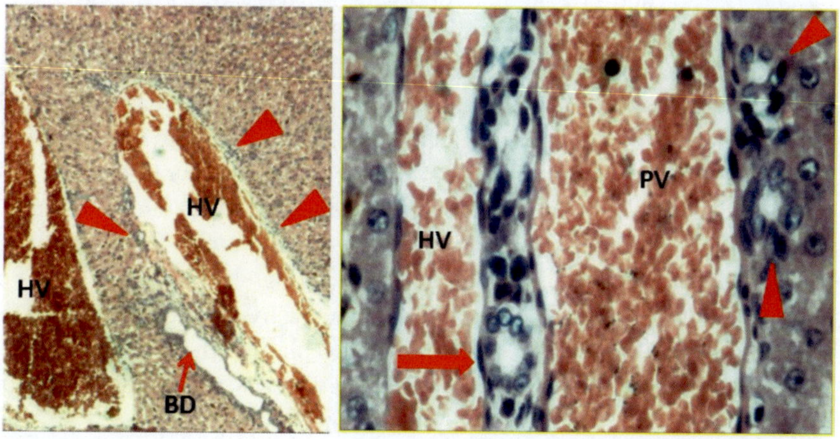

Figure 121. Rapprochement and Fusion of connective tissue spaces surrounding portal tract and hepatic vein tributaries. Bile ductule (arrow)in touch with tributary of hepatic vein (HV).The branch of portal vein (PV).Bile duct (BD); Periportal biliary plexus (arrowheads).Norm. H and E.X100, X200.

To understand the essence of bile ductules/DPs accompanying hepatic vein tributaries of different diameter it is ultimately important to clarify if these structures represent the existing (but unknown) compartment of the biliary tree or the newly-formed constructions.

It is considered that the appearance of new DPs, intralobullarly after CBDL in rodents, is caused by the proliferation of existed bile ducts (ductules) and/or biliary trans-differentiation of hepatocytes and/or proliferation of oval cells with formation of ductule-like structures (Desmet V., et al., 1995; Priester S., et al., 2010). All these three mechanisms may develop from the 2nd -3rd day after CBDL and maintained over several weeks (Georgiev P., et al., 2008; Roskams T., Desmet V., 1998).

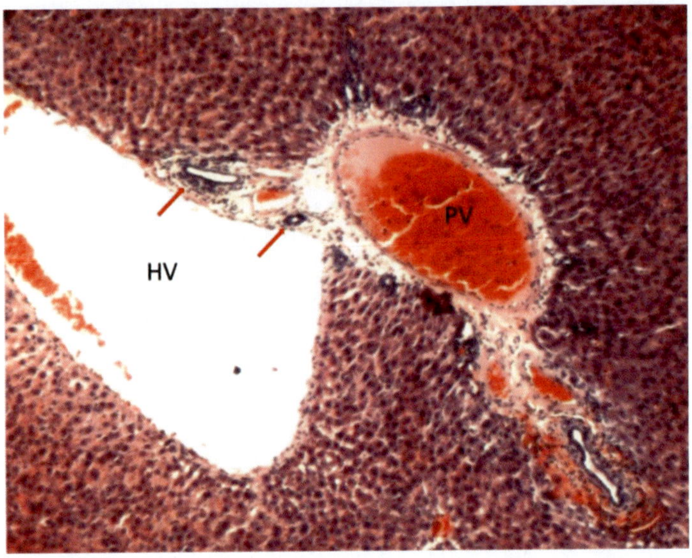

Figure 122. Fusion of connective tissue spaces surrounding the portal tract and hepatic vein tributaries (HV). Bile ductules (arrow) dislocated from the portal area toward the tributary of hepatic vein. The branch of portal vein (PV).Branch of hepatic artery (arrowhead).BDL-6. H and E.X100, X100, X200.

However, we have described the increased number of DP at the earliest stages of bile congestion - after 3, 6 and 12 hours following CBDL, when the above-mentioned mechanisms were not initiated yet. Thus, the DR observed at early stages following CBDL could be considered only as a result of widening and manifestation of already existing, but invisible by conventional methods, intralobullar biliary ductules (Azmaiparashvili E., et al., 2012). Similarly, the appearance of bile ductules (DPs) accompanying (attached to) the different caliber tributaries of hepatic veins also can't be associated with the processes of cell proliferation and/or transdifferentiation and must be explained by the widening–manifestation of the existing biliary structures. It is shown that several intralobular ductuli (Hering's ductuli) can penetrate deep into the lobule in a quite long distance from the Portal area (Theise N., et al., 1999; Saxena R., et al., 1999; Azmaiparashvili E., et al., 2012; Dezso K. et al., 2009; Dezso K., et al., 2009). Therefore, it is acceptable that the DPs directly attached to the central and sub-lobular veins represent the intersections of these deeply penetrated ductuli.

However, this presumption cannot explain the essence of ductules (ductular profiles) emerged in the connective tissue surrounding the large caliber tributaries of hepatic veins.

Based on the histological images shown above, we conclude that biliary ducts, accompanying hepatic vein branches, must originate from the classical portal ducts or periportal biliary plexi - in the areas where portal tracts and hepatic vein tributaries cross each other and merging their connective tissue sheaths. In these areas bile ducts/ductules can translocate from the periportal space towards the adjacent hepatic vein. It is established that in the human liver, the arterial branches sprouting from classical portal arteries can dislocate towards the hepatic veins in the areas of crossing of portal tracts with hepatic veins and the fusion of their connective tissue sheaths (Toidze Sh., Chanukvadze I., 1978; Chanukvadze I., 1989). The arteries supplying the central/sublobular and hepatic veins were also described in rats by Ekataskin W., Kaneda K. (1999).

Similar dislocation of nerves and lymphatic vessels is also described in the above-mentioned areas; The branches of vagal nerves dislocated perivenously from the portal tract participate in the innervation of the hepatic vein's system, while the dislocated lymphatics provide the communication between the portal lymph vessels and those accompanying hepatic veins (Chanukvadze I., 1989; Izraelashvili M., 1989).

The bile ducts in humans (and mammals in general having gallbladders) are supplied by mucosal biliary glands. The size and shape of these glands are quite variable. Small glands are situated within the walls of the bile duct (intramural glands), while large glands with different types of branching (alveolar-acinar glands) extend far beyond the lumina of bile ducts (extramural glands) and can be located in any area of the portal tract (Chanukvadze I., 2010; Kordzaia D., 1990). Furthermore, Sh. Toidze and I. Chanukvadze have described the extramural biliary glands dislocated from the portal area toward the hepatic vein in the areas of crossing portal tracts and hepatic vein tributaries and the fusion of their connective-tissue structures (Toidze Sh., Chanukvadze I., 1978; Chanukvadze I., 1989). Thus, the dislocation of tubular and/or fibrilar structures from the portal tract toward the hepatic vein tributary in the areas of their crossing can be considered as a typical feature.

We have described the similar fusion of connective tissue structures of portal tracts and hepatic veins in rats. Importantly, the intrahepatic bile ducts in rats are not supplied by extramural mucosal glands (rats like other laboratory animals without gallbladders have no mucosal glands or only few of them specifically supplying the common bile duct) (Andrews C., Andrews W., 1979).However, they are supplied by an interesting but rarely considered structure - periportal biliary plexus (PBP), which connects to the bile duct with one side, and with bile canaliculi and intralobular biliary ductules - with the other side, respectively. SEM of corrosion casts confirms that this plexus surrounds the branches of the portal vein and hepatic artery (Murakami T., et al., 2001; Yamamoto K., Phillips M., 1984).The smallest branches of this plexus, similarly the canals of Hering, are hardly observable not only by standard histology, but also by fluorescent microscopy (Ekataksin W., et al., 1997; Saxena R., et al., 1999). PBP probably has the reserving function and in normal condition doesn't involve bile flow, which makes it harder to visualize (Murakami T., et al., 2001; Yamamoto K., Phillips M., 1984; Roskams T., et al., 2004).

But even at the early stages following CBDL or retrograde injection of the biliary tract with different media under high pressure, the lumina of PBP may widen and become clearly visible, giving the picture of periportal DR (Azmaiparashvili E., et al., 2012; Kordzaia D., et al., 2012; Roskams T., et al., 2004).The fragments of periportal biliary plexi can also undergo the porto-venous dislocation in the areas of portal tracts and hepatic vein tributaries crossing - similarly the portal biliary branches. The finest ramifications of dislocated biliary structures may follow hepatic vein tributaries up to their smallest structures – central and sublobular veins. As a result of this, the small CK -19, CK-7 and OV6 - positive DPs adjacent to the lumina of central/ sublobular veins may appear on histological slices (Figures 118-120).

Thus we may consider that the ductular profiles accompanying the different caliber tributaries of hepatic veins represent the component of the common biliary network. It is additionally confirmed by the study of histological slices, which shows that the contrast medium injected into the biliary system via the Common Bile Duct appears not only in the lumina of classical compartments - portal bile ducts and bile canaliculi, but in the lumina of bile ducts/ductuli adjacent to the different caliber tributaries of the hepatic veins, which underlines the continuity of all three biliary structures mentioned above (Figure 123).

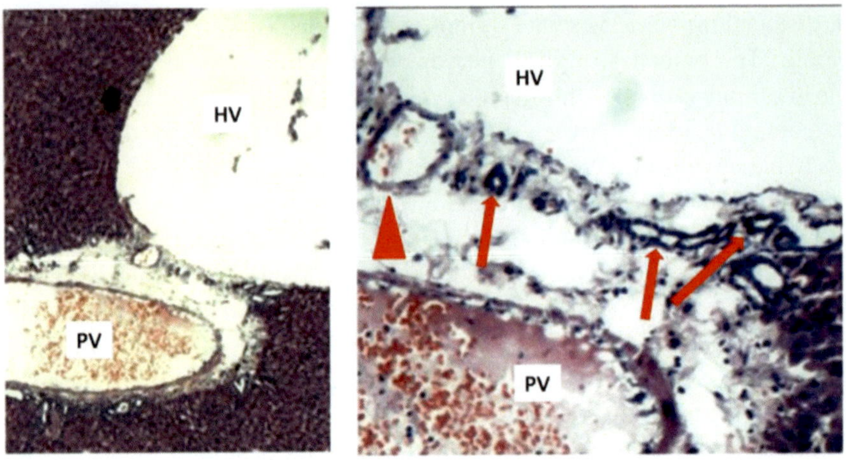

Figure 123. Fusion of connective tissue spaces surrounding portal tract and hepatic vein tributaries(HV). Bile ductules (arrow) dislocated from the portal area toward the tributary of hepatic vein. The branch of portal vein (PV).Branch of hepatic artery (arrowhead).BDL-6. H and E.X100, X100, X200.

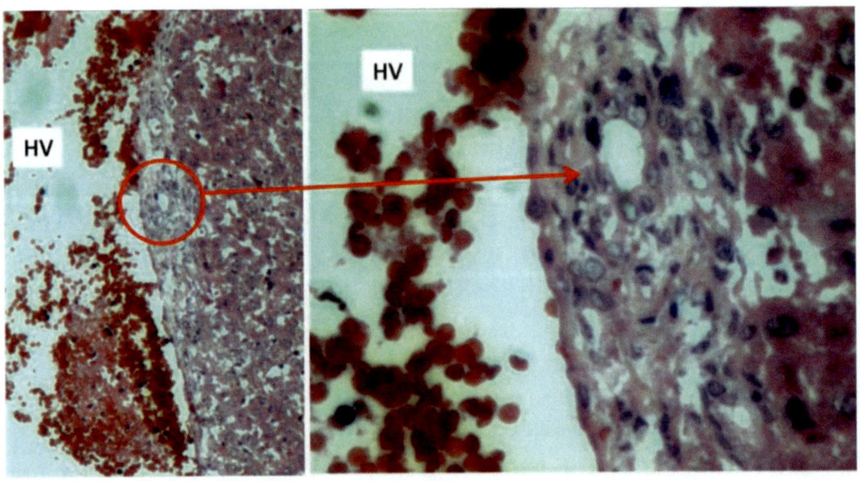

Figure 124. DPs (arrow) situated in connective tissue sheath (adventitia) of hepatic vein branches (HV).

The dislocated bile ducts and/or fragments of periportal biliary plexi accompanying hepatic vein tributaries and extending up to smallest sublobular/central veins logically should not be ended blindly.

It is "biologically" inexpedient. Presumably, they must have the contact with the lobular compartment of bile circulation (Azmaiparashvili E., et al., 2012). Otherwise, as passive reservoirs they may become the sites of biliary stasis and result in different pathological complications. The bile canaliculi, in fact, may be the only structures from which bile should flow into these atypical biliary ductuli located at the center of some lobuli. However, no similar communications are implicated yet in humans and/or other mammals. But, for example, entrancing of sinusoids at different levels of the hepatic venous tree (including sublobular and collecting veins) is described only in rat liver, while in humans and other mammals sinusoids drain only into the central veins (Gershbein L., Elias H., 1954).

It is not excluded that communication of bile canaliculi with atypically located bile ductuli also represents a specific feature of rat liver.

It may be concluded that bile from the bile canaliculi in the appropriate number of rat liver lobuli is drained in two directions: portal and caval.

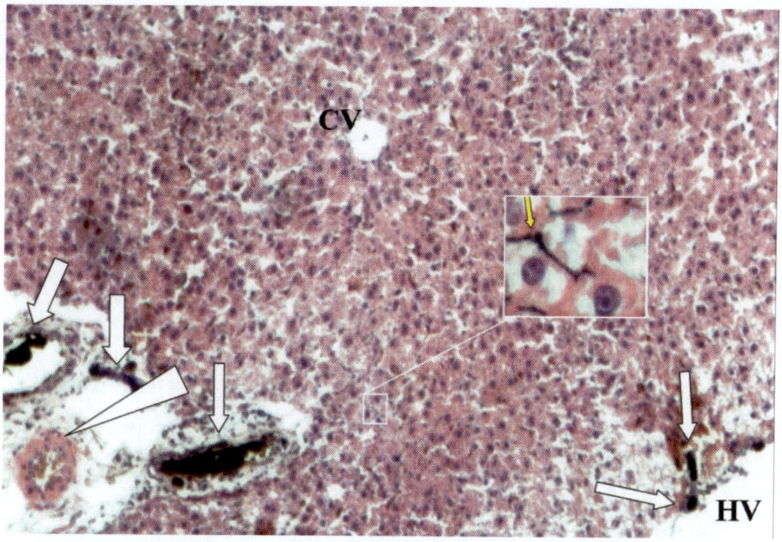

Figure 125. Ink injected through the common bile duct appears in portal bile ducts-periportal ductuli-bile canaliculi (arrows); The lumina of hepatic vein branch (HV), central vein (CV) and artery (arrowhead) are free from injected media.

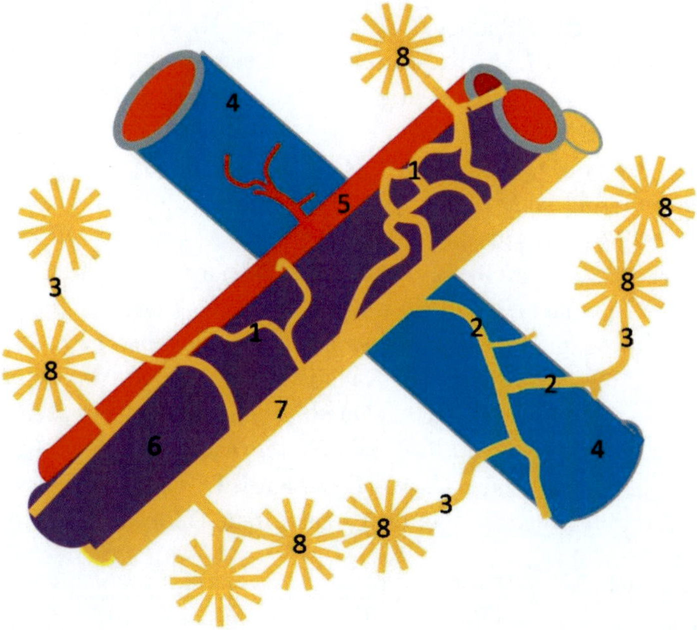

Figure 126. Scheme of bile circulation in the lobuli with central/sublobular veins are accompanied with the branches of dislocated bile ducts. 1-periportal biliary plexus; 2-dislocated bile duct/ductule; 3-interlobular bile ductule; 4-tributaries of hepatic vein; 5-artery; 6- portal vein; 7-bile duct; 8- bile canaliculi.

In portal areas the bile is collected by classical portal bile ducts/ductules, while centrilobularly it would be collected by atypical, dislocated ductules (Figure 124), originating from the sites of crossing of portal tracts and hepatic vein tributaries, fusing their connective-tissue sheaths.

Presumably, these dislocated ductuli have the reserve function and there is no active bile flow inside their lumina, which supports their invisibility in normal conditions. Bile drainage via these ductuli must be "switched on" in bile congestion and increased biliary pressure settings.

This phenomenon may account for additional adaptive mechanisms in bile congestion in rats, when the biliary tree is not provided either by the gallbladder or mucosal glands and therefore is more vulnerable to changes induced by biliary hypertension.

References

[1] Alekseev, B. V. (1984). *Surgery of Thoracic Duct* (4 ed.): Meditsina.

[2] Alpini, G., Glaser, S. S., Ueno, Y., Pham, L., Podila, P. V., Caligiuri, A., & LaRusso, N. F. (1998).Heterogeneity of the proliferative capacity of rat cholangiocytes after bile duct ligation. *Am. J. Physiol.,* 274(4 Pt 1), G767-775.

[3] Alpini, G., McGill, J. M.and Larusso, N. F. (2002). The pathobiology of biliary epithelia. *Hepatology,* 35(5), 1256-1268.doi: 10.1053/jhep.2002.33541.

[4] Andrews, C. J. and Andrews, W. H. (1979). The relation between structure and function of bile ducts in man, some laboratory animals and the Adelie penguin. *Q. J. Exp. Physiol. Cogn. Med. Sci.,* 64(2), 61-67.

[5] Aoki, T., Imamura, H., Sakamoto, Y., Hasegawa, K., Seyama, Y., Kubota, K., and Makuuchi, M. (2003). Bile duct of Luschka connecting with the cystohepatic duct: the importance of cholangiography during surgery. *AJR Am. J. Roentgenol.,* 180(3), 694-696. doi: 10.2214/ajr.180.3.1800694.

[6] Archer, S. B., Brown, D. W., Smith, C. D., Branum, G. D., and Hunter, J. G. (2001). Bile duct injury during laparoscopic cholecystectomy: results of a national survey. *Ann. Surg.,* 234(4), 549-558; discussion 558-549.

[7] Azmaiparashvili, E., Berishvili, E., Jangavadze, M., and Kordzaia, D. (2012). Study on the Origin of "Newductules" Appearing in the Rat Liver in Several Hours After Common Bile Duct Ligation. *Acta morphologica et anthropologica,* 18, 6.

[8] Azmaiparashvili, E., Berishvili, E., Kakabadze, Z., Pilishvili, O., Mikautadze, E., Solomonia, R., ... Kordzaia, D. (2012).Ductular reaction at the early terms of common bile duct ligation in the rats.*Acta Biologica Hungarica,* 63(3), 321-332.

[9] Azmaiparashvili, E., Kordzaia, D. and Dzidziguri, D. (2009). Biliary hypertension as the cell proliferation trigger in bile duct ligated rats. *Georgian Med. News* (168), 111-116.

[10] Bartos, V. and Brzek, V. (1973). [Significance of thoracic duct drainage in clinical medicine].*Chirurg,* 44(3), 110-114.

[11] Battezzati, M. (1975). [Decompression of the lymphatic system in portal hypertension]. *Minerva Chir.,* 30(7), 383-384.

[12] Benedetti, A., Bassotti, C., Rapino, K., Marucci, L., and Jezequel, A. M. (1996). A morphometric study of the epithelium lining the rat intrahepatic biliary tree. *J. Hepatol.*, 24(3), 335-342.

[13] Burden, V. G. (1925). Observations on the Histologic and Pathologic Anatomy of the Hepatic, Cystic, and Common Bile Ducts. *Ann. Surg.*, 82(4), 584-597.

[14] Burke, D. R. and McLean, G. K. (1989). Obstructions of the hepatic duct confluence: internal drainage of bilateral lesions with a single catheter. *Radiology,* 172(3 Pt 2), 1035-1038.doi: 10.1148/172.3.1035.

[15] Burt, A. D. and MacSween, R. N. (1993). Bile duct proliferation-its true significance? *Histopathology,* 23(6), 599-602.

[16] Cardinale, V., Wang, Y., Carpino, G., Cui, C. B., Gatto, M., Rossi, M., & Reid, L. (2011). Multipotent stem/progenitor cells in human biliary tree give rise to hepatocytes, cholangiocytes, and pancreatic islets. *Hepatology,* 54(6), 2159-2172.doi: 10.1002/hep.24590.

[17] Cardinale, V., Wang, Y., Carpino, G., Mendel, G., Alpini, G., Gaudio, E., & Alvaro, D. (2012).The biliary tree-a reservoir of multipotent stem cells. *Nat. Rev. Gastroenterol. Hepatol.* 9(4), 231-240. doi: 10.1038/nrgastro.2012.23.

[18] Carpino, G., Cardinale, V., Onori, P., Franchitto, A., Berloco, P. B., Rossi, M., & Gaudio, E. (2012). Biliary tree stem/progenitor cells in glands of extrahepatic and intraheptic bile ducts: an anatomical in situ study yielding evidence of maturational lineages. *J. Anat.*, 220(2), 186-199. doi: 10.1111/j.1469-7580.2011.01462.x.

[19] Champetier, J., Davin, J. L., Letoublon, C., Laborde, Y., Yver, R., and Cousset, F. (1982). [Choleperitoneum following perforation of the liver. The role of the vasa aberrantia].*Ann. Chir.*,36(4), 312.

[20] Champetier, J., Letoublon, C., Alnaasan, I., and Charvin, B. (1991). The cystohepatic ducts: surgical implications. *Surg. Radiol.Anat.*, 13(3), 203-211.

[21] Chanukvadze, I. (1975). About intrahepatic connective tissue structures. *Paper presented at the Challenging issues about liver and bile duct pathologies, Tbilisi.*

[22] Chanukvadze, I. (1979). *Construction and interactions of paravasal connective tissue structures in the liver.* (PhD), Tbilisi State Medical Institute.

[23] Chanukvadze, I. (2003). Intrahepatic portal channels and mucosal biliary glands. *Georgian Med. News* (3), 8.

[24] Chanukvadze, I. (2011). Anatomical substance for intra hepatic Porto-Caval bypass. *Paper presented at the Materials of Tbilisi Third International Simposium, Tbilisi, Georgia.*

[25] Chanukvadze, I. and Archvadze, V. (2003).[Surgical anatomy of main intrahepatic portal tracts].*Zentralbl. Chir.*,128 (11), 958-962. doi: 10.1055/s-2003-44809.

[26] Chanukvadze, I., Archvadze, V., Mgeliashvili, T. I., and Koberidze, G. (2013). Bilio-lymphatic connections of intrahepatic portal tracts.*Paper presented at the New Steps in Critical Care Medicine. Sixth National Conference. Tbilisi Fifth International Symposium.*

[27] Chanukvadze, I., Archvadze, V.and Soreli, M. (2012).Bilio-vascular architecture of main magistral portal tracts. *Paper presented at the New Steps in Critical Care Medicine. Materials of Tbilisi Fourth International Conference Tbilisi.*

[28] Chanukvadze, I.and Toidze, S. (1980). Intrahepatic porto-caval connective tissue junctions. *Paper presented at the I Ukrainian Congress of Anatomists, Histologists, Embryologists and Topographioanatomists.*

[29] Chanukvadze, I. M. (1989). [Structure and Connections of Fibrous Sheaths of Portal Complexes and Hepatic Veins]. *Collections of Scientific Works of Tbilisi State Medical Institute,* 1, 11.

[30] Chanukvadze, I. M. (2010).Surgical Anatomy of Main Intrahepatic Portal Tracts. *Proc. Georgian Nat. Acad. Sci., Biomed. Series,* 36(Supplement), 9.

[31] Chenderovitch, J. (1972). Secretory function of the rabbit common bile duct.*Am. J. Physiol.,* 223(3), 695-706.

[32] Choi, J. W., Kim, T. K., Kim, K. W., Kim, A. Y., Kim, P. N., Ha, H. K., and Lee, M. G. (2003). Anatomic variation in intrahepatic bile ducts: an analysis of intraoperative cholangiograms in 300 consecutive donors for living donor liver transplantation. *Korean J. Radiol.,* 4(2), 85-90.

[33] Choi, T. K., Fan, S. T., Lai, E. C., and Wong, J. (1988). Malignant hilar biliary obstruction treated by segmental bilioenteric anastomosis. *Surgery,* 104(3), 525-529.

[34] Cohen, P. J. (1964). The Renewal Areas of the Common Bile Duct Epithelium in the Rat. *Anat. Rec.,* 150, 237-241.

[35] Couinaud, C. (1954a). [Liver lobes and segments: notes on the anatomical architecture and surgery of the liver]. *Presse Med.,* 62(33), 709-712.

[36] Couinaud, C. (1954b). [Studies on intrahepatic bile ducts].*J. Chir.* (Paris), 70(4), 310-328.

[37] Counaud, C. (1989). Surgical anatomy of the liver revisited *Anatomy of the Dorsal Sector of the Liver. New considerations on liver anatomy* (pp. 26-39). Paris: Pers Ed.

[38] Counaud, C. L. F. (1957).*Etudes Anatomiques et Chirurgicales.* Paris: Masson.

[39] Dedo, D. D. (1973). A cannula for maintaining long-term thoracic duct fistulas. *Surgery,* 73(5), 791-794.

[40] Demetris, A. J., Sakamoto, T., Liu, Z., Yokomuro, S., Ezure, T., Murase, N., and Blakolmer, K. (1999). The ductular reaction in liver disease – emphasis on a type I response. In: W. E. Fleig (Ed.), *Normal and Malignant Liver Cell Growth* (pp. 156-170): Springer.

[41] Desmet, V., Roskams, T. and Van Eyken, P. (1995). Ductular reaction in the liver. *Pathol. Res. Pract.,*191(6), 513-524.

[42] Desmet, V. J. (1992). Modulation of the liver in cholestasis. *J. Gastroenterol. Hepatol.,* 7(3), 313-323.

[43] Desmet, V. J. (2011). Ductal plates in hepatic ductular reactions. Hypothesis and implications. I. Types of ductular reaction reconsidered. *Virchows Arch.,* 458(3), 251-259.doi: 10.1007/s00428-011-1048-3.

[44] Dezso, K., Paku, S., Papp, V., Turanyi, E., and Nagy, P. (2009). Architectural and immunohistochemical characterization of biliary ductules in normal human liver. *Stem. Cells Dev.,* 18(10), 1417-1422. doi: 10.1089/scd.2009.0110.

[45] Dirlik, M., Canbaz, H., Dusmez Apa, D., Caglikulekci, M., Yaylak, F., Balli, E., & Aydin, S. (2009). The monitoring of progress in apoptosis of liver cells in bile duct-ligated rats. *Turk. J. Gastroenterol.,* 20(4), 247-256.

[46] Dittmer, A. and Dittmer, J. (2006). Beta-actin is not a reliable loading control in Western blot analysis. *Electrophoresis,* 27(14), 2844-2845.doi: 10.1002/ elps.200500785.

[47] Dooley, J. and Sherlock, S. (2011). *Sherlock's diseases of the liver and biliary system* (12th ed.). Chichester, West Sussex; Hoboken, NJ: Wiley-Blackwell.

[48] Dutra, R. A., Dos Santos, J. S., de Araujo, W. M., Simoes, M. V., de Paixao-Becker, A. N., and Neder, L. (2008). Evaluation of hepatobiliary excretion and enterobiliary reflux in rats with biliary obstruction submitted to bilioduodenal or biliojejunal anastomosis. *Dig. Dis. Sci.,* 53(4), 1138-1145. doi: 10.1007/s10620-007-9955-5.

[49] Ekataskin, W., Kaneda, K. (1999). Liver Microvascular Architecture: An Insight Into The Pathophysiology of Portal Hypertension. *Seminars in Liver Disease*, 19(4), 359-382.doi: 10.1055/s-2007-1007126.

[50] Ekataksin, W., Zou, Z., Wake, K., Chunhabundit, P., Somana, R., Nishida, J., and McCuskey, R. (1997). The hepatic microcirculatory subunits: an over-threecentury-long search for the missing link between an exocrine unit and an endocrine unit in mammalian liver lobules. In: P. M. Motta (Ed.), *Recent Advances in Microscopy of Cells, Tissues and Organs.* (pp. 375-380). Rome: University of Rome La Sapienza Press.

[51] Elias, H. (1955). Liver Morphology. *Biological Reviews,* 30(3), 263-310.doi: 10.1111/j.1469-185X.1955.tb01210.x.

[52] Elias, H. and Petty, D. (1952). Gross anatomy of the blood vessels and ducts within the human liver.*Am. J. Anat.,* 90(1), 59-111. doi: 10.1002/aja.1000900104.

[53] Elias, H. and Sherrick, J. C. (1969). *Morphology of the liver*: Academic Press.

[54] Fishzon-Ryss Iu, I.and Postrelov, N. A. (1985). [Cholangitis]. *Klin. Med.* (Mosk.), 63(11), 121-127.

[55] Franchitto, A., Onori, P., Renzi, A., Carpino, G., Mancinelli, R., Alvaro, D., and Gaudio, E. (2012). Recent advances on the mechanisms regulating cholangiocyte proliferation and the significance of the neuroendocrine regulation of cholangiocyte pathophysiology. *Annals of Translational Medicine,* 1(3).

[56] Galperin, E. and Volkova, N. (1988). *Biliary tract disease after cholecystectomy*: Medicine.

[57] Gaudio, E., Franchitto, A., Pannarale, L., Carpino, G., Alpini, G., Francis, H., & Onori, P. (2006). Cholangiocytes and blood supply. *World J. Gastroenterol.,* 12(22), 3546-3552.

[58] Gautier, M., Jehan, P. and Odievre, M. (1976). Histologic study of biliary fibrous remnants in 48 cases of extrahepatic biliary atresia: correlation with postoperative bile flow restoration. *J. Pediatr.,* 89(5), 704-709.

[59] Georgiev, P., Jochum, W., Heinrich, S., Jang, J. H., Nocito, A., Dahm, F., and Clavien, P. A. (2008). Characterization of time-related changes after experimental bile duct ligation. *Br. J. Surg.,* 95(5), 646-656. doi: 10.1002/bjs.6050.

[60] Gerlovin, M. V. (1982). *Histogenesis and Differentiation of Digestive Glands*. Moscow: Meditsina.

[61] Gershbein, L. L. and Elias, H. (1954). Observations on the anatomy of the rat liver. *Anat. Rec.,* 120(1), 85-98.

[62] Glaser, S. S., Gaudio, E., Miller, T., Alvaro, D., and Alpini, G. (2009).Cholangiocyte proliferation and liver fibrosis. *Expert Rev. Mol. Med.,* 11, e7. doi: 10.1017/S1462399409000994.

[63] Glaser, S. S., Onori, P., Wise, C., Yang, F., Marzioni, M., Alvaro, D., & Gaudio, E. (2010). Recent advances in the regulation of cholangiocyte proliferation and function during extrahepatic cholestasis. *Dig.Liver Dis.,* 42(4), 245-252.doi: 10.1016/j.dld.2010.01.008.

[64] Gordeev, P. S. and Korneev, A. V. (1991). [Cystic transformation of the bile ducts]. *Khirurgiia* (Mosk.)(2), 145-148.

[65] Greenbaum, L. E. and Wells, R. G. (2011). The role of stem cells in liver repair and fibrosis. *Int. J. Biochem. Cell Biol.,* 43(2), 222-229. doi: 10.1016/j.biocel.2009.11.006.

[66] Gugushvili, L. (1972). *Hepatic Retrograde Blood Circulation and Portal Hypertension.* Moscow: Meditsina.

[67] Hayashi, S., Murakami, G., Ohtsuka, A., Itoh, M., Nakano, T., and Fukuzawa, Y. (2008).Connective tissue configuration in the human liver hilar region with special reference to the liver capsule and vascular sheath. *J. Hepatobiliary Pancreat. Surg.,* 15(6), 640-647.doi: 10.1007/s00534-008-1336-8.

[68] Healey, J. E., Jr. and Schroy, P. C. (1953). Anatomy of the biliary ducts within the human liver; analysis of the prevailing pattern of branchings and the major variations of the biliary ducts. *AMA Arch. Surg.,* 66(5), 599-616.

[69] Hjortsjo, C. H. (1951).The topography of the intrahepatic duct systems. *Acta Anat.*(Basel), 11(4), 599-615.

[70] Hopwood, D., Wood, R. and Milne, G. (1988). The fine structure and histochemistry of human bile duct in obstruction and choledocholithiasis. *J. Pathol.,*155(1), 49-59. doi: 10.1002/path.1711550109.

[71] Ishida, F., Terada, T. and Nakanuma, Y. (1989).Histologic and scanning electron microscopic observations of intrahepatic peribiliary glands in normal human livers. *Lab. Invest.,* 60(2), 260-265.

[72] Izraelashvili, M. S. (1989). [Topographic Anatomy of Lymphatic Vessels and Regional Lymph Nodes of Liver. The Applied Aspect.].*Collections of Scientific Works of Tbilisi State Medical Institute,* 1, 20.

[73] Jahan, M., Xiao, P., Go, A., Cheema, M., and Hameed, A. (2009). Intraductal and invasive adenocarcinoma of duct of Luschka, mimicking chronic cholecystitis and cholelithiasis. *World J. Surg. Oncol.,*7, 4. doi: 10.1186/1477-7819-7-4.

[74] Jenkins, M. A., Ponsky, J. L., Lehman, G. A., Fanelli, R., and Bianchi, T. (1994). Treatment of bile leaks from the cystohepatic ducts after laparoscopic cholecystectomy. *Surg. Endosc.,* 8(3), 193-196.

[75] Jeong, J. Y., Kang, D. Y. and Noh, S. M. (1993). A morphologic study on the bile duct changes induced by common bile duct ligation in rats.*Korean Journal of Pathology,* 27(6), 618-629.

[76] Kartashova, O.and Maksimova, L. (1979).*Functional Morphology of Liver*: Zinatne.

[77] Ko, K., Kamiya, J., Nagino, M., Oda, K., Yuasa, N., Arai, T., & Nimura, Y. (2006). A study of the subvesical bile duct (duct of Luschka) in resected liver specimens. *World J. Surg.,* 30(7), 1316-1320. doi: 10.1007/s00268-005-0469-z.

[78] Kochnev, O. S., Davletkil'deev, F. A. and Kim, B. (1979). [Measured drainage of the thoracic lymphatic duct in emergency surgery]. *Khirurgiia* (Mosk.)(3), 90-93.

[79] Kogure, K., Ishizaki, M., Nemoto, M., Kuwano, H., Yorifuji, H., Ishikawa, H., & Makuuchi, M. (2007). Close relation between the inferior vena cava ligament and the caudate lobe in the human liver. *J. Hepatobiliary Pancreat. Surg.,* 14(3), 297-301.doi: 10.1007/s00534-006-1148-7.

[80] Konstantinov, B. A., Got'e, S. V., Tsirul'nikova, O. M., and Filin, A. V. (2000). [liver portion transplantation from living donor: pilot clinical experience]. *Khirurgiia* (Mosk.)(3), 4-9.

[81] Kordzaia, D. (1990). *Extrahepatic cholestasis*. Tbilisi, Georgia: Ganatleba.

[82] Kordzaia, D. (1994). *Plasticity of Bile Ducts, Validation of Therapeutic and Surgical Strategy in Extrahepatic Cholestasis.* (Doct. Med. Sci.), TSMU, Tbilisi.

[83] Korolev, B. and Pikovskiy, D. (1990). *Emergency surgery of the biliary tract*: Medicine.

[84] Kovanov, V. V.and Anikina, T. I. (1967). *Surgical Anatomy of Human Fasciae and Tissue Spaces* (2 ed.). Moscow: Meditsina.

[85] Kovanov, V. V., Anikina, T. I. and Razumnaia, T. A. (1973). [Surgical Significance of the Connective Tissue Structures of the Posterior Part of Human Liver] *Scientific Methodological Problems of Soft Tissue Studying* (pp. 137-146). Gorkyi: Kirov Medical Institute.

[86] Lavdovsky, M. and Ovsyanikov, T. (1888). *The causes changing the microscopic anatomy of humans and animals* (Vol. II). S-Pietersburg: Publishing House of Karl Piker.

[87] Lee, J., Tschai, H., Lee, S., and Tu, Y. (1981).Liver Histologic Changes in Bile Ligated Rats.*Med. Sci.,* 4(2), 1179-1187.

[88] Libbrecht, L., Desmet, V., Van Damme, B., and Roskams, T. (2000). The immunohistochemical phenotype of dysplastic foci in human liver: correlation with putative progenitor cells. *J. Hepatol.,*33(1), 76-84.

[89] Liu, Z., Sakamoto, T., Ezure, T., Yokomuro, S., Murase, N., Michalopoulos, G., and Demetris, A. J. (1998). Interleukin-6, hepatocyte growth factor, and their receptors in biliary epithelial cells during a type I ductular reaction in mice: interactions between the periductal inflammatory and stromal cells and the biliary epithelium. *Hepatology,* 28(5), 1260-1268.doi: 10.1002/hep.510280514.

[90] Loginov, S. and Aruin, L. I. (1985). *Clinical Morphology of the Liver*. Moscow Meditsina.

[91] Mallet-Guy. (1970). *Kestens Syndrome post-cholécystectomie.* Paris: Masson.

[92] Mancinelli, R., Onori, P., Gaudio, E., DeMorrow, S., Franchitto, A., Francis, H., & Alpini, G. (2009). Follicle-stimulating hormone increases cholangiocyte proliferation by an autocrine mechanism via cAMP-dependent phosphorylation of ERK1/2 and Elk-1. *Am. J. Physiol. Gastrointest. Liver Physiol.,* 297(1), G11-26.doi: 10.1152/ajpgi.00025.2009.

[93] Marinozzi, G. and et al. (1977). Scanning electron microscope observations of intrahepatic biliary tree. I. Canaliculo-ductular junction. Bile ductules and ducts. *J. Submicrosc. Cytol.,*9(12).

[94] Marucci, L., Baroni, G. S., Mancini, R., Benedetti, A., Jezequel, A. M., and Orlandi, F. (1993). Cell proliferation following extrahepatic biliary obstruction. Evaluation by immunohistochemical methods.*J. Hepatol.,*17(2), 163-169.

[95] McMinn, R. M. and Kugler, J. H. (1961). The glands of the bile and pancreatic ducts: autoradiographic and histochemical studies. *J. Anat.,* 95, 1-11.
[96] McQuillan, T., Manolas, S. G., Hayman, J. A., and Kune, G. A. (1989). Surgical significance of the bile duct of Luschka.*Br. J. Surg.,* 76(7), 696-698.
[97] Michalopoulos, G. K., Barua, L.and Bowen, W. C. (2005). Transdifferentiation of rat hepatocytes into biliary cells after bile duct ligation and toxic biliary injury. *Hepatology,* 41(3), 535-544.doi: 10.1002/hep.20600.
[98] Mori, S.and Kasahara, M. (2001). Papillary adenocarcinoma of the subvesical duct.*J. Hepatobiliary Pancreat.Surg.,* 8(5), 494-498.
[99] Morikawa, H., Hachiya, K., Mizuhara, H., Fujiwara, H., Nishiguchi, S., Shiomi, S., & Kaneda, K. (2000). Sublobular veins as the main site of lymphocyte adhesion/transmigration and adhesion molecule expression in the porto-sinusoidal-hepatic venous system during concanavalin A-induced hepatitis in mice. *Hepatology,* 31(1), 83-94.doi: 10.1002/hep.510310115.
[100] Motta, P. M., Fujita, T. and Muto, M. (1978). *The Liver: An Atlas of Scanning Electron Microscopy*: Igaku-Shoin.
[101] Murakami, T., Sato, H., Nakatani, S., Taguchi, T., and Ohtsuka, A. (2001). Biliary tract of the rat as observed by scanning electron microscopy of cast samples. *Arch. Histol. Cytol.,* 64(4), 439-447.
[102] Nakano, S., Haratake, J. and Hashimoto, H. (1995).Alterations in bile ducts and peribiliary microcirculation in rats after common bile duct ligation. *Hepatology,* 21(5), 1380-1386.
[103] Nakanuma, Y., Katayanagi, K., Terada, T., and Saito, K. (1994).Intrahepatic peribiliary glands of humans. I. Anatomy, development and presumed functions. *J. Gastroenterol. Hepatol.,*9(1), 75-79.
[104] Nakanuma, Y., Sasaki, M., Terada, T., and Harada, K. (1994).Intrahepatic peribiliary glands of humans. II. Pathological spectrum. *J. Gastroenterol. Hepatol.,*9(1), 80-86.
[105] Nechai, A. I. and Novikov, K. V. (1991). [Causes and predisposing factors of accidental (iatrogenic) injuries of the bile ducts during cholecystectomy and gastrectomy].*Vestn. Khir. Im. I. I. Grek.,*146(1), 15-22.
[106] Niederle, B. V. and Keclík, M. (1981). *Surgery of the biliary tract: old problems, new methods, current practice*: M. Nijhoff B.V., Medical Division.
[107] Nishikawa, Y., Doi, Y., Watanabe, H., Tokairin, T., Omori, Y., Su, M., & Enomoto, K. (2005). Transdifferentiation of mature rat hepatocytes into bile duct-like cells in vitro. *Am. J. Pathol.,* 166(4), 1077-1088. doi: 10.1016/S0002-9440(10)62328-0.
[108] Ostroverchov, G. S. and Zabrodskaiya, V. F. (1972). *Surgical Anatomy of Liver and Biliary Tract.Abdominal Surgical Anatomy*. Leningrad: Meditsina.
[109] Ostroverchov, G. S., Zabrodskaiya, V. F. and Aliev, A. Z. Compensatory Role of Lymphatic System in Choledochal and Cystic Duct Obstruction in Experiment. *The Works of M.M.I.* 2, 18, 6.
[110] Pavlinov, B. G. (1969). *Structure and Development of Fibrous Tissue around Hepatic Blood Vessels and Bile Ducts.* (PhD), Omsk Medical State Institute, Omsk.
[111] Pereira-Lima, L. (1992). Biliary reconstruction in benign postoperative stricture with transhepatic tubes. *Am. J. Surg.,* 164(2), 124-128.

[112] Priester, S., Wise, C. and Glaser, S. S. (2010).Involvement of cholangiocyte proliferation in biliary fibrosis.*World J. Gastrointest. Pathophysiol.,*1(2), 30-37. doi: 10.4291/wjgp.v1.i2.30.

[113] Purtokas, A. I. (1983). [Biorhythmic function and adaptive organization of the bile secreting system after cholecystectomy].*Khirurgiia* (Mosk.)(8), 90-95.

[114] Racanelli, V.and Rehermann, B. (2006).The liver as an immunological organ. *Hepatology,* 43(2 Suppl. 1), S54-62.doi: 10.1002/hep.21060.

[115] Ravensky, I. A. (1977).*The Scanning Electron Microscopy of Normal and cancer Cells*: Meditsina.

[116] Razumnaiya, T. A. (1979).*Morphological and Topographical Peculiarities of Fixative System of Human Liver.* (PhD), Sechenov Medical Institute, Moscow.

[117] Roskams, T. and Desmet, V. (1998).Ductular reaction and its diagnostic significance. *Semin. Diagn. Pathol.,*15(4), 259-269.

[118] Roskams, T., van den Oord, J. J., De Vos, R., and Desmet, V. J. (1990). Neuroendocrine features of reactive bile ductules in cholestatic liver disease. *Am. J. Pathol.,*137(5), 1019-1025.

[119] Roskams, T. A., Libbrecht, L.and Desmet, V. J. (2003). Progenitor cells in diseased human liver. *Semin. Liver Dis.,* 23(4), 385-396.doi: 10.1055/s-2004-815564.

[120] Roskams, T. A., Theise, N. D., Balabaud, C., Bhagat, G., Bhathal, P. S., Bioulac-Sage, P., West, A. B. (2004). Nomenclature of the finer branches of the biliary tree: canals, ductules, and ductular reactions in human livers. *Hepatology,* 39(6), 1739-1745.doi: 10.1002/hep.20130.

[121] Sareli, M., Chanukvadze, I., Valeanu, A., Zippel, D. B., Shapiro, R., and Papa, M. Z. (2009). The posterior intrahepatic approach to the left portal pedicle using the ligamentum venosum: anatomical basis. *Surg. Radiol. Anat.,* 31(10), 809-813.doi: 10.1007/s00276-009-0530-y.

[122] Saxena, R. and Theise, N. (2004). Canals of Hering: recent insights and current knowledge. *Semin. Liver Dis.,* 24(1), 43-48.doi: 10.1055/s-2004-823100.

[123] Saxena, R., Theise, N. D.and Crawford, J. M. (1999). Microanatomy of the human liver-exploring the hidden interfaces. *Hepatology,* 30(6), 1339-1346.doi: 10.1002/hep.510300607.

[124] Schneck, C. (1994). Embryology, histology, gross anatomy, and normal imaging anatomy of the gallbladder and biliary tract. In: A. C. Friedman and A. H. Dachman (Eds.), *Radiology of the liver, biliary tract, and pancreas* (1st ed., pp. 355-376). St. Louis: Mosby.

[125] Sheung-To, C.and Gibson, J. B. (1970). The histochemistry of biliary mucins and the changes caused by infestation with Clonorchis sinensis. *J. Pathol.,*101(2), 185-197. doi: 10.1002/path.1711010213.

[126] Shibayama, Y. (1990). Factors producing bile infarction and bile duct proliferation in biliary obstruction. *J. Pathol.,* 160(1), 57-62. doi: 10.1002/path.1711600112.

[127] Sirica, A. E., Gainey, T. W., Harrell, M. B., and Caran, N. (1997). Cholangiocarcinogenesis and biliary adaptation responses in hepatic injury. In: A. E. Sirica and D. S. Longnecker (Eds.), *Biliary and pancreatic ductal epithelia: pathobiology and pathophysiology* (pp. 229-290). New York: M. Dekker.

[128] Sirica, A. E.and Longnecker, D. S. (1996). *Biliary and Pancreatic Ductal Epithelia: Pathobiology and Pathophysiology*: Taylor and Francis.

[129] Slott, P. A., Liu, M. H.and Tavoloni, N. (1990). Origin, pattern, and mechanism of bile duct proliferation following biliary obstruction in the rat. *Gastroenterology,* 99(2), 466-477.

[130] Snegirevskaiya, E.and Veselov, V. (1986).Changes in Plasmogenic Hepatocytes and their Specific Sites of Intercellular Junctions in Complicated Forms of Cholelithiasis. *Arkhiv Anatomii, Gistologii, Embriologii,* 1, 12-15.

[131] Solomonia, R. O., Apkhazava, D., Nozadze, M., Jackson, A. P., McCabe, B. J., and Horn, G. (2008). Different forms of MARCKS protein are involved in memory formation in the learning process of imprinting. *Exp. Brain Res.,* 188(2), 323-330.doi: 10.1007/s00221-008-1428-3.

[132] Spitz, L.and Petropoulos, A. (1979). The development of the glands of the common bile duct.*J. Pathol.,* 128(4), 213-220. doi: 10.1002/path.1711280407.

[133] Sulaberidze, G. D., Kardzaia, D. D., Kikalishvili, L. A., and Khomeriki, Ts., T. (2006). [Common intralobular microcirculatory module peculiarities in cholestasis in white rats].*Georgian Med. News* (132), 100-105.

[134] Tanaka, K., Uemoto, S., Tokunaga, Y., Fujita, S., Sano, K., Nishizawa, T., et al. (1993). Surgical techniques and innovations in living related liver transplantation. *Ann. Surg.,* 217(1), 82-91.

[135] Terada, T., Kida, T.and Nakanuma, Y. (1993). Extrahepatic peribiliary glands express alpha-amylase isozymes, trypsin and pancreatic lipase: an immunohistochemical analysis. *Hepatology,* 18(4), 803-808.

[136] Terada, T.and Nakanuma, Y. (1990). Pathological observations of intrahepatic peribiliary glands in 1,000 consecutive autopsy livers. III. Survey of necroinflammation and cystic dilatation. *Hepatology,* 12(5), 1229-1233.

[137] Terada, T.and Nakanuma, Y. (1992). Pathologic observations of intrahepatic peribiliary glands in 1,000 consecutive autopsy livers: IV. Hyperplasia of intramural and extramural glands. *Hum. Pathol.,*23(5), 483-490.

[138] Terada, T. and Nakanuma, Y. (1997). Pathobiologyof Human Intrahepatic Peribiliary Glands. In: A. E. Sirica and D. S. Longnecker (Eds.), *Biliary and pancreatic ductal epithelia: pathobiology and pathophysiology* (pp. 291-321). New York: M. Dekker.

[139] Terada, T., Nakanuma, Y.and Ohta, G. (1987).Glandular elements around the intrahepatic bile ducts in man; their morphology and distribution in normal livers. *Liver,* 7(1), 1-8.

[140] Terasaki, S., Nakanuma, Y., Unoura, M., Kaneko, S., and Kobayashi, K. (1997). Involvement of peribiliary glands in primary sclerosing cholangitis: a histopathologic study. *Intern. Med.,* 36(11), 766-770.

[141] Teutsch, H. F. (2005). The modular microarchitecture of human liver. *Hepatology,* 42(2), 317-325.doi: 10.1002/hep.20764.

[142] Theise, N. D., Saxena, R., Portmann, B. C., Thung, S. N., Yee, H., Chiriboga, L., Crawford, J. M. (1999). The canals of Hering and hepatic stem cells in humans.*Hepatology,* 30(6), 1425-1433.doi: 10.1002/hep.510300614.

[143] Toidze, S.and Chanukvadze, I. (1978). *Interactions Among Liver Paravascular Fibrous Structures.* Paper presented at the Matherials of Transcaucasian Conference of Morphologists, Baku.

[144] Toidze, S., Kevanishvili, S.and Danelian, M. (1976). Intrahepatic Biliary tract Changes in Elders. *Scientific Works. Tbilisi Medical Institute.,*26, 9.

[145] Toidze, S. and Kordzaia, D. (1988). Regarding the interaction of intrahepatic bile ducts and lymphatic vessels in cholestasis. *General Regularity of Morphogenesis and Regeneration* (pp. 323-326). Tbilisi: Metsniereba.

[146] Venediktov, A. (1946). *Glands of gross bile ducts of human and some domestic animals studied by macro-microscopic methods.* (PhD), Kuibishev.

[147] Vinogradov, V., Tshakaya, Z. and Pautkin, Y. (1991).*Biliary tract surgery.* Tbilisi: Sakartvelo.

[148] Virenkov, Y. and Kataev, S. (1983). Hepatic Microcirculatory Flow According to the Evidences of Electronic Microscopy. *Arkhiv Anatomii, Gistologii, Embriologii,* 4, 21-24.

[149] Virenkov, Y., Makarenko, E.and Martirosova, M. (1971). Hepatic Lymphocirculation in Biliary Hypertension.*Khirurgiya,* 2, 35-40.

[150] Vitebsky, I. D. (1988). *The valve anastomoses in digestive tract surgery*: Meditsina.

[151] Wright, J. E.and Braithwaite, J. L. (1964). The Effects of Interruption of a Lobar Bile Duct in the Rat. *J. Anat.,* 98, 219-225.

[152] Yamada, K. (1970). The glands of the common bile duct in the rat and mouse. An electron microscope study. *Acta Anat.*(Basel), 77(3), 438-453.

[153] Yamamoto, K., Fisher, M. M. and Phillips, M. J. (1985). Hilar biliary plexus in human liver. A comparative study of the intrahepatic bile ducts in man and animals. *Lab. Invest.,*52(1), 103-106.

[154] Yamamoto, K., Itoshima, T., Tsuji, T., and Murakami, T. (1990). Three-dimensional fine structure of the biliary tract: scanning electron microscopy of biliary casts. *J. Electron. Microsc. Tech.,* 14(3), 208-217.doi: 10.1002/jemt.1060140303.

[155] Yamamoto, K. and Phillips, M. J. (1984). A hitherto unrecognized bile ductular plexus in normal rat liver. *Hepatology,* 4(3), 381-385.

[156] Yoshida, K., Yasuda, M., Nasu, T., and Murakami, T. (2010). Scanning electron microscopic study of vascular and biliary casts in chicken and duck liver. *J. Vet. Med. Sci.,* 72(7), 925-928.

[157] Zatolokin, V. D. (1974). *[Anatomical Resections of Hepatic Lobe].* (PhD), Moscow.

[158] Zemskov, V. S., Skiba, V. V., Khmel'nitskii, S. I., Gichka, S. G., and Cheverdiuk, D. A. (1992). [A new approach to the intraoperative diagnosis of cholangitis and to the choice of surgical procedure in operations on the bile ducts]. *Klin. Khir.* (9-10), 2-6.

In: Bile Duct
Editor: Miguel Ángel Mercado

ISBN: 978-1-63321-771-3

Chapter 2

Anatomy of the Extrahepatic Biliary Tract: Variations of the Bile Ducts and Arterial Blood Supply

Beata Jabłońska
Department of Digestive Tract Surgery,
University Hospital of the Medical University of Silesia,
Katowice, Poland

Abstract

The chapter is a review of the literature concerning anatomical variations of the extrahepatic biliary tract and its arterial blood supply, including the literature regarding arterial vascularization of all segments of the extrahepatic biliary system and aspects that are most important and essential for a surgeon. Different variations of formation, number and position of the gallbladder, hepatic ducts and common bile duct are reported in 1,6 to 47,2% of cases.

The arterial blood supply of the extrahepatic biliary tract is different in particular parts. The gallbladder and cystic duct are supplied by a cystic artery. The blood supply to the right and left hepatic ducts and the upper portion of the common hepatic duct is from the cystic artery and the right and left hepatic arteries. The supraduodenal common bile duct is supplied by arterial branches from the right hepatic, cystic, posterior superior pancreaticoduodenal and retroduodenal arteries. The blood supply to the retroduodenal and intrapancreatic common bile duct is from the posterior superior pancreaticoduodenal and retroduodenal arteries. The proximal (hilar) part of the extrahepatic biliary tract has a very rich arterial blood supply. The arterial vascularization of the supraduodenal common bile duct is poor, in most cases as axial distribution (3- and 9- o'clock arteries), or less frequently - ladder distribution. It is a critical segment, in which most postoperative complications, such as biliary duct strictures, occur.

A surgeon should remember about the variability of the extrahepatic bile ducts and biliary tract arterial vascularization, in their particular parts, during surgical procedures, particularly such as cholecystectomy, biliary and biliary-alimentary anastomoses, pancreatoduodenectomy, liver transplantation and other procedures performed within the hepatoduodenal ligament. This knowledge will help avoid many serious postoperative complications.

Introduction

Knowledge of anatomy of the extrahepatic biliary tract is indispensable for a surgeon in the safe performance of operative procedures in this region. Biliary anomalies, including anatomical variations of bile ducts and arterial blood supply, most frequently are asymptomatic and recognized intraoperatively. Therefore, it is important to know proper biliary anatomy as well as different ductal and vascular variations in this region.

1. Anatomy of the Extrahepatic Biliary Tract

1.1. Typical Anatomy and Embryonic Development of the Extrahepatic Biliary Tract

The biliary tree (BT) is divided into intra- and extrahepatic bile ducts. Knowledge of the extrahepatic biliary tract (EBT) is particularly essential for a surgeon. The extrahepatic biliary system consists of the common hepatic duct (CHD) formed by the union of the right and left hepatic ducts (formed by the union of the segmental ducts), the gallbladder, the cystic duct and the common bile duct (CBD) which is formed by the union of the common hepatic and cystic ducts. The CBD joins the main pancreatic duct and enters the major papilla of the descending part of the duodenum. Different radiological investigations are used in the imaging of the biliary tract and their pathologies, including ultrasonography (USG), computed tomography (CT); direct cholangiographic methods like endoscopic retrograde cholangiopancreatography (ERCP), percutaneous transhepatic cholangiography (PTC), intravenous cholangiography and T-tube cholangiography, as well as indirect methods like magnetic resonance cholangiopancreatography (MRCP) or cholescintigraphy. USG and CT play a limited role in diagnostics of EBT, because only dilatation of the intra- and extrahepatic bile ducts can be visualized in these investigations. Cholangiographic investigations are the most useful diagnostic methods for the biliary tree imaging [1-6].

The embryonic development of the extrahepatic biliary tract is following: At the end of the intrauterine life 4th week, entoderm cells of the middle portion of the duodenal bud grow into the ventral mesenterium forming the hepatic bud. The hepatic bud divides into the right and left parts, from which the hepatic lobes are formed. The biliary ducts - hepatic ducts and CBD originate from the upper entoderm wall of the hepatic bud, the gallbladder and the cystic duct originate from the lower entoderm wall of the hepatic duct. At the 5th week, the liver begins to secrete the bile [1-4].

There are a lot classification systems of biliary anatomy according to Couinaud (1957), Huang (1996), Karakas (2008), Choi (2003), Champetier (1994), and Ohkubo (2004) in the literature [1, 7-12].

Different variations of formation, number and position of the gallbladder, hepatic ducts and common bile duct are reported in 1,6 to 47,2% of cases [1, 2, 13].

1.2. Anatomical Variants and Anomalies of the Gallbladder

There are different types of the shape, the number and the position among the gallbladder (GB) anomalies [1, 2].

1.2.1. Anomalies of the Gallbladder Shape

The most common (18%) anomaly of the GB shape is the „phrygian cap" that occurs in the each age, commonly in women [1,14]. This variant of the GB structure is caused by an infolding of a septum between the body and the fundus of the gallbladder. The another shape variations of the gallbladder are as follows: the bilobed gallbladder (asymptomatic), the hourglass gallbladder (asymptomatic in adults, but it can be the cause of the chronic cholecystitis in children), the diverticulum of the gallbladder (clinically asymptomatic, but it can lead to the cholelithiasis with the acute cholecystitis, even with the gallbladder wall perforation), Hartmann's pouch – the particular variant of the diverticulum, located in the infundibulum or the neck of the gallbladder, the rudimentary gallbladder (it can be the cause of the chronic cholecystitis and fibrosis in adults) [1, 15].

1.2.2. Anomalies of the Gallbladder Number

Anomalies of the GB number are: absent or the accessory gallbladder. More than 200 cases of the gallbladder agenesis have been reported (occurrence frequency 0,01-0,06%) [1, 2, 16, 17].

Three groups of patients, based on clinical presentation of this variation, have been distinguished in the literature. Asymptomatic patients belong to the first group (35%). The second group contains the patients with clinical manifestation of this anomaly, due to cholangiectasia and extrahepatic biliary ducts calculus. The most common clinical symptoms are: the right epigastric pain (90%), dyspepsia (30%), nausea and vomiting (66%), fat intolerance (37%) and jaundice (35%). The third group is represented by the children with multiple congenital anomalies of the respiratory system (pulmonary agenesis), cardiovascular system (Fallot's tetralogy), digestive system, urinary-reproductive system and skeletal system (anomalies of the extremities). In this group, the survival rate is 15-16% and most patients die before 6 months of age [1, 16, 17].

A double gallbladder (GB duplication) occurring in approximately in 1/4000 patients is clinically asymptomatic and it requires no treatment [1, 2]. This anomaly is associated with an increased risk of cholelithiasis and occurrence of other malformations within the bile ducts [18].

Anatomic variants of GB duplication differentiated according to Boyden's classification are presented in Table 1 [23-25].

A triple gallbladder has been also reported in the literature [26, 27]. In patients with GB triplication, all three gallbladders should be removed (laparoscopic cholecystectomy is a possible and safe procedure) in order to avoid reoperation.

1.2.3. Anomalies of the Gallbladder Position

Variations of GB position are: the intrahepatic gallbladder described in 3% of cases (cholelithiasis occurs in 60% of them), and the "floating" gallbladder with its own mesenterium (it occurs in 5% of persons, commonly in women older than 60 years of age).

Table 1. Boyden's classification (anatomic variants of the gallbladder duplication)

Type	Description
Vesica fellea divisa	Bilobed or bifid gallbladder. Double gallbladder with a common neck.
Vesica fellea duplex	Double gallbladder with two cystic ducts.
Y-shaped type	The two cystic ducts uniting before entering the common bile duct.
H-shaped type	Ductular type, the two cystic ducts entering separately into the biliary tree.

In the "floating" type, a risk of gallbladder torsion occurs with clinical symptoms such as: an acute right epigastric pain, nausea and vomiting. Torsion of the gallbladder requires urgent operative detorsion and cholecystectomy (the gallbladder may be infarcted due to occlusion of its blood vessels) [1, 19]. The another position variant occurring in 2% of cases is the bipartite (bifid) gallbladder with the neck situated under the hepatoduodenal ligament [1, 19]. Presence of mesenterium facilitates surgical procedure but intrahepatic position may be the cause of severe intraoperative complications as a result of the CBD or the portal vein injuries [1, 19]. The another anomaly is the left-sided gallbladder or GB sinistroposition. In this situation, the gallbladder is located on the undersurface of the left hepatic lobe, most commonly in segment 3. This site type may be accompanied by the situs inversus [1, 20] or it occurs as a single anomaly [1, 20]. In these cases, the cystic duct joins the CHD in the usual location or less frequently it joins the left hepatic duct. Situs inversus totalis, when all abdomino-thoracic organs are transposed, occurs in 1/10000. A left-sided gallbladder without situs inversus occurs in 0.04-0.3%.

Two types of gallbladder malposition have been distinguished in the literature: medioposition and transposition. Medioposition is present when the GB is shifted medially to the base of segment 4 but still is located to the right of the round ligament. In sinistroposition, the GB is located to the left of the round ligament and either at the base of segment 3 or between segments 3 and 4. Patients with this anomaly commonly present with typical biliary colic and cholecystitis symptoms. The abnormal location might not be recognized during the cholecystectomy. Therefore, careful dissection and proper identification of biliary anatomy is very important during surgery in order to avoid bile duct injuries [22, 23]. A rare anomaly is the transverse gallbladder which is situated horizontally in the transverse fissure of the liver and displacement of the gallbladder to the other part of the hepatic underface or position with the GB fundus directed posteriorly, partially within the retroperitoneum [1, 2].

1.3. Anatomical Variants of a Cystic Duct and Hepatic Ducts

In 1975, Jesipowicz et al. [19] described three basic types of the cystic duct opening to the CHD: high (4.5%), middle (88%) and low (7.5%). In the high type, the cystic duct drains into the right, the left or the common hepatic ducts just below the hepatic ducts union. This type is difficult technically during a surgical procedure, during preparation of the cystic duct terminal portion accompanied by the inflammatory reaction. In the middle type, the cystic duct comes to the supraduodenal part of the main biliary tract. In these cases, it is well visible and relatively easy for dissection. Only these cases, in which the cystic duct opens on the posterior or the left surface of the CHD (in 5.5% of cases), may be the cause of difficulties. The low opening is difficult during surgical procedures. In these cases, the cystic duct runs parallel to the CHD on the long distance. Frequently, these ducts are connected by the connective tissue. Dissection of the cystic duct from the supraduodenal portion of the main biliary tract is very difficult. Bleeding from multiple small vessels reduces the visible surgical area and may be indirect cause of the CBD and the duodenal wall injury [1, 19].

In 1976, Benson and Page [28] described five essential for a surgeon anatomical variants of the bile ducts concerning the length, the course and the insertion of the cystic duct into the common hepatic duct (Table 2). According to the authors, the course of the cystic duct may be parallel (15%) or spiral (8%) in relation to the common hepatic duct [1, 28].

According to Kocoń, the cystic duct joins the common hepatic duct at an acute angle (87%), a right angle (9.2%) or runs spirally around the CBD (3.7%). The cystic duct opens the most frequently on the right wall of the CHD (72.2%), on the right posterior wall (13%), on the posterior left wall (1.8%). The cystic duct entering the CHD at the acute angle, may run close to the CHD, in the shorter or longer distance. Parallel course occurs in 42.6% of cases. In 38.8% the common wall separating the CHD and the cystic duct lumens occurs, so called carina [1, 29].

The fact is that the cystic duct may open on the right, posterior, anterior or even the left wall of the common biliary tract and it obligates to careful and precise preparation up to the opening. Abiding by this, we avoid leaning of the too long stump which may be the cause of certain complications. This dissection must be particularly careful and precise if the cystic duct in its terminal portion runs parallel to the CHD. Then division of existing loose or even solid adhesion of both these ducts should be performed in order to ligate the cystic duct properly. A carina can make the instrumental control of the proximal CBD by the cystic duct be very difficult or impossible, with necessity of choledochotomy. The presence of the long carina may also narrow ducts in this site.

Table 2. Anatomical variants of bile ducts according to Benson and Page

No	A anatomical variant type.
1	Long cystic duct running parallel to the CHD with low fusion with CHD.
2	High insertion of the cystic duct into the CHD – at the level of right and left hepatic ducts fusion (trifurcation).
3	Accessory hepatic duct draining into the CHD, above cystic duct.
4	Cystic duct entering the right hepatic duct.
5	Cholecystohepatic duct.

The lumen stenosis may be the place where the concrements occur or stop, or it may make bile outflow more difficult [1, 29].

Moreover, the cystic duct draining into the right and left hepatic ducts, cases of double cystic duct and very short or total absence of the cystic duct have been described in the literature [13, 30, 31]. During ligation of a short cystic duct (occurs in 5-10%) care must be taken not to damage the CBD wall. The risk of this injury is increased during excessive traction of the gallbladder neck during preparation. In case of total agenesis of the cystic duct, the gallbladder opens directly on the CBD which may be mistaken for the cystic duct [1, 2, 13].

1.4. The Other Anomalies of the Gallbladder, Cystic and Hepatic Ducts

Ortiz et al. [32] described a case of CHD draining into the gallbladder with the CBD agenesis – a kind of the persistent hepatocystic duct. In this case, hepaticojejunostomy was performed after cholecystectomy [1]. Picardi et al. [33] described the right hepatic duct coming to the infundibulum of the gallbladder, without confluence with the left hepatic duct [1]. Walia et al. [32] and Nikolov et al. [35] described the right and the left hepatic ducts draining into the gallbladder, with absence of the CHD and with the cystic duct replacing the CBD, coming to the major duodenal papilla [1].

The right hepatic duct draining into the cystic duct was also noted. It is associated with a rising risk of the right hepatic duct division during cholecystectomy. In the case of the intraoperative bile duct injury, primary reconstruction or biliary-intestine anastomosis gives usually good results [1, 36, 37]. The cases of hepatic ducts coming to the gallbladder are the argument of gallbladder removal inferiorly, in the direction of its neck. The not-recognized and ligated, divided right hepatic duct draining into the gallbladder or the cystic duct is particularly dangerous, because it may lead to functional defect of the large liver surface (drained by this duct), jaundice and ascending cholangitis [1, 36].

1.5. The Aberrant and Accessory Hepatic Ducts

The presence of the accessory hepatic ducts is described in about 10% of cases [1, 2]. The contradictory data concerning precise frequency of their occurrence – from 2% to even 30% can be found in the literature (according to some authors it is the commonest type of biliary tract anomalies) (1, 13, 19, 36]. Contradiction of these data may be associated with their not-uniform definition. According to Kocoń, accessory hepatic ducts are the small ducts joining the gallbladder or the cystic duct, and also small supernumerary ducts from particular segments of the liver and not forming the lobar duct [1, 38]. They arise from the surface of the liver (usually from the singular segments) and drain into the right, the left hepatic ducts, the cystic duct, the CBD or the gallbladder [1, 2]. A case of the accessory duct draining into the pancreatic duct [39] and the lesser curvature of the stomach [40] has been also described. In most cases, they arise from the right hepatic lobe, more rarely from the left or the caudate lobe of the liver. They are remaining, aberrant in the embryogenesis process hepatic cords. They are usually delicate, thin structures (diameter to 2 mm), which may be easily overlooked during the operative procedure, although sometimes they may reach the cystic duct sizes.

They often course within the hepatocystic triangle and may be injured during preparation of this region [1, 2, 19].

Some authors [41, 42, 43] have differentiated between ''major'' aberrant duct and a ''minor'' accessory duct. In this differentiation, a major aberrant bile duct does not communicate with other biliary segments and is the only bile duct draining a particular segment of the liver. On the other hand, an accessory or ''minor'' bile duct intercommunicates with other biliary segments and is an additional bile duct draining the same area of the liver. This division is significant in surgery, because ligation of an accessory or ''minor'' bile duct may not cause recurrent cholangitis or focal fibrosis of the liver because of the existence of another draining bile duct, whereas ligation of the aberrant or ''major'' bile duct results in serious complications. The differentiation between the two types can be made on the basis of preoperative or intraoperative cholangiography [43].

Balija et al. [44] distinguished three groups of clinically important accessory bile ducts. First group involves accessory bile ducts between the gallbladder and the respective site of the low hepatic surface. This group includes: so called Luschka's accessory bile ducts and hepatocystic ducts. The hepatocystic ducts are the small biliary ducts coursing directly to the gallbladder from the surface of the liver. The hepatocystic duct draining bile from the large hepatic area is particularly dangerous, because a high risk of this duct injury during dissection exists [45, 46]. The cut recognized hepatocystic duct during preparation of the gallbladder from the lower hepatic surface should be ligated in order to avoid postoperative bile leakage [1, 2, 45, 46]. According to some authors, this type anomaly may play a role in pathogenesis of cholecystitis caused by disturbances of bile drainage with its stasis [11].

Second group comprises accessory bile ducts located within the hepatocystic triangle, draining into the cystic duct or one of the hepatic ducts. This group contains: hepatocystic ducts running from the liver parenchyma to the cystic duct, hepatohepatic ducts draining bile from the liver part to the CHD and so called anastomotic ducts connecting the cystic duct with one of the hepatic ducts or the hepatic ducts with each other [44].

Third group contains (includes) hepatocystic ducts running from the liver parenchyma to different sites within the gallbladder [44]. Diwadkar et al. [47] described the accessory duct connecting the lateral and the medial segments of the left hepatic lobe.

Accessory hepatic ducts accidentally injured during surgical procedure may be the source of postoperative bile leakage. Iso et al. [48] described a case of bile peritonitis after Bilroth I partial gastrectomy for a cancer, due to bile leakage from the injured accessory hepatic duct coursing along the free edge of the left triangular ligament. Within the upper end of the left hepatic lobe – so called appendix fibrosa hepatic, the small bile ducts so called aberrant vessels occur, being rudimentary primarily further situated liver tissue. In case of intraoperative cutting of appendix fibrosa hepatic, it should be ligated in order to avoid postoperative bile leakage and relaparotomy [1, 48]

The cases of postoperative bile leakage from accidentally damaged another accessory hepatic ducts: Luschka's duct (arising from the gallbladder fossa of the liver) and the accessory cholecystohepatic duct have been described in the literature [49]. Careful preparation of the bile ducts allows proper identification and ligation of the accessory hepatic duct and it allows to avoid postoperative bile leakage [1, 48].

Differentiation between Lushka's ducts and cholecystohepatic ducts is important for a surgeon. Lushka's ducts are defined as small bile ducts lying in the gallbladder fossa, either as blind ducts emerging from the right hepatic lobe, or ducts that run subserosally to join one of the main biliary channels later. They do not enter the gallbladder lumen that is different from the true cholecystohepatic ducts [50]. The true cholecystohepatic ducts occur rarely (0.9-2%). They are formed by the atypical resorption of the initially plexiform pattern of hepatic ducts during embryogenesis [51].

Also a right hepatic duct draining into a cystic duct has been described in the literature. It is an extremely rare anomaly of the biliary tract, with an incidence below 1% [52, 53].

1.6. Anomalies of the Common Bile Duct

Anomalies concerning the CBD position and number belong to rare anatomical variations. Recognition of their presence is very important for the surgeon in the prevention of iatrogenic bile duct injuries during surgical procedures. According to Jesipowicz et al., in 52.5% of cases, the CBD enters the major papilla in the middle portion of the descending part of the duodenum, on its posterior wall. In remaining cases not-typical position of Vater's papilla occurs: higher (4%) or lower (43.5%). In 68% of cases, the CBD forms with the pancreatic duct, before entering the duodenum, the hepatopancreatic ampulla (connection of the CBD and the pancreatic duct occurs in the preduodenal portion). In 32% of cases, the CBD courses within the Vater's papilla above the pancreatic duct and the both ducts enter near each other at the apex of the papilla [1, 19].

Some variations of abnormal position (malposition) or duplication of the CBD draining into the pylorus or the prepyloric part of the stomach have been noted in the literature. Kubik et al. [54] described the bile duct originating in the superior area of the lateral segment of the liver, passing through the pyloric sphincter to the submucosa of the superior part of the duodenum. Other anomalies of the CBD are the following: a single duct opening into the pylorus or antrum, a single duct opening into the gastric fundus, a single duct entering the duodenum independently of the pancreatic duct, two separate ducts entering the duodenum 1 cm apart, a bifurcating duct with one branch entering the duodenum and the other one entering the stomach, a bifurcating duct with both branches entering the duodenum, septated (divided by a septum) CBD, with two openings of the single duct into the duodenum [1, 2].

A very rare congenital anomaly that it is clinically important is the ectopic opening of bile ducts to the third and fourth parts of the duodenum, the pyloric channel, the bulbus and the stomach is very much unusual.

Table 3. Kanematsu's classification of the congenital anomalies associated with ectopic biliary drainage

Type	Description
I	One septated draining duct, which enters the stomach.
II	Division of the common bile duct in 2 separate junctions, one of which enters the normal position of the papilla of Vater, whereas the second one enters the stomach.
III	Presence of two independent draining ducts, one of which enters the normal position of the papilla of Vater, whereas the second one enters the stomach.
IV	Presence of two independent draining ducts, one of which enters the normal position of the papilla of Vater, whereas the second one enters the stomach and share one or more intercommunications.

In patients with this anomaly, recurrent cholangitis due to increased rate of choledocholithiasis and gastric outlet obstruction due to duodenal ulcer formation induced by duodenogastric reflux of bile components are observed [55, 56].

Kanematsu et al. [57] distinguished four types of the congenital anomalies associated with ectopic drainage of the biliary tract. This classification is presented in Table 3.

A double common bile duct (DCBD) is an extremely rare anomaly. It is often associated with biliary lithiasis, choledochal cyst, pancreaticobiliary maljunction (PBM), and upper gastrointestinal tract malignancies. The first case of this anomaly was reported by Vesarius in 1543. Since this time, no more 90 cases have been reported in the world literature. It is interesting that two-thirds of them are Asian people, most frequently from Japan [57].

Also, a double papilla of Vater has been reported in the literature. In this extremely rare anomaly, two independent and separate orifices of bile and pancreatic ducts are found. According to the literature, it does not predispose to any pancreatobiliary diseases [58].

2. Arterial Blood Supply of the Extrahepatic Biliary Tract

2.1. An Anatomical Division of Arterial Blood Supply of the Extrahepatic Biliary Tract

Arterial blood supply of the extrahepatic biliary tract is based on its topographical division that was presented in Table 4 [59, 60].

2.2. Arterial Blood Supply of the Gallbladder and the Cystic Duct

The gallbladder and the cystic duct are supplied with the arterial blood by the cystic artery (CA). The cystic artery usually arises as a single branch of the right hepatic artery (RHA) (a right branch of the proper hepatic artery) within the hepatocystic triangle [59, 61-69]. The hepatocystic triangle is formed by: the common hepatic duct – medially, the cystic duct – laterally and the inferior margin of the right lobe of the liver – superiorly. This description of the hepatocytic triangle differs from the original Calot's definition. In 1891, Calot defined a triangle-shaped anatomic area formed by the common hepatic duct medially, the cystic duct laterally and the cystic artery superiorly [70].

Table 4. Topographical division of the extrahepatic biliary tract according to arterial blood supply

Type	Description
I	The gallbladder and the cystic duct.
II	The right and the left hepatic ducts – the hilar part.
III	The common hepatic duct and the common biliary duct (CBD) (in its supra- and retroduodenal portion) – the supra- and retroduodenal part.
IV	The common biliary duct (in its pancreatic part).

The primary (described by Calot in De la Cholecystectomie, t.2) and currently used definition of Calot's triangle differ from each other in only one – superior boundary. It is proposed to reserve the name „hepatocystic triangle" for the primary definition. The current definition of the hepatocystic triangle (with the upper boundary within the inferior margin of the right lobe of the liver) is more significant for a surgeon. In some cases, the accessory bile ducts, draining into the cystic duct or the common hepatic duct, run within this triangle. The accessory or replaced hepatic artery originating from the superior mesenteric artery usually courses through the medial part of the triangle. Therefore, visualization of this area and identification of all structures is very important during cholecystectomy [59, 61, 62, 66, 71, 72].

In approximately 80% of cases, the cystic artery (CA) arises from the right hepatic artery within the hepatocystic triangle. All variants of the CA origins are presented in Table 5 [59, 62, 66, 70]. The cystic artery may arise from the proximal right hepatic artery or from the common hepatic artery and may run close to the hepatic duct, which may be injured when the artery is ligated [61, 62]. Within of the hepatocystic triangle, the cystic artery supplies the cystic duct with one or more small arterial branches. Near the gallbladder, the cystic artery usually divides into a superficial branch and a deep branch. The superficial branch of the cystic artery courses along the anterior surface of the gallbladder, and the deep branch passes between the gallbladder and liver within the cystic fossa [59, 61, 62, 64, 65, 73, 74].

Anatomic variations of the hepatic and cystic arteries are described in approximately 50% of cases [59]. An accessory or double cystic artery occurs in 15-20% of cases [61, 63, 75]. These arteries usually arise from the right hepatic artery within the hepatocystic triangle. During dissection of the hepatocystic triangle, it is important to remember about the possibility of the accessory cystic artery occurrence. If it is present, the vessel should be ligated, in order to avoid bleeding. A triple cystic artery occurs very rarely – 0,3% of cases [63]. The cystic artery may course anteriorly to the common bile duct or the common hepatic duct. In this location, the cystic artery is the first structure encountered during dissection within the lower margin of the hepatocystic triangle. Such artery should be ligated and divided in the early phase of dissection during cholecystectomy in order to proper visualisation of the cystic duct [59, 62]. In 5-15% of cases, the right hepatic artery courses through the hepatocystic triangle close to the cystic duct before turning upward to enter the hilum of the liver.

Table 5. Anatomical variants of origins of the cystic artery

Origin artery	Incidence
Right hepatic artery	80%
Left hepatic artery	5.9%
Proper hepatic artery	11.5%
Common hepatic artery	3.8%
Superior pancreaticoduodenal artery	0.15%
Superior mesenteric artery	0.9%
Celiac trunk	0.3%

In such situation, the cystic artery arises from the convex aspect of the angled or humped portion of the hepatic artery. This „caterpillar hump" right hepatic artery may be easily mistaken for the cystic artery and divided during cholecystectomy. The cystic artery arising from such hepatic artery may be easily avulsed from the hepatic artery during excessive traction of the gallbladder [59, 61, 62].

2.3. Arterial Blood Supply of the Hilar Part of the Extrahepatic Biliary Tract

2.3.1. The Hepatic Arteries

The hilar part of the extrahepatic biliary tract has a very rich arterial blood supply from the right and left hepatic arteries. In 85% of cases, the right hepatic artery passes posteriorly to the common hepatic duct, and in the remaining 15% of cases it courses anteriorly to the common hepatic duct [59, 61, 62]. The accessory or replaced (aberrant) right hepatic artery originates from the superior mesenteric artery and courses through the hepatocystic triangle. The aberrant hepatic artery supplies a liver instead of the proper hepatic artery. The accessory hepatic artery supplies a liver segment independently of the proper hepatic artery. The aberrant replaced hepatic artery is the sole blood supply of a liver, without the proper hepatic artery. Aberrant hepatic arteries are recognized in 12-26% of cases. In 75-85% of cases, the aberrant right hepatic artery is a replaced vessel, which accidental ligation could be the cause of the segmental liver necrosis. The aberrant right hepatic artery usually arises from the superior mesenteric artery, but it may also arise from the celiac trunk, the aorta, the gastroduodenal artery and left hepatic artery. The aberrant left hepatic artery usually originates from the left gastric, rarely from the gastroduodenal or the common hepatic artery. It passes through the hepatoduodenal ligament and supplies the left liver lobe [59, 61, 63, 75-78].

2.3.2. The Hilar Plexus

Vellar described an arterial plexus between the branches of the left and right hepatic arteries that was found on the inferior surface of the "hilar plate". The hilar plate is a condensation of the connective tissue lining the hilum of the liver and forming a roof over the contents of the hilum, separating these structures from the liver parenchyma. The hilar plexus is formed by collateral vessels bridging between the right and left hepatic arteries. The hilar arterial plexus plays a role not only in the arterial supply of the hepatic ducts confluence. It is an important place of collateral circulation between branches of the right and the left hepatic arteries. Branches originating from the hilar plexus also supply the caudate lobe and process of the liver. The most branches to the hilar plexus originate from the right and left hepatic arteries, and they ascend posterior to the right and left hepatic ducts [59, 79, 80].

2.4. Arterial Blood Supply of the Pancreatic Part of the Extrahepatic Biliary Tract

The pancreatic part of the CBD has also very rich arterial blood supply. It is supplied with the arterial blood by the posterior superior pancreatic artery (PSPDA.) mainly, and supra- and retroduodenal arteries [59, 62, 81]. The PSPDA usually arises from the gastroduodenal artery (GDA) 1-2 cm below its origin from the common hepatic artery (CHA) at the level of the superior margin of the first part of the duodenum. Less frequently, the PSPDA may arise from: the superior pancreaticoduodenal artery (as its posterior branch), the common hepatic artery, the proper hepatic artery, the left hepatic artery, the replaced or accessory right hepatic artery, the superior mesenteric artery, the dorsal pancreatic artery or the splenic artery. The course of the PSPDA is descending. At the beginning, it runs transversely to the right, crossing anteriorly the space between the common bile duct and the portal vein at the level of the superior margin of the pancreatic head and the lowest portion of the pancreatic part of the common bile duct. Next, it turns around the right side of the common bile duct, reaching the posterior surface of the pancreas, between the gland and the Treitz' layer. From this location, it runs to the left, crossing posteriorly the intrapancreatic portion of the common bile duct, and ends anastomosing with the inferior pancreaticoduodenal artery (IPDA). The PSPDA has very characteristic course in relation to the CBD. It surrounds CBD spirally. This spiral descending course was called the "vascular arch of Gregoire" (Peri et al.) [82]. The PSPDA crosses the supraduodenal part of the CBD anteriorly, and next it crosses the pancreatic part of the CBD posteriorly. In posterior crossing, the CBD and PSPDA lie at close range, separated from each other only by a layer of pancreatic parenchyma in thickness of 3-12 mm. Variations of the course of the PSPDA have been described in the literature. Before anterior crossing of the CBD, the PSPDA may descend along its left margin in length of 1 cm. Sometimes, instead of anterior crossing of the suprapancreatic part of the CBD, the PSPDA crosses it posteriorly [59, 83]. According to Woodburne and Olsen [84] and Vandamme [85], the course of this type occurs when the PSPDA arises from the accessory right hepatic artery originating from the superior mesenteric artery or from the dorsal pancreatic artery. In these cases, the artery is situated behind the pancreas from its beginning. The relation between the origin of the PSPDA and the CBD is also variable. In 80% of the cases, the proximal part of the PSPDA is situated on the left side of the CBD and in 10-20% of the cases on the right side. In the second case, the anterior crossing of the suprapancreatic portion of the CBD does not occur [59, 83]. The vascular arch of the PSPDA around the CBD is the consequence of the embryologic development. At the age of 5 weeks, when the ventral pancreatic bud develops, the PSPDA lies anteriorly to the CBD and the ventral pancreatic bud. During rotation of the CBD, the anterior surface of the CBD and the ventral pancreatic bud turn posteriorly and to the right following them pulling at the PSPDA which takes a lateral position to both of these structures. After finished rotation of the pancreas, the PSPDA has a spiral course around the CBD, entering the posterior surface of the ventral pancreatic bud. The PSPDA, as the vessel supplying the CBD and the ventral pancreatic bud, follows them during the embryological development and takes the spiral course. Because of this spiral PSPDA course around the CBD, this artery is the main source of the arterial blood supply in its intrapancreatic portion. Two main branches to the CBD (one ascending and the second descending) frequently originate at the level of anterior crossing with the CBD. The ascending branch passes to the superior along the anterior surface of the CBD, the descending branch passes along its right margin [59, 83].

The supraduodenal artery usually arises from the gastroduodenal artery or the posterior superior pancreaticoduodenal artery. It crosses anteriorly the CBD, runs through the hepatoduodenal ligament and supplies the supraduodenal part of the CBD [63, 59, 83].

The retroduodenal artery usually is a branch of the gastroduodenal artery or the posterior superior pancreaticoduodenal artery. It supplies with the arterial blood the supraduodenal and pancreatic parts of the CBD [59, 62, 63].

2.5. Arterial Blood Supply of the Supraduodenal Part of the Extrahepatic Biliary Tract

The supraduodenal part of the extrahepatic biliary tract is supplied with the arterial blood very poorly [60, 62, 86]. The vascularization of the supraduodenal CBD, within the hepatoduodenal ligament, is critical. In 1948, Shapiro and Robilland [87] concluded that the CBD is poorly supplied by several end-type arteries, and their damage would surely lead to biliary stricture and bile leakage [59, 87]. In the same year 1948, Douglass and Carter [88] described a rich vascular plexus around the CBD (peri-choledochal plexus). Therefore, in the authors' opinion, even skeletonization would not lead to complete damage of the biliary tract vascularization [59, 88]. In 1978, Northover and Terblanche [89] described the axial type of vascularization of the supraduodenal part of the CBD, formed by two main arterial vessels: the 3 o'clock artery and 9 o'clock artery, running along the lateral margins of the CBD [59, 89]. These arteries course parallelly to the supraduodenal CBD. The 3 o'clock artery runs around the left margin of the CBD, and 9 o'clock artery runs around the right margin of the CBD. Small arteries join the main axial vessels from above and below. The supraduodenal part of the CBD has three main sources of the arterial blood supply. The axial supply of the supraduodenal part of the CBD comes mainly from below – 60%, from above – 38%, from left – 2%. Approximately 60% of the blood supply to the supraduodenal bile duct originates inferiorly from the pancreaticoduodenal and retroduodenal arteries, and 38% of the blood supply originates superiorly from the right hepatic artery and cystic artery. Only 2% of the arterial blood supply of the supraduodenal CBD is not axial, but segmental. These small segmental arterial branches arise from the common hepatic artery, in the portion of its course within the hepatoduodenal ligament at close range with the CBD [59, 60, 62, 89].

In 1978, Northover and Terblanche described the third marginal artery – so called the retroportal artery (the 12 o'clock artery), running along the posterior surface of the CBD [59, 60, 89]. This vessel arises posteriorly from the celiac trunk or the superior mesenteric artery. It runs to the right, posteriorly to the portal vein and the pancreatic head entering the inferior end of the CBD. From this point, the further course of the artery occurs in two variations. In the first type, the artery ends joining the retroduodenal artery at the level of the inferior portion of the supraduodenal CBD. In this type, small branches originating from the trunk of the portal artery pass on the posterior surface of the CBD. In the second variety, the retroportal artery runs superiorly and posteriorly to the supraduodenal part of the CBD and joins the right hepatic artery posterior to the common hepatic duct (as third axial 12 o'clock artery). The first type of the retroportal artery supplies only the inferior portion of the supraduodenal duct, and the second type of retroportal artery plays a important role in arterial supplying to all the duct from inferior as far to its superior level [59, 60, 89].

In 1993, Rath et al. [86] described three main types of arterial vascularization of the extrahepatic biliary tract: axial, ladder and mixed type. The axial type occurs most frequently. It is formed by a single, two or three vascular arches of marginal arteries running around the CBD (3-, 9-, 12 o'clock arteries). The less common (less than 10%) is the ladder type with a single (at left border) or double ladder (at left and right borders). In this type, the choledochal arteries origin at the different levels, run horizontally and transversely to the margins of the CBD and divide at the left border of the bile duct into ascending and descending branches which anastomose with each other. In the mixed type, both the vascular arches and ladders are present – in different combinations [59, 86].

Also, Rath et al. [86] linked a zone of overlap between superior and inferior sources of extrahepatic biliary tract vascularization. According to authors', this zone is situated at the level of the inferior border of the cystic duct, which is a kind of the boundary zone between the ascending (from below) and descending (from above) circulations. The each area, situated out of this zone, has its own blood supply source: the common hepatic duct is supplied by an axis of the right hepatic and cystic artery, and the CBD – by an axis of the gastroduodenal and PSPD artery. Based on this theory, in liver transplantation, a proposed level of the CBD transection is the junction of the inferior border of the cystic duct with the common hepatic duct, in both donor and recipient [59, 86].

2.6. Anatomical Variations oOf tThe Hepatic Arteries

Hiatt et al. [90] distinguished six types of arterial hepatic anatomy presented in Table 6.

3. Clinical Implications of Biliary Anatomy for Surgery

Knowledge of anatomy of the extrahepatic biliary tract is very important for safe surgery within the hepatoduodenal ligament, most frequently during cholecystectomy which is the commonest surgical procedure.

Table 6. Hiatt's classification of arterial hepatic anatomy

Type	Definition
I	Normal pattern: the common hepatic artery arises from the celiac axis to form the gastroduodenal and proper hepatic arteries; the proper hepatic artery divides distally into the right and left branches.
II	A replaced or accessory left hepatic artery arises from the left gastric artery.
III	A replaced or accessory right hepatic artery originates from the superior mesenteric artery.
IV	A double replaced pattern: the right hepatic artery arises from the superior mesenteric artery and the left hepatic artery as a branch of the left gastric artery.
V	The entire common hepatic artery originates as a branch of the superior mesenteric artery.
VI	The common hepatic artery takes direct origin from the aorta.

3. Clinical Implications of Biliary Anatomy for Surgery

Knowledge of anatomy of the extrahepatic biliary tract is very important for safe surgery within the hepatoduodenal ligament, most frequently during cholecystectomy which is the commonest surgical procedure.

Most biliary anomalies are disclosed by the surgeon during dissection of the bile ducts on cholecystectomy performed for cholelithiasis. Intraoperative cholangiography may be helpful in precise description and supporting of the bile ducts variants. Accidental and not reported during surgical procedure cutting of the bile ducts may be the cause of postoperative bile leakage, that may lead to bile peritonitis and requires relaparotomy. Lesion of the normal or accessory bile duct is the cause of increased frequency of postoperative morbidity and mortality. Therefore, careful dissection of the bile ducts and identification of all the anatomical structures before their cutting and ligation are such essential. In the case of intraoperative cutting of the small accessory bile duct, it should be ligated, in order to avoid postoperative bile leakage. The large duct should be anastomosed, if possible, to the cystic duct (after cholecystectomy with the duct stump), common hepatic duct, duodenum or Roux-en-Y jejunal loop. Not recognized divided biliary ducts are the cause of bile leakage in the postoperative period, which may lead to complications such as follows: bile peritonitis, subphrenic abscess, an external biliary fistula or postoperative stricture of the CBD (as a result of inflammatory reaction to bile leakage) [1, 13].

Knowledge of arterial blood supply of the extrabiliary biliary tract is very useful in reconstructive biliary surgery [59, 91-97]. Terblanche et al. [91] analyzed 19 patients undergoing postoperative repairs of bile duct strictures. They concluded that repair of extrahepatic biliary tract injuries and strictures should involve anastomoses to the well-vascularized upper common hepatic duct tissue. This study supported the hypothesis of an ischaemic basis for recurrent biliary strictures [59, 97]. Based on the arterial blood supply of the biliary tract, a high hepaticojejunostomy (less than 2 cm below the hepatic duct confluence) should be used to repair biliary strictures. Biliary strictures less frequently occur in a high hepaticojejunostomy than in a low hepaticojejunostomy (more than 2 cm below the hepatic duct confluence) or choledochojejunostomy, because the proximal segment of the common hepatic duct has a better blood supply than its distal part or the CBD. This principle is also used in creating biliary anastomoses in hepatic and pancreatic surgery [59, 97].

Anatomical anomalies of the bile ducts and hepatic arteries significantly increase the risk of iatrogenic bile duct injuries (IBDI). The most frequent cause of IBDI is the misidentification of bile ducts as a cystic duct in cases of anomalies of the cystic duct insertion into the common hepatic duct. About 70-80% of all IBDI are a consequence of the misidentification of biliary anatomy before clipping, ligating and dividing structures. Excessive dissection along the common bile duct margins during open cholecystectomy can lead to the biliary stricture due to damage of the 3 o'clock and 9 o'clock axial arteries and their branches to the pericholedochal plexus. According to the literature, distal IBDI are accompanied by damage of axial arteries (10-15%) and proximal IBDI are usually associated with damage of the proper hepatic artery and its branches (40-60%). Complex IBDI involving the bile ducts and hepatic arteries are more serious and difficult to repair [98-104].

Conclusion

Knowledge of biliary anatomy including variations and arterial blood supply of the extrahepatic biliary tract is very important for surgeons. It may be helpful to perform safe surgical procedures and to avoid many serious postoperative complications.

References

[1] Jabłońska B., Bałuka D. Anatomical variations of the extrahepatic biliary tract - surgical significance. *Pol. J. Surg*., 2005; 77(9): 994-1006.

[2] Gadacz T. R. Anatomy, Embriology, Anomalies, and Physiology of the Gallbladder and Biliary Ducts. W: Zuidema G. D., Yeo Ch. J. Shackelford's Surgery of the Alimentary Tract. Vol III. 5th edition. WB Saunders Company, Philadelphia 2002, 143-150.

[3] Linder H. H. Embriology and anatomy of the biliary tree. In Way, LW, and Pellegrini, CA (eds). Surgery of the Gallbladder and Bile Ducts. Philadelphia, WB Saunders 1987: 3.

[4] Frierson H., Jr. The gross anatomy and histology of the gallbladder, extrahepatic ducts, vaterian system and minor papilla. *Am. J. Surg. Pathol*., 1989; 13: 146.

[5] Bockman D. E., Freeny P. C. Anatomy and anomalies of the biliary tree. *Laparosc. Surg*., 1992; 1:92.

[6] Onder H., Ozdemir M. S., Tekbaş G., Ekici F., Gümüş H., Bilici A. 3-T MRI of the biliary tract variations. *Surg. Radiol. Anat*., 2013; 35(2): 161-7.

[7] Couinaud C. Le foie: etudes anatomiques et chirurgicales. Paris: Masson & Cie; 1957: 530–32.

[8] Huang T. L., Cheng Y. F., Chen C. L., Lee T. Y. Variants of the bile ducts: clinical application in the potential donor of living-related hepatic transplantation. *Transplant. Proc*., 1996; 28: 1669–70.

[9] Karakas H. M., Celik T., Alicioglu B. Bile duct anatomy of the Anatolian Caucasian population: Huang classification revisited. *Surg. Radiol. Anat.,* 2008; 30: 539–45.

[10] Champetier J. Les voies biliaires. In: Chevrel J. P., (ed). Anatomie Clinique, Le tronc. Paris: Springer; 1994: 416–7.

[11] Ohkubo M., Nagino M., Kamiya J., Yuasa N., Oda K., Arai T., Nishio H., Nimura Y. Surgical anatomy of the bile ducts at the hepatic hilum as applied to living donor liver transplantation. *Ann. Surg*., 2004; 239: 82–6.

[12] Deka P., Islam., Jindal D., Kumar N., Arora A., Negi S. S. An analysis of biliary anatomy according to different classification systems. *Indian J. Gastroenterol*., 2014; 33(1): 23-30.

[13] Lamah M., Dickson G. H. Congenital anatomical abnormalities of the extrahepatic biliary duct: a personal audit. *Sur. Radiol. Anat*., 1999; 21(5): 325-327.

[14] Boyden E. "Phrygian cap" in cholecystography: a congenital anomaly of the gallbladder. *AJR Am. J. Roentgenol*., 1935; 33:589.

[15] Davies E., Harding H. E. The pouch of Hartmann. *Lancet,* 1942; 1:193.

[16] Vijay K. T., Kocher H. H., Koti R. S., Bapat R. D. Agenesis of gall bladder – a diagnostic dilemma. *J Postgrad. Med.,* 1996; 42: 80-82.

[17] Marin-Pineda R., Arnaud-Carreno C., Leyva-Ramos A., Marín-Domínguez R. Accessory gallbladder. Diagnosis by ERCP. *Rev. Gastroenterol. Mex.,* 2002; 67(2): 100-102.

[18] Malde S. Gallbladder agenesis diagnosed intra-operatively: a case report. *J. Med. Case Rep*., 2010; 4: 285.

[19] Jesipowicz M., Karski J., Kurylcio L. Chirurgiczne problemy związane ze zmiennością budowy zewnątrzwątrobowych dróg żółciowych. *Pol. Przegl. Chir*., 1975; 47(1): 7-11.

[20] Korn O., Csendes A., Bastias J. Anomalies of extrahepatic biliary duct and gallbladder associated with intestinal malrotation: a case report. *Surgery*, 1988; 103(4): 496-498.

[21] Idu M., Jakimowicz J., Iuppa A., Cuschieri A. Hepatobiliary anatomy in patients with transposition of the gallbladder: implications for safe laparoscopic cholecystectomy. *Br. J. Surg.,* 1996; 83(10): 1442-1443.

[22] Moo-Young T. A., Picus D. D., Teefey S., Strasberg S. M. Common bile duct injury following laparoscopic cholecystectomy in the setting of sinistroposition of the galladderand biliary confluence: a case report. *J. Gastrointest. Surg.*, 2010; 14(1): 166-70.

[23] Boyden E. A. The accessory gallbladder: an embryological and comparative study of aberrant biliary vesicles occurring in man and the domestic mammals. *Am. J. Anat.,* 1926; 38: 177–231.

[24] Lamah M., Karanjia N. D., Dickson G. H. Anatomical variations of the extrahepatic biliary tree: review of the world literature. *Clin. Anat.*, 2001; 14(3): 167–172.

[25] Desolneux G., Mucci S., Lebigot J., Arnaud J. P., Hamy A. Duplication of the gallbladder. A case report. *Gastroenterol. Res. Pract.*, 2009; 2009: 483473.

[26] Nanthakumaran S., King P. M., Sinclair T. S. Laparoscopic excision of a triple gallbladder. *Surg. Endosc.*, 2003; 17(8): 1323.

[27] Schroeder C., Draper K. R. Laparoscopic cholecystectomy for triple gallbladder. *Surg. Endosc.*, 2003; 17(8): 1322.

[28] Benson E., Page R. E. A practical reappraisal of the anatomy of the extrahepatic bile ducts and arteries. *Br. J. Surg*., 1976; 63: 853.

[29] Kocoń T. Niektóre odmiany anatomiczne dróg żółciowych i ich znaczenie w praktyce chirurgicznej. *Pol. Przegl. Chir*., 1988; 60(10): 801-807.

[30] Gergely M., Csipo L., Gyory-Kiss F. Interposition of the gall bladder: a rare congenital malformation of the extrahepatic bile ducts. *Acta. Chir. Acad. Sci. Hung.,* 1979; 20(4): 335-340.

[31] Augustyniak E., Kocoń T., Zając S. Rzadki przypadek podwójnego przewodu pęcherzykowego. *Folia Morphol*., 1968; 27(1): 75-77.

[32] Ortiz V. N., Vidal E., Padilla J. S. Surgical significance of persistent cholecystohepatic ducts. *Bol. Asoc. Med. P. R.,* 1989; 81(9): 355-358.

[33] Picardi N., Monti M., Pasta V., Nudo R., Costantini D., Cassano C. Rare malformation of the bile ducts of surgical interest. *Ann. Ital. Chir*., 1989; 60(5): 399-403.

[34] Walia H. S., Abraham T. K., Baraka A. Gall-bladder interposition: a rare anomaly of the extrahepatic ducts. *Int. Surg*., 1986; 71(2): 117-121.

[35] Nikolov K., Chobanov G., Belchev B., Donev S. A rare case of gallbladder interposition In the extrahepatic bile ducts. *Khirurgiia (Sofiia),* 1994; 47(6):52-53.

[36] Prinz R. A., Howell H. S., Pickleman J. R. Surgical significance of extrahepatic biliary tree anomalies. *Am. J. Surg.,* 1976; 131(6): 755-757.

[37] Hashimoto M., Hashimoto M., Ishikawa T., Iizuka T., Matsuda M., Watanabe G. Right hepatic duct emptying into the cystic duct: report of a case. *Surg. Endosc*., 2002; 16(2): 359.

[38] Kocoń T. Odmiany anatomiczne połączenia przewodów wątrobowych w obrazie cholangiograficznym. *Pol. Przegl. Chir*., 1968; 40(6): 654-660.

[39] Atlas H., Jacquemin J. P. Rare abnormality of the extrahepatic bile ducts. Accessory hepatic duct opening into the middle of Wirsung's duct. *J. Chir. (Paris),* 1972; 104: 591-594).

[40] Mascarenhas R., Varadarajan R., Mathias J., Traynor O., Geoghegan J. Accessory left biliary duct draining into the lesser curve of the stomach. *Gut,* 2002; 51(6):884.

[41] Hirao K., Miyazaki A., Fujimoto T., Isomoto I., Hiyashi K. Evaluation of aberrant bile ducts before laparoscopic cholecystectomy: helical CT cholangiography versus MR cholangiography. *AJR*, 2000; 175:713–720.

[42] Izuishi K., Toyama Y., Nakano S., Goda F., Usuki H., Masaki T., Macta H. Preoperative assessment of the aberrant bile duct using multislice computed tomography cholangiography. *Am. J. Surg.,* 2005; 189:53–55.

[43] Lal R., Behari A., Hari R. H., Sikora S. S., Yachha S. K., Kapoor V. K. Variations in biliary ductal and hepatic vascular anatomy and their relevance to the surgical management of choledochal cysts. *Pediatr. Surg. Int.*, 2013; 29(8): 777-86.

[44] Balija M., Huis M., Szerda M., Bubnjar J., Stulhofer M. Laparoscopic cholecystectomy – accessory bile ducts. *Acta. Med. Croatica*, 2003; 57(2): 105-109.

[45] Champetier J., Letoublon C., Arvieux C., Gerard P., Labrosse P. A. Variations of division of the extrahepatic bile ducts: significance and origin, surgical implications. *J. Chir. (Paris),* 1989; 126(3): 147-154.

[46] Losanoff J. E., Jones J. W., Richman B. W., Rangnekar N. J. Hepatocystic duct: a rare anomaly of the extrahepatic biliary system. *Clin. Anat.*, 2002; 15(4): 314-315.

[47] Diwadkar G. B., Schwaitzberg S. D. An extrahepatic biliary anomaly. *Laparoendosc. Adv. Surg. Tech. A.,* 2003; 13(1): 41-43.

[48] Iso Y., Kusaba I., Matsumata T. Postoperative bile peritonitis caused by division of an aberrant bile duct In the left triangular ligament of the liver. *Am. J. Gastroenterol.,* 1996; 91(11): 2428-2430.

[49] Pisanu A., Altana M. L., Piu S., Uccheddu A. Bile leak from the accessory biliary duct following laparoscopic cholecystectomy. *G. Chir.,* 2003; 24(4): 115-118.

[50] Schofield A., Hankins J., Sutherland F. A case of cholecystohepatic duct with atrophic common hepatic duct. *HPB (Oxford)*, 2003; 5(4): 261-3.

[51] Gandy R. C., Hargreaves W., Fenton-Lee D. Images for surgeons. Aberrant cholecystohepatic duct. *ANZ J. Surg*., 2010; 80(6): 455-6.

[52] Lampe P., Jabłońska B., Bałuka D., Alli-Balogun A., Baron J. Difficulties in recognition of rare biliary tract anomalies. *Pol. J. Surg*., 2006; 78(12): 1490-1497.

[53] Kostov D. V., Kobakov G. L. Accessory right hepatic duct in which a cystic duct drains. *HPB (Oxford)*, 2011; 13(5): 364.

[54] Kubik S., Groscurth P. Rare anomaly of the extrahepatic bile duct and the V. Coronaria ventriculi. *Chirurg.*, 1977; 48(2): 77-80.

[55] Saritas U., Senol A., Ustundag Y. The clinical presentations of ectopic biliary drainage into duodenal bulbus and stomach with a thorough review of the current literature. *BMC Gastroenterol*., 2010; 10: 2.

[56] Sezgın O., Altintaş E., Uçbılek E. Ectopic opening of the common bile duct into the stomach. *Turk. J. Gastroenterol.*, 2010;21(2):163-7.

[57] Chen G., Wang H., Zhang L., Li Z., Bie P. Double common bile duct with choledochal cyst and cholelithiasis: report of a case. *Surg. Today*, 2014; 44(4): 778-82.

[58] Katsinelos P., Chatzimavroudis G., Fasoulas K., Katsinelos T., Pilpilidis I., Lazaraki G., Terzoudis S., Kokonis G., Patsis I., Zavos C., Kountouras J. Double major papilla of Vater - a rare endoscopic finding during endoscopic retrograde cholangiopancreatography: a case report. *Cases J.*, 2009;2:163.

[59] Jabłońska B. The arterial blood supply of the extrahepatic biliary tract - surgical aspects. *Pol. J. Surg.,* 2008; 80(6): 593-604.

[60] Northover J., Terblanche J. A new look at the arterial blood supply of the bile duct in man and its surgical implications. Br. J. Surg 1979; 1979; 66: 379-384.

[61] Adams D. B. The importance of extrahepatic biliary anatomy in preventing complications of laparoscopic cholecystectomy. *Surg. Clin. North Am.*, 1993; 73: 861-871.

[62] Gadacz T. R. Anatomy, Embriology, Anomalies, and Physiology of the Gallbladder and Biliary Ducts. W: Zuidema G. D., Yeo Ch. J. Shackelford's Surgery of the Alimentary Tract. Vol III. 5th edition. WB Saunders Company, 2002: 150-152.

[63] Michels N. A. The hepatic, cystic and retroduodenal arteries and their relations to the biliary ducts: With samples of entire celiacal blood supply. *Ann. Surg.*, 1992; 215: 203-208.

[64] Sarkar A. K., Roy T. S. Anatomy of the cystic artery arising from the gastroduodenal artery arising from the gastroduodenal artery and its choledochal branch – a case report. *J. Anat.,* 2000; 197; 503-506.

[65] Ding Y. M., Wang B., Wang W. X., Wang P., Yan J. S. New classification of the anatomic variations of cystic artery during laparoscopic cholecystectomy. *Word J. Gastroenterol.,* 2007; 13(42): 5629-5634.

[66] Bergamaschi R., Ignjatovic D. More than two structures in Calot's triangle. A postmortem study. *Surg. Endosc.*, 2000; 14(4): 354-357.

[67] Chen T. H., Shyu J. F., Chen C. H., Ma K. H., Wu C. W., Lui W. Y., Liu J. C. Variations of the cystic artery in Chinese adults. *Surg. Laparosc. Endosc. Oercutan. Tech.*, 200, 10(3): 154-157.

[68] Suzuki M., Akaishi S., Rikiyama T., Naitoh T., Rahman M. M., Matsuno S. Laparoscopic cholecystectomy. Calot's triangle, and variations in cystic arterial supply. *Surg. Endosc.*, 2000; 14(2): 141-4.

[69] Saidi H., Karanja T. M., Ogengo J. A. Variant anatomy of the cystic artery in adult Kenyans. *Clin. Anat.*, 2007; 20(8): 943-945.

[70] Calot J. F. De la Cholecystectomie (Ablation de las Vesicule Biliare). G. Steinheil, ed. Paris, University of Paris: 41.

[71] Muirhead W. R., O'Leary P. Calot's triangle: Loose interpretation or respectful accuracy? *The American Surgeon*, 1999; 65: 186-187.

[72] Michalewski K. Przypadek odejścia tętnicy pęcherzykowej (arteria cystica) od tętnicy krezkowej górnej. *Folia Morphol.*, 1965; 24(4): 401-403.

[73] Nowak M. Variation of the cystic artery in man. *Folia Morphol.*, 1977; 36(2): 98-98.

[74] Kędzior E., Kuś J. Naczynia krwionośne pęcherzyka żółciowego. *Folia Morphol.*, 1965; 24(4): 393-403.

[75] Benson E., Page R. E. A practical reappraisal of the anatomy of the extrahepatic bile ducts and arteries. *Br. J. Surg.,* 1976; 63: 853.

[76] Audio E., Franchitto A., Pannarale L., Carpino G., Alpini G., Francis H., Glaser S., Alvaro D., Onori P. Cholangiocytes and blood supply. *Word J. Gastroenterol.*, 2006; 12(22): 3546-3552.

[77] Guni H., Cho A., Tohma T., Okazumi S., Makino H., Shuto K., Mochizuki R., Matsubara K., Hayano K., Mori C., Murakami G., Ochiai T. The blood supply of the hilar bile duct and its relationship to the communicating arcade located between the right and left hepatic arteries. *Am. J. Surg.*, 2006; 192(3): 276-280.

[78] Eisedrath D. N. Anomalies of the bile ducts and blood vessels as the cause of accidents in biliary surgery. *JAMA,* 1918; 71: 864-867.

[79] Vellar I. D. The blood supply of the biliary ductal system and its relevance to vasculobiliary injuries following cholecystectomy. *Aust. NZJ Surg*., 1999; 69: 816-820.

[80] Kawarada Y., Das B. C., Taoka H. Anatomy of the hepatic hilar area: the plate system. *J. Hepatobiliary Pancreat. Surg*., 2000; 7(6): 580-586.

[81] Osemblak J., Siwek R. The arterial supply of the extrahepatic biliary ducts in newborns and infants. *Folia Morphol.,* 1984; 42(2): 137-143.

[82] Peri G., Veralli E., Trivellini G. La vascularizzazione del pancreas. *Arch. It. Chir.,* 1969; 95: 287-300.

[83] Bertelli E., Di Georgio F., Bertelli L., Civeli L., Mosca S. The arterial blood supply of the pancreas: a review II. The posterior superior pancreaticoduodenals artery. An anatomical and radiological study. *Surg. Radiol. Anat.,* 1996; 18: 1-9.

[84] Woodburne R. T., Olsen L. L. The arteries of the pancreas. *Anat. Rec.,* 1951; 111: 255-270.

[85] Vandamme J. P., Van der Schueren G., Bonte J. Vascularization du pancreas: proposition de nomenclature PNA et angioarchitecture des ilots. *CR ASS Anat.,* 1967; 137: 1184-1189.

[86] Rath A. M., Zhang J., Bourdelat D., Chevrel J. P. Arterial vascularization of the extrahepatic biliary tract. *Surg. Radiol. Anat.,* 1993; 15: 105-111.

[87] Shapiro A. L., Robilland G. L. The arterial supply of the common and hepatic bile ducts with reference to the problem of common duct injury and repair. *Surgery*, 1948; 23: 1-11.

[88] Douglass T. C., Cutter W. W. Arterial blood supply of the common bile duct. *Arch. Surg.,* 1948; 57: 599-612.

[89] Northover J., Terblanche J. Bile duct blood supply: its importance in human liver transplantation. *Tranplantation,* 1978; 26: 67-69.

[90] Hiatt J. R., Gabbay J., Busuttil R. W. Surgical anatomy of the hepatic arteries in 1,000 cases. *Ann. Surg.,* 1994; 220:50–52.

[91] Hoekstra H., Porte R. J., Tian Y., Jochum W., Stieger B., Moritz W., Slooff M. J.,.Graf R., Clavien P. A. Bile salt toxity aggravates cold ischaemic injury of bile ducts after liver transplantations in Mdr2+/- mice. *Hepatology,* 2006; 43(5): 1022-1031.

[92] Gupta N., Solomon H., Fairchild R., Kaminski D. L. Management and outcome of patients with combined bile duct and hepatic artery injuries. *Arch. Surg*., 1998; 133: 176-181.

[93] Hart R. S., Passi R. B., Wall W. J. Long term outcome after repair of major bile duct injury created during laparoscopic cholecystectomy. *HPB Surg.,* 2000; 2: 325-332.

[94] Johnson S. R., Koehler A., Pennington L. K., Hanto D. W. Long-term results of surgical repair of bile duct injuries following laparoscopic cholecystectomy. *Surgery,* 128; 668-677.

[95] Koffron A., Ferrario M., Parsons W., Nemcek A., Saker M., Abecassis M. Failed primary management of iatrogenic biliary injury: Incidence and significance of concomitant hepatic arterial disruption. *Surgery,* 2001; 130: 722-731.

[96] Lillemoe K. D., Melton G. B., Cameron J. L., Pitt H. A., Campbell K. A., Talamini M. A., Sauter P. A., Coleman J., Yeo C. J. Postoperative bile duct strictures: management and outcome in the 1990s. *Ann. Surg.*, 2000; 232: 430-441.

[97] Terblanche J., Worthley Ch. S., Krige J. E. J. High or low hepaticojejunostomy for bile duct strictures? *Surgery*, 1990; 108: 828-834.

[98] Jabłońska B., Lampe P. Iatrogenic bile *World J. Gastroenterol.*, 2009 Sep. 7;15(33):4097-104.

[99] Connor S., Garden O. J. Bile duct injury in the era of laparoscopic cholecystectomy. *Br. J. Surg.*, 2006; 93: 158-168.

[100] Flum D. R., Cheadle A., Prela C., Dellinger E. P., Chan L. Bile Duct Injury During Cholecystectomy and Survival in Medicare Beneficiares. *JAMA*, 2003; 290(16): 2168-2173.

[101] Schmidt S. C., Settmacher U., Langrehr J. M., Neuhaus P. Management and outcome of patients with combined bile duct and hepatic arterial injuries after laparoscopic cholecystectomy. *Surgery*, 2004; 135: 613-618.

[102] Buell J. F., Cronin D. C., Funaki B., Koffron A., Yoshida A., Lo A., Leef J., Millis J. M. Devastating and Fatal Complications Associated With Combined Vascular and Bile Injuries During Cholecystectomy. *Ann. Surg.*, 2002; 137: 703-710.

[103] Li J., Frilling A., Nadalin S., Broelsch C. E., Malago M. Timing and risk *J. Gastrointest. Surg.*, 2012; 16(4): 815-20.

[104] Jabłońska B. Hepatectomy for bile *World J. Gastroenterol.,* 2013; 19(38): 6348-6352.

In: Bile Duct
Editor: Miguel Ángel Mercado

ISBN: 978-1-63321-771-3

Chapter 3

Assessment of the Biliary Duct: Advancement of Imaging Modalities

Reiji Sugita, MD*
Department of Radiology, Sendai City Medical Center,
Miyagino-ku, Sendai, Miyagi, Japan

Abstract

Various imaging modalities, invasive and noninvasive, are useful for the assessment of bile duct anatomy in pre-surgical evaluation. In this chapter, I present characteristics of each modality and the new technical developments in this field. Assessment of the functional anatomy of the bile duct is important in evaluation of the risk factors affecting bile duct cancer. I show that MRI is the most appropriate modality for this purpose, because MRI facilitates analysis of bile and pancreatic juice flow, which may have associations with carcinogenesis in bile duct tumors. Although flow analysis of the bile duct with MRI has focused on continuous MRCP examination after secretin injection, a new method (time-SLIP imaging) is available for easier and faster flow analysis. I present various cases and clinical management approaches based on this new technique (time-SLIP imaging). I present how various radiological modalities can be used to help differentiate between benignity and malignancy, stage tumors, select surgical candidates, and guide surgical planning when biliary disease is suspected. I also discuss how recent developments in imaging modalities contribute to the diagnosis of bile duct disease.

Introduction

The biliary tree consists of an intricate thin wall ductal system and has complicated anatomical and functional connections with the neighboring organs, including the liver,

* Corresponding author to: Reiji Sugita, MD; Sendai City Medical Center; 5-22-1, Tsurugaya, Miyagino-ku, Sendai, Miyagi, JAPAN; Tel: +81-252-1111, Fax: +81-252-9431; E-mail:rsugita@openhp.or.jp.

pancreas, and duodenum. Therefore, imaging modalities for visualization of the biliary tree in pre-and post-operative evaluations must provide morphological information with high spatial resolution as well as functional information.

In this chapter, I discuss how various imaging modalities, invasive and noninvasive, play roles in the assessment of bile duct anatomy in pre-surgical evaluation and clarify the characteristics of each modality and new technical developments in this field. I also discuss methods for functional assessment of the bile duct, such as the visualization of bile duct leakage after surgery. Moreover, I point out the importance of functional anatomy assessment of the bile duct in the evaluation of patients with risk factors affecting bile duct cancer. I show that magnetic resonance imaging (MRI) is a very appropriate modality for this purpose, because MRI enables evaluation of bile and pancreatic juice flow, which may be related to carcinogenesis in bile duct tumors. A new MRI method (time-SLIP imaging) allows easier and faster flow analysis. I present various cases and clinical management approaches based on this new method.

I also discuss how various radiological modalities can be used to help differentiate between benignity and malignancy, stage tumors, select surgical candidates, and guide surgical planning when biliary disease is suspected.

Bile Duct Anatomy in Pre- and Post-Surgical Evaluations: Various Modalities

During pre- and post-surgical evaluations of bile duct anatomy, the optimal imaging studies provide the required information about not only bile duct anatomy but also the neighboring structures, including the vascular anatomy (portal system, arteries, etc.) and organs (liver, gallbladder, pancreas, etc.). Moreover, functional assessment of the bile duct is often required, such as in monitoring for bile leakage after surgery and in the evaluation of bile secretion and excretion [1]. In addition, functional anatomy assessment is necessary in identifying patients with morphologically normal bile duct anatomy, but with hidden risk factor affecting malignancy [2].

Various imaging modalities, invasive and noninvasive, are used in pre-surgical planning and post-surgical evaluation [3-5]. The invasive methods include endoscopic retrograde cholangiopancreatography (ERCP), percutaneous transhepatic cholangiography (PTC), endoscopic ultrasonography (EUS), intraductal ultrasonography (IDUS), and optical coherence tomography. Noninvasive imaging methods include ultrasonography (US), intravenous computed tomography (CT) cholangiography, oral contrast agent-enhanced CT cholangiography, intravenous contrast-enhanced MR cholangiography (c MRC), and MR cholangiography (MRC).

ERCP and PTC are not used as diagnostic tools alone because of the invasive nature, the inability to demonstrate vascular anatomy and neighboring organs, and the risk of complications. Nowadays ERCP is used for interventions such as biopsy, drainage, and EUS/IDUS. US, EUS, and IDUS are useful techniques for screening for biliary diseases particularly gallbladder disease; however, their efficacy depends on operator skill and experience.

Multi-detector CT (MDCT) is an accurate and useful imaging technique for the evaluation of biliary diseases. MDCT offers detailed information about the biliary tree and surrounding structures; however, disadvantages include ionizing radiation and adverse reactions to intravenous contrast materials. Intravenous CT cholangiography and oral contrast agent-enhanced CT cholangiography have been evaluated for visualization of the biliary tree. In conjunction with MDCT, these methods are accurate and useful imaging techniques for the evaluation of biliary duct anatomy.

MRI is a reliable noninvasive imaging tool, which is commonly available, for the diagnosis and pre-surgical evaluation of bile duct diseases. MRI has many advantages over other modalities: [1] It is completely noninvasive, does not require exposure to ionizing radiation, and does not cause patient discomfort. [2] It does not require expert technicians with sophisticated technical skills. Therefore, MRI has become an important diagnostic tool for bile duct diseases. In particular, MRC does not use contrast medium, which avoids the possibility about adverse reactions. Therefore, MRC is a reliable noninvasive common available imaging tool for pre-surgical evaluation of the bile duct tree and has become an important diagnostic tool for bile duct diseases. However, from the view point of spatial resolution, CT cholangiography enabled significantly better visualization than MRC.

c-MRC appeared relatively recently because the hepatobiliary-specific agents used for c-MRC have only been available for the past two decades [6]. Although these contrast agents are aimed at detection of focal liver lesions, researchers noticed visualization of the biliary tree by the excretion of these agents via the biliary tree. Thus, c-MRC allows visualization of the anatomy of the biliary tree together with functional assessment with the excretion of contrast agent.

Nowadays remarkable technical advances in MR technology have increased the clinical applications of MRI for diagnosing biliary diseases [4, 7-9]. The new time-SLIP technique, used in vascular studies, has the potential for direct visualization of biliary and pancreatic juice flow. As a result, this technique may enable evaluation of the functional anatomy of the biliary tree.

Functional Assessment and Functional Anatomy Assessment of the Bile Duct

(a) Functional Assessment of the Bile Duct

Functional assessment of the bile duct comprises [1] preoperative assessment, for anatomical assessment of the biliary tree, prevention of involuntary bile injury in laparoscopic cholecystectomy, and complex surgical procedures such as biliary enteric anastomosis and liver transplantation; [2] postoperative assessment, for the biliary tree evaluation after surgery when complications such as bile leakage and involuntary biliary tree stricture or ligation are suspected; and [3] evaluation of bile secretion/excretion.

Although various modalities are used for evaluation of function of the bile duct, CT and MRI are two typical non-invasive modalities. MDCT including CT cholangiography is superior to MRI with regard to spatial resolution and is thus the primary imaging tool for pre- and post-operative evaluations [10]. However, for assessment of the biliary tree, especially functional assessment, MRI is considered superior because CT has several drawbacks: restriction of biliary CT contrast agents in certain countries, mandatory delayed examination due to drip infusion of biliary contrast agent, and high risk of adverse reactions.

MRI including MR cholangiopancreatography (MRCP) is another imaging modality used for assessment of the biliary tree. Although MRCP enable totally non-invasive delineation of the biliary tree, visualization of the intrahepatic biliary tree is less effective. Moreover functional assessment of the biliary duct as described earlier is impossible.

In recent years, intravenous contrast-enhanced MR cholangiography has attracted attention with regards to functional assessment of the biliary tree [1, 6, 11-14] in Figure 1. Several contrast agents are available for use in biliary contrast-enhanced MR, such as mangafodipir trisodium (Mn-DPDP), gadolinium-ethoxybenzyl-diethylenetriamine-pentaacetic-acid (Gd-EOB-DPTA), and gadobenate dimeglumine (Gd-BOPTA), which are excreted through the biliary tree after accumulation by the hepatocytes, causing T1 shortening of bile. Of these biliary MR contrast agents, only a small fraction (3%-5% of the injected dose) of Gd-BOPTA is excreted into the biliary tree, while with Mn-DPDP and Gd-EOB-DTPA, about half of the injected dose (50%-60% and 50%, respectively) is excreted into the biliary tree [13].

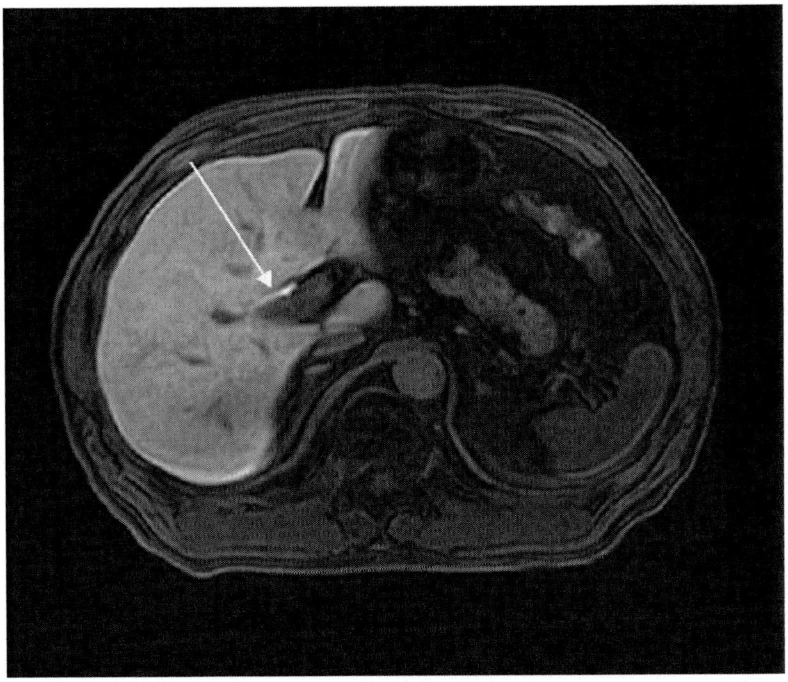

Figure 1. Functional MR cholangiography with hepatobiliary-phase imaging with Gd-EOB-DTPA. A 25-year-old male patient with suspected liver tumor. Coronal T1-weighted Gd-EOB-DTPA-enhanced image shows excreted contrast in the biliary ducts (arrow).

c-MRC is considered useful for preoperative anatomic assessment because visualization of intrahepatic ducts and anatomic variants with c-MRC is superior to conventional MRCP. Thus, preoperative knowledge of bile duct anatomic variants lessens the risk of bile leakage, which is a major cause of morbidity in living donor liver transplantation and in tumor resection, particularly when surgery involves the left lobe of the liver. c-MRC may also prevent inadvertent ligation or transection of aberrant bile ducts in laparoscopic cholecystectomy by knowledge of the anatomic variants.

c-MRC is also very valuable procedure for postoperative assessment of the biliary tree, particularly, when bile leakage or inadvertent biliary duct ligation or stricture is suspected. c-MRC is superior to conventional MRCP because c-MRC can provide functional information regarding biliary excretion and the site of bile leakage.

In functional assessment, c-MRC can provide functional information about the flow of bile just like scintigraphy. c-MRC is superior to scintigraphy regarding radiation exposure, spatial resolution, and evaluation of partial obstruction. Diagnosis of acute cholecystitis and chronic cholecystitis, and evaluation of obstruction in a dilated biliary tree, can be detected with c-MRC as effectively as with scintigraphy.

(b) Functional Anatomy Assessment of the Bile Duct

Abnormal arrangement of the pancreaticobiliary ductal system (AAPB) is a congenital anomaly defined as location of the junction of the pancreatic and bile ducts outside the duodenal wall. As the contraction of the sphincter of Oddi within the duodenal wall does not functionally affect the junction in patients with this congenital abnormality, continuous pancreaticobiliary reflux occurs, resulting in a high incidence of biliary cancer [2, 15, 16]. This anatomical abnormality can be detected with ERCP, EUS, and MRCP.

Recently, several case series have been published on the reflux of pancreatic juice into the bile duct without a morphological AAPB, and the correlation of such cases with biliary diseases, particularly biliary malignancies, is drawing attention [15, 17-21]. These cases could not be detected with existing imaging modalities based on morphological change. Thus, functional anatomy assessment is anticipated to extract and diagnose these patients.

Several reports have shown that high amylase levels in bile samples on ERCP, which indicate reflux of pancreatic juice, were found in 26% of patients with normal pancreaticobiliary duct anatomy. However, ERCP is a slightly invasive modality and is not suitable for screening [2, 22].

In addition, it is reported that MRCP can be used to detect pancreatic juice reflux in these patients. In patients without AAPB, reflux of pancreatic juice into the common bile duct can be indirectly observed with secretin-stimulating MRCP [23, 24]. However, this cannot reveal direct pancreatic juice movement. As a result, reports differ about the validity of measurement of pancreatic juice movement by this method [17, 25, 26]. Thus, a robust method for assessment of pancreatic juice movement is required.

Recently, Sugita et al. developed a new MR method for the direct visualization of pancreatic juice flow based on a time-SLIP technique [27]. The technique has been applied for visualization of flow in various regions, and they have proved that this method can be used to detect pancreatic juice flow reflux in morphologically normal patients.

Detailed procedures of the time-SLIP examination are as follows. A flow-out technique, comprising of a non-selective inversion recovery pulse immediately followed by a spatially selective inversion labeling (tag) pulse, is applied, whereas in some cases, a subtraction technique added to a flow-out technique are also performed to validate visualization of pancreatic juice movement with time-SLIP imaging. Subtraction images are made by subtracting one labeled image from one control (unlabeled) image. The non-selective inversion recovery pulse is applied to null the background signals and the selective labeling pulse is applied to observe the movement of the labeled pancreatic juice in Figure 2, 3.

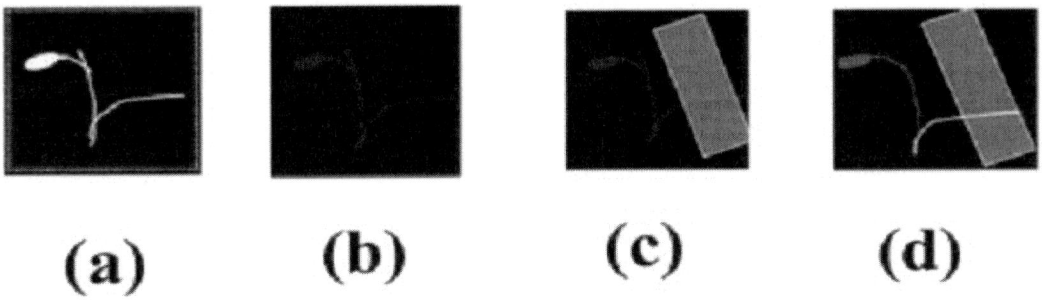

Figure 2. Schema of the time-SLIP technique. (a) MR cholangiopancreatography image. (b) Background signal depression. (c) Labeling with an inversion pulse at a labeling site located upstream. (d) Pancreatic juice visualization is acquired by scanning the pancreas a few second after labeling.

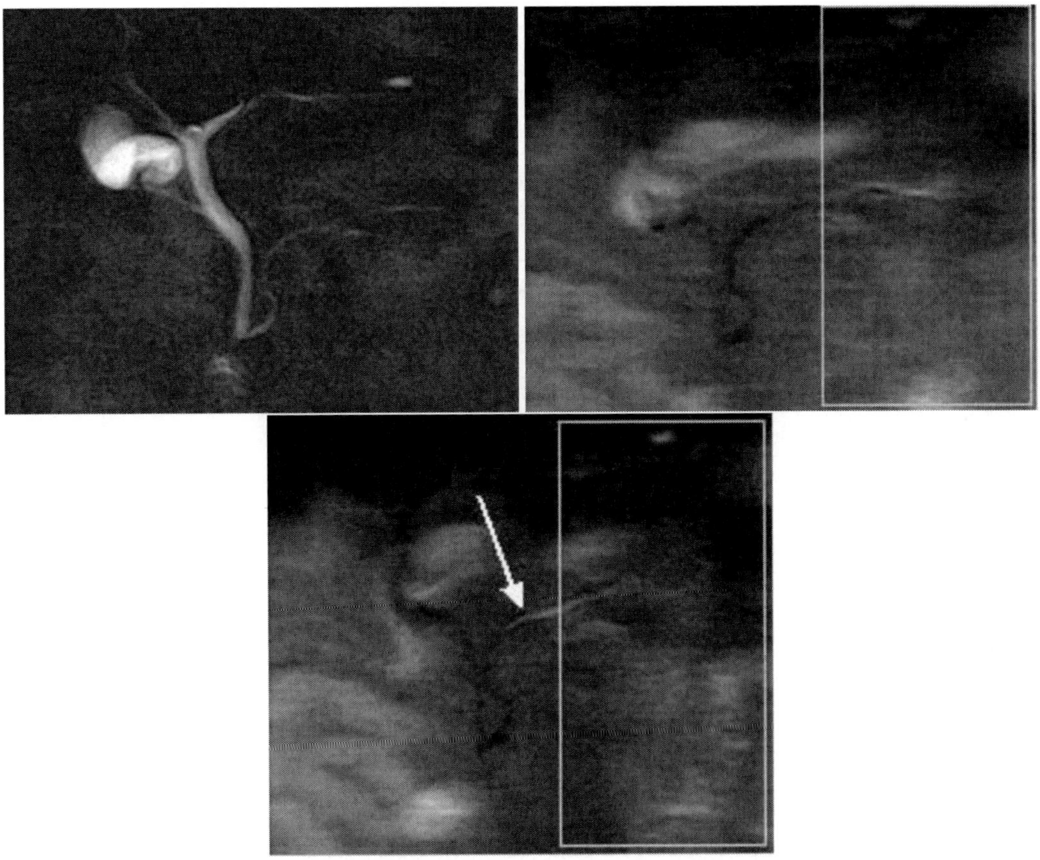

Direct pancreatic juice visualization method. (a) MRCP image. (b) Time-SLIP image obtained by applying labeling pulse (box surrounding by lines) in body and caudal portion of the main pancreatic duct, not showing movement. (c) Flow of pancreatic juice from body of the pancreas into head of pancreas is noted by high signal intensity (arrow).

For clinical examination, patients eat meals to promote pancreatic juice excretion 1-2 hours before the examination firstly. Then, 30 minutes before the examination, 600 mg of ferric ammonium citrate (Feriselz, Otuka Pharmaceutical, Tokushima, Japan) is taken orally with 300 ml of water to reduce the signal of the bowel content. Next, a thick-slab two-dimensional MRCP image is obtained prior to the time-SLIP study for determination of labeling pulse placement. Then, an ECG preparation acquisition with a series of two-dimensional oblique-coronal half-Fourier FSE is performed along the main pancreatic duct with various inversion recovery times. This procedure is repeated several times for delineating an irregular pancreatic juice movement due to an irregular secretion. Total acquisition time is about 10 minutes.

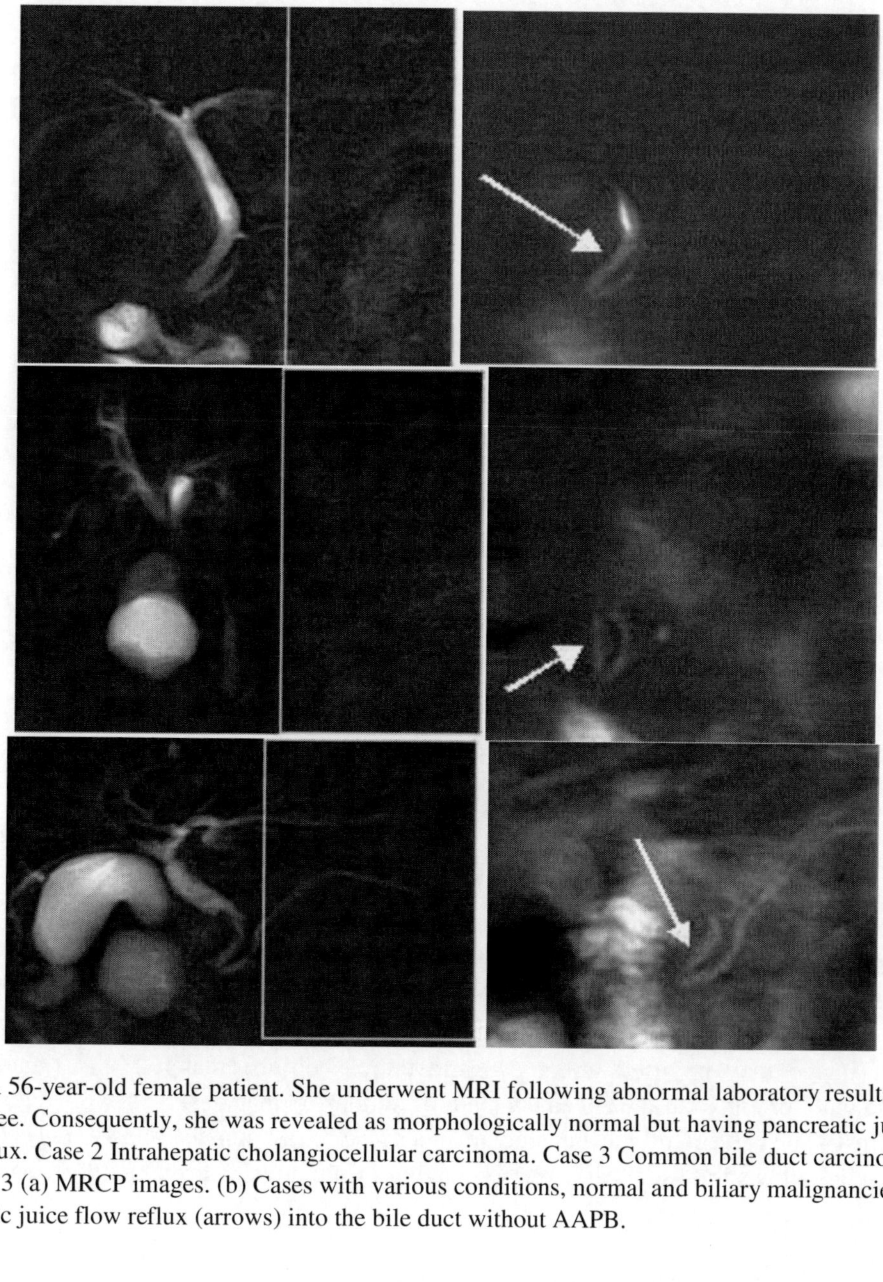

Case 1 A 56-year-old female patient. She underwent MRI following abnormal laboratory results of the biliary tree. Consequently, she was revealed as morphologically normal but having pancreatic juice flow reflux. Case 2 Intrahepatic cholangiocellular carcinoma. Case 3 Common bile duct carcinoma. Cases 1- 3 (a) MRCP images. (b) Cases with various conditions, normal and biliary malignancies, show pancreatic juice flow reflux (arrows) into the bile duct without AAPB.

This new technique enables noninvasive visualization of the pancreatic juice movement in Figure 4. The technique employs tagged pancreatic juice as an intrinsic tracer, providing precise information about direction and velocity of the flow of pancreatic juice without the influence of bile flow. Additionally, the technique allows repeated studies because of its noninvasive nature and as well as observation of pancreatic juice movement under physiological conditions. Therefore, the method can be easily added to a routine MR examination protocol and may reveal more information on the rate of pancreaticobiliary reflux in the population with normal biliary anatomy, enabling determination of whether this phenomenon is associated with an increased incidence of biliary malignancy. In addition, this technique can allow examination of the bile flow as well as pancreatic juice analysis and may facilitate functional assessment of the biliary tree before and after surgery without the use of contrast agent.

Imaging of the Bile Duct Disease

(a) Imaging Technique of the Bile Duct Disease

When biliary disease is suspected, optimal imaging studies provide the required information for differentiating between benign and malignant tumors, tumor staging, selection of surgical candidate, and surgical planning of bile duct cancer. Various imaging modalities, invasive and noninvasive, are employed in diagnosis and staging of bile duct tumors. Generally US, CT and MRI are dedicated for these examinations exclusively.

A multi-detector row CT is used in most institute for evaluation of the bile duct disease. Rapid scanning, thinner sections of this multi-detector row CT enable the evolution from section-based to volume-based technique. Thus, after examination, post-processing analysis of coronal and sagittal reconstruction images is performed on workstation. The advent of contrast agent (extravascular or biliary specific) is normally required to delineate lesion and surrounding structure. Extravascular contrast agent examination allows the usual early-phase imaging of the arterial, portal, and venous phases. Biliary specific contrast agents need to administrate for 30 minutes before the initiation of 1 hour of scanning.

The examination of MRI requires a number of preparations. A pre-procedural fasting is recommended for gallbladder distension and gastric emptying. When fluid is present in the stomach and duodenum, visualization of the bile duct may be obscured by interposition of bowel loop. Therefore administration of oral contrast agent (iron oxide particles, blueberry juice or pineapple juice) is recommended. Most institutes may perform MR examinations at 1.5 T with a torso coil. Although imaging at 3 T can improve the signal-to-noise ratio and spatial resolution, it may be hampered by dielectric effects, banding, and other pulse sequence-related effects. The pulse sequences used for MRI of the bile duct are usually axial T1- and T2- weighted imaging, MRCP, and axial diffusion-weighted imaging (DWI). T1-weighted image may be used under an intravenous contrast material. Most gadolinium contrast agents produce an enhancement pattern similar to that observed with iodine-based CT contrast. The advent of the hepatocyte-specific contrast agents (Gd-EOB-DTPA, Gd-BOPTA, etc.) allows the usual early-phase imaging of the arterial, portal, and venous phases, plus delayed-phase hepatic parenchymal and biliary imaging, taking advantage of the fact that about 50% of injected dose of these contrast agents are excreted via the biliary system.

MRCP use 2 varieties of T2-weighted sequences. One is obtained with a single-shot TSE T2-weighted sequence by using a long echo time to selectively display the fluid filled bile ducts. The other is obtained by using a navigator-based respiratory-triggered three-dimensional (3D) acquisition sequence with a longer acquisition time. The differences of both are small, and thus either or both are used for MRCP accordingly.

DWI can obtain additional information derived from the microscopic motion of proton in water, which is not possible by using conventional MRI. DWI is a sensitive sequence for the detection of tumors and inflammation of the bile ducts. It has the advantage of quantitative data analysis through the generation of apparent diffusion coefficient (ADC) maps, which can contribute to objective disease assessment and monitoring of response to therapy.

(b) Benign Biliary Disease

The most common disorders of the bile duct are related to biliary stones and include symptomatic cholelisthiasis, and acute and chronic cholecystitis. Generally, US is considered the first-choice modality in these diseases settings, and it is not difficult to diagnose these diseases with clinical and imaging information. However, malignant disease is sometimes obscured by these diseases. Therefore, careful examination is required when diagnosing these diseases.

Gallbladder wall thickening due to acute cholecystitis and chronic cholecystitis is difficult to differentiate from malignant disease even with multiple modern diagnostic modalities. Differentiation between benignity and malignancy may be difficult with US because thickening of the gallbladder wall is nonspecific. On the other hand, MDCT and MRI can provide beneficial information for differentiating between gallbladder carcinoma and benign diseases.

Primary sclerosing cholangitis (PSC) is a chronic cholestatic liver disease of possible autoimmune origin, characterized by intra- and extrahepatic bile duct inflammation and fibrosis [28-33]. PSC is the most common risk factor for cholangiocarcinoma in Western countries, with a prevalence of cholangiocarcinoma ranging from 8% to 25% [28]. The diagnosis of PSC has been based on characteristic cholangiographic findings in combination with clinical, biochemical, and histologic features, and ERCP has been considered the standard method for diagnosis of PSC. However, owing to developments in MR technology, MRCP has become accepted as another important modality [34-43], and the result of a meta-analysis showed that MRCP had high sensitivity and very high specificity for the diagnosis of PSC [35]. However, the radiological characteristics of PSC mimic those of cholangiocarcinoma [44], which makes differential diagnosis problematic even with current diagnostic modalities including MRI.

(c) Biliary Malignancies

Bile duct malignancies are relatively rare, estimated at 2% of all cancers with prevalence of 0.01%-0.04% in autopsy series [3]; however, the prevalence is rising worldwide [45-46].

In general, the diagnosis of biliary tumors, particularly early detection and differential diagnosis, is still challenging, although many sensitive direct and indirect techniques have been adopted.

Cholangiocarcinoma arise from the epithelial cells lining the biliary tree. CT and MRI with MRCP have generally been considered the modalities of choice for the diagnosis of cholangiocarcinomas. CT can demonstrate bile duct dilatation and a tumor mass as well as bile duct wall thickening. Hyper-enhancement of the stenosed duct after contrast enhancement has been considered a sign of malignancy but has low specificity (19%) as a single finding [47]. Several studies have shown that both sensitivity and specificity of MRI exceed 90% [48], but the ability to differentiate between benign and malignant obstruction is low and variable.

Primary carcinoma of the gallbladder is the most common malignancy of the biliary tract. Spread of gallbladder carcinoma to the liver is common because of the thinness of the smooth muscular layer of the gallbladder and the proximity to the liver, allowing spread to lymphatic channels. Usually, US is used as an initial diagnostic modality, and CT, MRI with MRCP, and traditional cholangiography are often used for obtaining additional information. Comparative studies of CT and MRI with MRCP are desirable.

Ampullary carcinoma tends to appear as a small mass that causes biliary obstruction. Although ampullary carcinoma can be detected with CT and MRI, this tumor is difficult to diagnose because of the small size and difficulty of differentiating between the tumor tissue and surrounding normal structures. MRI, including MRCP, has been reported to be more accurate than CT [49, 50]. MRI has a high sensitivity and low specificity in the diagnosis of ampullary carcinoma [51]. EUS and ERCP are usually used to identify ampullary carcinoma.

Conclusion

Modern imaging modalities provide promising non-invasive imaging techniques for evaluating biliary lesions in pre- and post-operative evaluations. These modalities allow visualization of not only morphological anatomy but also functional assessment and functional anatomy assessments of the biliary tree.

References

[1] Seale MK, Catalano OA, Saini S, Hahn PF, Sahani DV. (2009). Hepathobiliary-specific MR contrast agents: role in imaging the liver and biliary tree. *Radiographics*, 29, 1725-1748.

[2] Kamisawa T, Anjiki H, Egawa N, Kurata M, Honda G, Tsuruda K. Diagnosis and clinical implication of pancreatobiliary reflux. (2008). *World J. Gastroenterol.*, 14,6622-6626.

[3] Ganeshan D, Moron FE, Szklaruk J. Extrahepatic biliary cancer: new staging classification. (2012). *World J. Radiol.*, 4,345-352.

[4] Ajiffry M, Walsh MJ, Molinari M. Advances in diagnosis, treatment and palliation of cholangiocarcinoma: 1990-2009. (2009). *World J. Gastroenterol.*, 15,4240-4262.

[5] Sugita R. MR evaluations of biliary malignancy and condition at high-risk for biliary malignancy: current status. *World J. Hepatol.* In press.

[6] Smith AD, Venierto JC.Gd-EOB-DTPA as a functional MR cholangiography contrast agent: imaging gallbladder filling in patients with and without hepatobiliarydysfunction. (2011). *J. Comput. Assist. Tomogr.*, 35,439-445.

[7] Chung YE, Kim MJ, Park YN, Choi JY, Pyo JY, Kim YC, Cho HJ, Kim KA, Choi SY. Varying appearances of cholangiocarcinoma: radiologic-pathologic correlation. (2009). *Radiographics*, 29,683-700.

[8] Matos C, Serrao E, Antonieta M. Magnetic resonance imaging of biliary tumors. (2010). *Magn Reson Imaging Clin. N Am.*, 18,477-496.

[9] Manfredi R, Barbaro B, Masselli G, Vecchioli A, Marano P. Magnetic resonance imaging of cholangiocarcinoma. (2004). *Semin. Liver Dis*, 24:155-164.

[10] Kitami M, Takase K, Murakami G, Ko S, Tsuboi M, Saito H, Higano S, Nakajima Y, Takahashi S. Types and frequencies of biliary tract variations associated with a major portal venous anomaly: analysis with multi-detector row CT cholangiography. (2006). *Radiology.* 238,156-166.

[11] Lee MS, Lee JY, Kim SH, Park HS, Kim SH, Lee JM, Han JK, Choi BI. Gadoxetic acid disodium-enhanced magnetic resonance imaging for biliary and vascular comparison with gadobenate dimeglumine-enhanced MRI. (2010). *JMRI.* 33,149-159.

[12] Tamrazi A, Vasanawala SS. Functional hepatobiliary MR imaging in children. (2011). *Pediatr Radiol.* 41,1250-1258.

[13] Bae K, Na JB, Choi DS, Cho JM, Choi HC, Jeon K-N, Park MJ, Choi HY, Kim JE, Chung SH. Contrast-enhanced MR cholangiography: comparison of Gd-EOB-DTPA and Mn-DPDP in healthy volunteers. (2012). *BJR.* 85, 1250-1254.

[14] Lee NK, Kim S, Lee JW, Lee SH, Kang DH, Kim GH, Seo HI. Biliary MR imaging with Gd-EOB-DTPA and its clinical applications. (2009). *Radiographics.* 29,1707-1724.

[15] Sai JK, Suyama M, Kubokawa Y, et al. Occult pancreatobiliary reflux in subjects with a normal pancreaticobiliary junction. (2003). *Gastrointest Endosc.* 57,364-368.

[16] Nagata E, Sakai K, Kinoshita H, Kobayashi Y. The relation between carcinoma of the gallbladder and an anomalous connection between the choledochus and the pancreatic duct. (1985). *Ann Surg.* 202,182-190.

[17] Horaguchi J, Fujita N, Noda Y, Kobayashi G, Ito K, Takasawa O, Obana T, Endo T, Nakahara K, Ishida K, Yonechi M, Hirasawa D, Suzuki T, Sugawara T, Ohhira T, Onochi K, Harada Y. Amylase levels in bile inpatients with a morphologically normal pancreaticobiliary ductal arrangement. (2008). *J. Gastroenterol.*.43,305-311.

[18] Motosugi U, Ichikawa T, Araki T, et al. Secretin-stimulating MRCP in patients with pancreatobiliary maljunction and occult pancreatobiliary reflux: direct demonstration of pancreatobiliary reflux. (2007). *Eur. Radiol.* 17,2262-2267.

[19] Sai JK, Ariyama J, Suyama M, Kubokawa Y, Sato N. Occult regurgitation of pancreatic juice into the biliary tract: diagnosis with secretin injection magnetic resonance cholangiopancreatography. (2002). *Gastrointest Endosc.* 56,929-932.

[20] Anderson MC, Hauman RI, Suriyapa C, Schiller WR. Pancreatic enzyme levels in the bile of patients with extrahepatic biliary tract disease. (1979). *Am. J. Surg.* 137,301-306.

[21] Itokawa F, Itoi T, Nakamura K, Sofuni A, Kakimi K, oriyasu F, Tsuchida A, Aoki T. Assessment of occult pancreatobiliary reflux in patients with pancreaticobiliary disease by ERCP. (2004). *J. Gastroenterol.* 39,988-994.

[22] Beltran MA. Current knowledge on pancreaticobiliary reflux in normal pancreaticobiliary junction. (2012). *Int. J. Surg*. 10,190-193.

[23] Matos C, Metens T, Deviere J, et al. Pancreatic duct: Morphologic and functional evaluation with dynamic MR pancreatography after secretin stimulation. (1997). *Radiology*. 203,435-441.

[24] Matos C, Nicaise N, Deviere J, et al. Choledochal cysts: comparison of findings at MR cholangiopancreatography and endoscopic retrograde cholangiopancreatography in eight patients. (1998). *Radiology*. 209,443-448.

[25] Song HK, Kim MH, Lee SK, et al. Progressive bile duct and gallbladder dilatation on MRCP after secretin stimulation: physiologic or pathologic finding? (2003). *Gastrointest Endosc*. 58,165.

[26] Kanno N, LeSage G, Glaser S, et al. Regulation of cholangiocyte bicarbonatic secretion. (2001). *Am. J. Physiol. Gastrointest Liver Physiol*. 281,612-625.

[27] Sugita R, Furuta A, Horaguchi J, Ito K, Kobayashi G, Noda Y, Fujita N, Shimizu S, Miyazaki M, Takahashi S. Visualization of pancreatic juice movement using unenhanced MR imaging with spin labeling: preliminary results in normal and pathologic conditions. (2012). *J. Magn Reson Imaging*. 35,1119-1124.

[28] Khan SA, Thomas HC, Davidson BR, Robinson SDT. Cholangiocarcinoma. (2005). *Lancet.* 366,1303-1314.

[29] Ajiffry M, Renfrew PD, Walsh MJ, Laryea M, Morinari M. Analytical review of diagnosis and treatment strategies for dominant bile duct strictures in patients with primary sclerosing cholangitis. (2011). *HPB.* 13,79-90.

[30] Mendes FD, Lindor KD. Primary sclerosing cholangitis. (2004). *Clin. Liver Dis*. 8,195-211.

[31] Rosen CB, Nagorney DM, Wesner RH, Coffey RJ, Larusso NF. Cholangiocarcinoma complicating primary sclerosing cholangitis. (1991). *Ann. Surg*. 213,21-25.

[32] Lutz HH, Tischendorf JJ. Management of primary sclerosing cholangitis. (2011). *WJH.* 3,137-141.

[33] Lichtenstein DR. Hepatobiliary complication of inflammatory bowel disease. (2011). *Curr Gastroenterol Rep*. 13,495-505.

[34] Vitellas KM, Keagan MT, Freed KS, Enns RA, Sprinzer CE, Baillie JM, Nelson RC. Radiologic manifestations of sclerosing cholangitis with emphasis on MR cholangiopancreatography. (2000). *Radiographics.* 20,959-975.

[35] Deve M, Elmunzer BJ, Dwarmena BA, Higgins PR. Primary sclerosing cholangitis: meta analysis of diagnostic performance of MR cholangiopancreatography. (2010). *Radiology* 256,387-396.

[36] Vitellas KM, El-Dieb A, Vaswani KK, Bennet WF, Tzalonikou M, Mabee C, Kirkpatrick R, Bova JG. MR cholangiopancreatography in patients with primary sclerosing cholangitis: interobserver variability and comparison with endoscopic retrograde cholangiopancreatography. (2002). *AJR*. 179,399-407.

[37] Wieber C, Kuhlencordt R, Grotteluesschen R, Wedegaertner U, Ang TL, Adam G, Soehendra N, Seltz U. Magnetic resonance cholangiopancreatography in the diagnosis of primary sclerosing cholangitis. (2008). *Endoscopy*. 40,739-745.

[38] Vitellas KM, Enns RA, Keogan MT, Freed KS, Spritzer CE, Baillie J, Nelson RC. Comparison of MR cholangiopancreatographic techniques with contrast-enhanced cholangiography in the evaluation of sclerosing cholangitis. (2002). *AJR.* 178,327-334.
[39] Berstad AE, Aahakken L, Smith HJ, Aasen S, Baberg KM, Schrumpf E. Diagnostic accuracy of magnetic resonance and endoscopic retrograde cholangiography in primary sclerosing cholangitis. (2008). *Clin. Gastroenterol. Hepatol.* 4,514-520.
[40] Fulcher AF, Turner MA, Franklin KJ, Shiffman ML, Sterling RK, Luketic VAC, Sanyal AJ. Primary sclerosing cholangitis: evaluation with MR cholangiography- a case control study. (2000). *Radiology.* 215,71-80.
[41] Ferrara C, Valeri G, Salvolmi L, Giiovagnoni A. Magnetic resonance cholangiopancreatography in primary sclerosing cholangitis in children. (2002). *Pediatr Radiol.* 32,413-417.
[42] Textor HJ, Flacke S, Pauleit D, Keller E, Neubrand M, Terjung B, Gieseke J, Scheurlen C, Sauerbrucg T, Schild HH. Three-dimensional magnetic resonance cholangiopancreatography with respiratory triggering in the diagnosis of primary sclerosing cholangitis: comparison with endoscopic retrograde cholangiography. (2002). *Endoscopy.* 34,984-990.
[43] Meagher S, Yusuff I, Kennedy W, Murtel M, Adam V, Burkun A. The role of magnetic resonance and endscopic retrograde cholangiopancreatography (MRCP and ERCP) in the diagnosis of patients with suspected sclerosing cholangitis; a cost-effectiveness analysis. (2007). *Endoscopy.* 39,222-228.
[44] Manias CO, Surabhi VR, Prasad SR, Wang HL, Narra VR, Chintapalli KN. Mimics of cholangiocarcinoma: spectrum of disease. (2008). *Radiographics.* 28:1115-1129.
[45] Shaib Y, El-Serag HB. The epidemiology of cholangiocarcinoma. (2004). *Semin Liver Dis.* 24:115-125.
[46] Watanapa P. Cholangiocarcinoma in patients with opsthorchiasis. (1996). *Br. J. Surg.* 83,1062-1064.
[47] Kim SJ, Lee JM, Lee JY, Kim SH, Han JK, Choi BI, Choi JY. Analysis of enhancement pattern of flat gallbladder wall thickening on MDCT to differentiate gallbladder cancer from cholecystitis. (2008). *AJR.* 191,765-771.
[48] Van Beers BE. Diagnosis of cholangiocarcinoma. (2008). *HPB* (Oxford). 10,87-93.
[49] Anderson M, Kostic S, Johansson M, Londell L, Asztely M, Hellstrom M. MRI combined with MR cholangiopancreatography versus helical CT in the evaluation of patients with suspected periampullary tumors: a prospective comparative study. (2005). *Acta Radiol.* 46,16-27.
[50] Wu DS, Chen WX, Wang XD, Acharya R, Jiang XH. Pancreticobiliary duct changes of periampullary carcinomas: quantitative analysis at MR imaging. (2012). *Eur. J. Radiol.* 81,2112-2117.
[51] Chung YE, Kim MJ, Kim HM, Park MS, Choi JY, Hong HS, Kim KW. Differentiation of benign and malignant ampullary obstruction on MR imaging. (2011). *Eur. J. Radiol.* 80,198-203.

In: Bile Duct
Editor: Miguel Ángel Mercado
ISBN: 978-1-63321-771-3

Chapter 4

The Spectrum of Injuries and Their Classification

Miguel Ángel Mercado, MD[1], Daniel Zamora, MD[2], Alan Contreras, MD[2], Marco A. Tapia, MD[2], Santiago Mier-y-Teran, MD[2] and Bruno A. González-Nolasco, MD[2]
[1]Department of Surgery, National Institute of Medical Sciences and Nutrition of Mexico "Salvador Zubiran", Mexico
[2]National Institute of Medical Sciences and Nutrition of Mexico "Salvador Zubiran", Mexico

Introduction

In general, complete circumferential sections of the biliary tract, with or without tissue loss, are classified in the literature as complex lesions.

It is important to point out that the initial injury class is upgraded to a higher one as suggested by Bismuth, because the ischemic and/or inflammatory component leads to necrosis of the duct and may even compromise the confluence. Likewise, injury of the middle third of the hepatic duct may subsequently be upgraded due to the ischemic component.

Many classifications have been created before and after the laparoscopic era. Before the introduction of this technique, the Bismuth-Corlette classification was, and perhaps still is, the most popular one. This classification only includes [1] the complete section of the duct and the length of the stump of the proximal biliary tract.

Other classifications have been developed since the advent of laparoscopy. The mechanisms leading to injury are different albeit leading to the same results as open lesions, in most cases. [2-5]

In our opinion, the most complete classification describing laparoscopic injuries is Strasberg's. [6] It is an easy to understand classification (once it has been studied). Its sole disadvantage is the inclusion of random and not necessarily iatrogenic lesions, such as bile leaks in the gallbladder bed. Aside from injuries, it also describes every possible variant. It includes five groups classified by letters in alphabetical order and in which the 5th group (E) includes the various types of injury referred to in Bismuth's classification. Among the injuries studied by our group, only the isolated injury of the left hepatic duct has not been included in this very thorough classification.

Other classifications stand between Bismuth's and Strasberg's classifications and, one way or another, they include all forms of injury.

Lesions are individual to each patient and their final outcome depends on many factors. Frequently, a non-complex injury becomes complex after the first failed repair attempt (i.e. dehiscent hepatoduodenal anastomosis). In other cases, an inflammatory and/or infectious process in the hepatic hilum leads to a higher injury (including the confluence), upgrading its classification.

In different reports of iatrogenic injuries, classifications are used with the fundamental purpose of presenting reproducible results in terms of groups of injury.

Injuries encompassing the diameter of the biliary duct are the only ones not included in these classifications. In those cases, if the biliary tract is dilated and the confluence is preserved, their prognosis is excellent in the hands of surgeons well-acquainted with these procedures.

Strasberg Classification [6]

It classifies injuries into five groups whereby in the first group (A), there is biliary leak from the cystic duct stump or from an accessory duct originating in the gallbladder bed where the cystic duct could have ended. In both cases, the duct is continuous with the biliary tract. In the second group (B), the accessory duct is divided or non-continuous with the biliary tract. The third group (C) includes injuries with duct leaks with no communication with the biliary tract; the fourth group (D) is a partial section of a bile duct with no complete loss of continuity with the rest of the bile duct system; the fifth group (E) encompasses all injuries with complete section of the biliary tract and that in turn, are sub-classified into different grades according to the length of the stump (E1-E5), including those involving the confluence; this group also includes confluence injuries in association with an accessory duct (Figure 1).

Stewart-Way Classification [7]

This classification is divided into 4 strata based on the underlying mechanism and anatomy of the injury (Figure 2).

Class I injury refers to the incision or incomplete transection of the common bile duct without tissue loss. These injuries develop for two reasons: the first mechanism is mistaking the common bile duct with the cystic duct (most frequent), which can be solved resulting in only a small loss of tissue with no complete section of the bile duct; the second mechanism is the lateral injury of the duct due to an extension of the cystic opening when attempting to perform a cholangiography. In some of these cases, the right hepatic artery is also injured (5% of cases).

According to the literature, 72% of the injuries are caused by the first mechanism and 28% by the second. This type of injury accounts for 7% of all injuries.

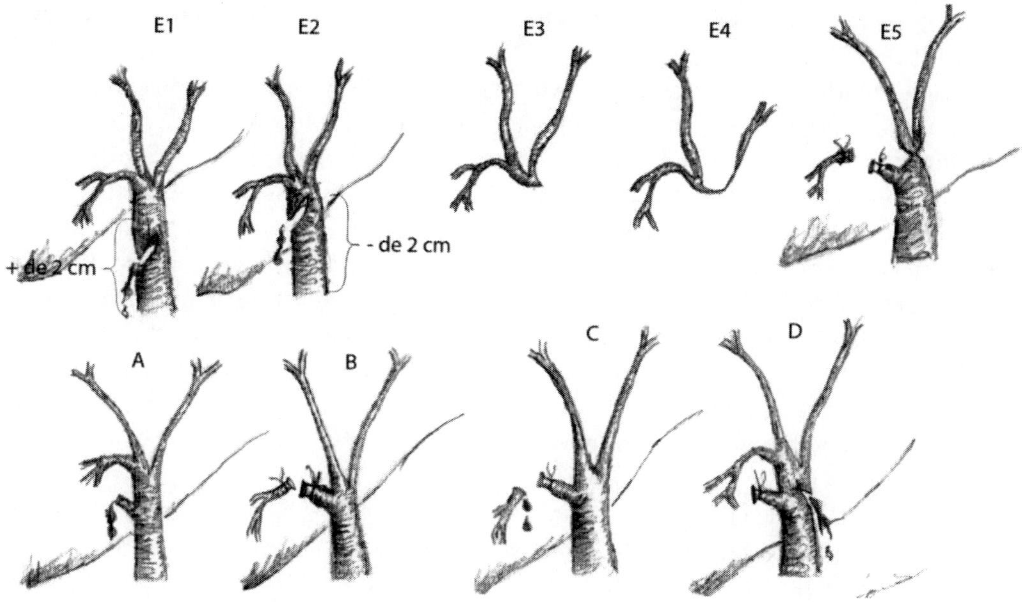

Figure 1. Strasberg classification.

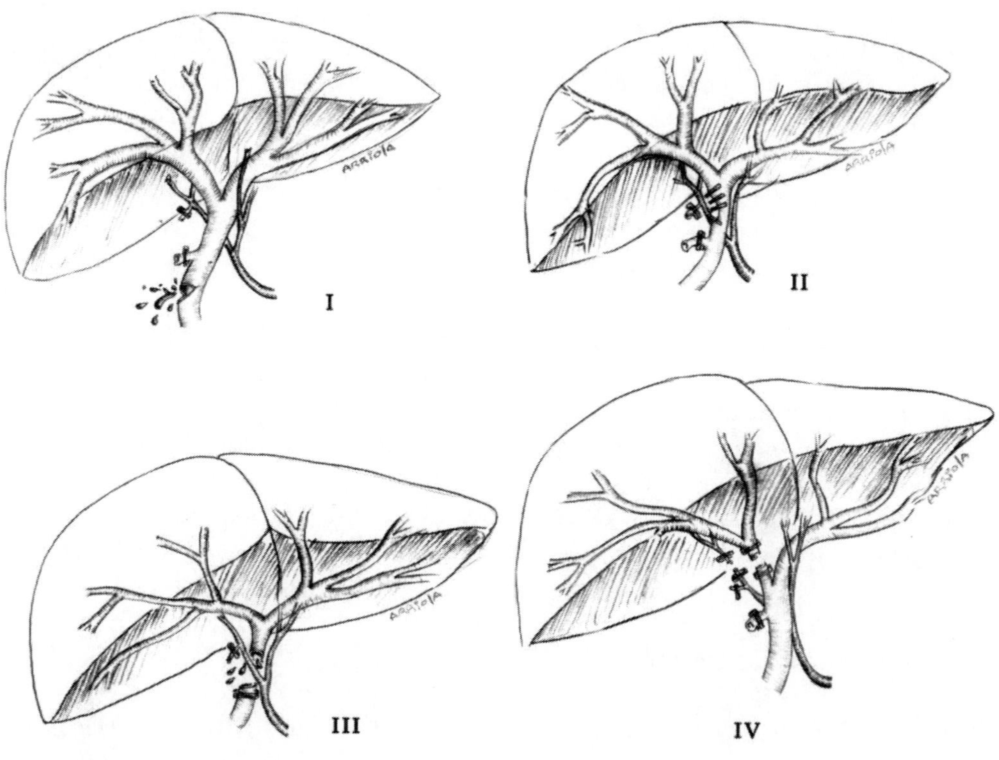

Figure 2. Stewart-Way classification.

Class II injuries refer to the lateral injury of the common hepatic duct leading to stricture and/or fistula formation. It results from placing staples in the duct or, occasionally, from thermal damage due to cauterization in an attempt to control hemorrhages. Their calculated frequency in the literature is around 2%. There may be a simultaneous injury to the hepatic artery in 18% of cases.

Class II injuries include cases in which a T-tube is misplaced after biliary tract exploration. T-tubes were the most useful in past decades (when endoscopic biliary tract exploration was unavailable) and perhaps, their placement was a little forceful leading to injury of the bile duct. Many surgeons perform an excessive dissection of the duct in order to place the tube, some others use tubes that are too large or too big, and others use inadequate materials to close the choledocotomy along with an inadequate suturing technique. In isolated cases, all three mistakes occur in the same patient. The purpose of the T-tube is to decrease ductal pressure after exploration. At some point, it allowed the removal of residual stones. It should be of small caliber, with short branches, placed through the anterior portion of the duct after a small longitudinal incision (well identified), carefully watching the lateral vasculature. The choledocotomy should be performed with small caliber (5-0) hydrolysable sutures, approximating only its edges.

An appropriate distance between sutures as well as a proper approximation of the ducts prevents the leakage of bile, but the choledocotomy should not be sealed too tightly since this could translate into damage to the biliary tract. Any bile leakage is resolved by maintaining the T-tube open.

Class III injuries, the most common according to this classification, representing 61% of all cases according to the literature, refer to the complete transection of the duct and excision of the duct proximal to the first transection (generally including the hepato-cystic union). It is further divided into sub-groups, including:

- IIIa: patients with a remnant common duct
- IIIb: patients with transection at the confluence level
- IIIc: patients with loss of confluence
- IIId: patients with injuries above the confluence and section of secondary ducts.

This type of injury occurs when the duct is mistaken for the cystic duct and, upon gallbladder removal, section of the common hepatic duct inevitably occurs. Concomitant lesion of the right hepatic artery occurs in 27% of cases.

Class IV injuries refer to lesions of the right main (68%) or accessory (28%) hepatic duct plus injury to the right hepatic artery in 60% of cases. This type of injury accounts for 10% of all injuries according to the authors. Occasionally, injury of the right accessory duct may also include injury to the main duct at the confluence level (4% of cases).

Corlette-Bismuth Classification

This classification was described in 1981 before the advent of laparoscopic cholecystectomy. It resulted from a national French survey that analyzed over 600 cases of postoperative biliary strictures (Figure 5. 3). Its use is widespread and it is based on the length of the biliary stump, which, according to the authors, is the most important factor in deciding whether or not it should be repaired. It is important to emphasize that this classification was created before the use of laparoscopy, and according to the mentioned technical factors, the mechanisms of injury are different according to the type of injury. However, many cases do lead to stricture, obstruction or both. These events may be included in this classification but they represent a sub-type of the Strasberg (E) and Stewart-Way (III-IV) classifications.

Type I refers to a low injury with a stump measuring over 2 cm. Type II is a mid-level injury with a stump length under 2 cm. Type III refers to high injuries with no viable and/or available common hepatic duct but with a preserved confluence. Type IV is an injury involving the confluence with no communication between the right and left hepatic ducts; a fibrous plaque exists between them. Type IV is a combined injury of the common duct as well as injury of an accessory duct, with separation of both.

Hannover Classification [8]

This classification, published in 2007, has had limited applications in the literature (particularly due to unawareness and inappropriate diffusion). It is a combination of the other classifications.

It classifies injuries according to their position (low, at level, high) in relationship to the confluence, and it also includes vascular injuries (injury to the right hepatic artery). It differs from the Stewart-Way classification because, as previously mentioned, that classification is based on the injury mechanism. It is divided into 5 types identified with the letters A to E, and it also includes sub-classifications. Class A refers to cystic and/or gallbladder bed leaks; B, to complete or incomplete stenosis caused by staples; C, to lateral tangential injuries (right); and D, to complete section of the common bile duct emphasizing its distance to the confluence. A sub-classification for the various arteries injured in the hilum (right, left, common) or the portal vein is also described. Class E refers to late stenosis at different levels.

References

[1] Bismuth H. Postoperative strictures of the bile ducts. En Blumgart LH, ed. The biliary Tract V. New York: Churchill-Livingstone INC; 1982: 209-18.

[2] Martin R. F., Rossi R. L. Bile duct injuries: spectrum, mechanism of injury and their prevention. *Surg. Clin. North Am.,* 1994; 74: 781-803.

[3] Muhas P., Schmidt Sc., Hintze R. E., Adler A., Veltzkc W., Raakow R., Langrehr J. M., Bechstein W. O. Classification and treatment of bile duct injuries after laparoscopic cholecystectomy. *Chirurg.,* 2000; 71: 166-73.

[4] Olsen D. Bile duct injuries during laparoscopic cholecystectomy. *Surg. Endosc.*, 1997; 11: 133-38.

[5] Richardson M. C., Bell G., Fullarton G. M. and the West of Scotland Laparoscopic Cholecystectomy Audit Group. Incidence and nature of bile duct injuries following laparoscopic cholecystectomy: an audit of 5913 cases. *Br. J. Surg.,* 1996; 83: 1356-60.

[6] Strasberg S. M., Hertl M., Soper N. J. An analysis of the problem of biliary injury during laparoscopic cholecystectomy. *J. Am. Coll. Surg*., 1995; 180: 101-25.

[7] Way L. W. Stewart L., Gantert W., Liu K., Lee Cm. Whang K., Hunter J. G. Causes and prevention of laparoscopic bile duct injuries. *Ann. Surg*., 2003; 237: 460-69.

[8] Bektas H., Schrem H., Winny M., Klempnauer J. Surgical treatment and outcome of iatrogenic bile duct lesions after cholecystectomy and the impact of different clinical classification systems. *Br. J. Surg*., 2007; 94: 1119-27.

In: Bile Duct
Editor: Miguel Ángel Mercado
ISBN: 978-1-63321-771-3

Chapter 5

Therapeutic Alternatives

Miguel Ángel Mercado, MD[1], Mario Vilatoba, MD[2] Daniel Zamora, MD[2], Ismael Domínguez, MD[2], Santiago Mier-y-Teran, MD[2] and Bruno A. González-Nolasco, MD[2]

[1]Department of Surgery, National Institute of Medical Sciences and Nutrition "Salvador Zubiran", Mexico

[2]National Institute of Medical Sciences and Nutrition "Salvador Zubiran", Mexico

Abstract

The Strasberg's classification of iatrogenic biliary injury includes all variables and possible injuries, and thus it is a comprehensive basis to determine which therapeutic approach is chosen depending on the type of injury. In the case of type A injury, an endoscopic approach is preferred.

Type B injuries, which require a right biliary tract anatomical variant, are generally managed symptomatically until the hepatic subsector becomes atrophic as a result of secondary biliary cirrhosis. Type C, in which a biliary fistula is presented, appropriate subhepatic drainage will prevent the formation of collections, and the duct may spontaneously occlude, leading to secondary biliary cirrhosis of the sector.

Type D injuries are basically exclusive of laparoscopic cholecystectomy, in which the treatment depends on the severity of the damage; suture with placement of a T tube, endoscopic approach and biliodigestive derivation are feasable. The different type E injuries are usually managed through a Roux-en-Y hepaticojejunal anastomosis. Partial resection of segments of IV and V may be necessary to allow duct identification and execution of the anastomosis.

The Strasberg's classification includes most variables and possible iatrogenic biliary injuries, thus we chose it as the basis for the design of potential treatment options.

Type A Strasberg Injury

This is the most common type of injury in all series and, in essence, many authors do not consider it an iatrogenic injury. The section of an accessory duct within the gallbladder bed with consequent bile leak as well as leakage from the cystic duct stump is included in this type of injuries. The injured ducts remain communicated to the biliary tract. Leaks develop when the occlusion of the cystic duct is incomplete or when the common bile duct is obstructed, leading to increased ductal pressure and subsequent leak (Figure 1).

The same mechanism applies to the gallbladder bed accessory duct; if a leak develops, it will further increase if the pressure is elevated. It is manifested as a subhepatic accumulation of variable magnitude and, occasionally, it may be associated with symptoms of peritoneal irritation secondary to biliperitoneum. Some patients develop fever and postoperative pain; the collection is visualized by ultrasound and, in sporadic cases, it is an incidental finding. In general, liver function tests are normal unless there is biliperitoneum; in that case, mixed hyperbilirrubinemia may be detected.

This type of injury is difficult to prevent unless common bile duct obstruction has been documented and the cystic stump is under increased pressure. In these cases, preoperative sphincterotomy with stone extraction and/or endoprosthesis placement will prevent the development of this complication since in both cases (gallbladder bed and cystic stump), the decrease in ductal pressure will minimize the leak. [2]

When this type of injury develops, an endoscopic approach is preferred. Percutaneous and/or surgical drainage is rarely necessary. If the biliperitoneum is extensive, it is recommended to surgically drain it in order to obtain an adequate lavage. If the site of the leakage can be identified, occlusion may be attempted, although the risk of it failing is high as long as the ductal pressure is not decreased.

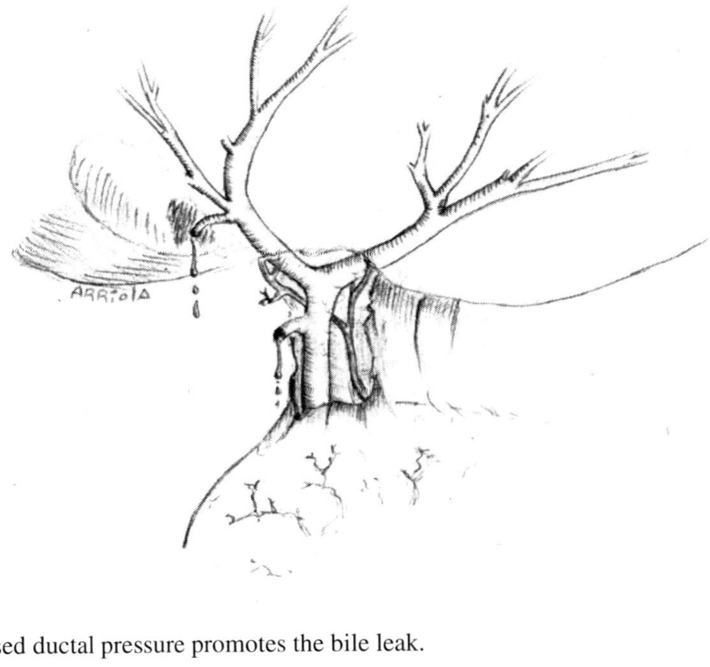

Figure 1. Increased ductal pressure promotes the bile leak.

If an endoscopist and/or the appropriate infrastructure are not available, and surgical drainage is chosen, placement of a T-tube of a suitable caliber and with adequate suture of the choledocotomy may solve the problem.

If such a procedure cannot be done, a subhepatic drainage may be placed in order to create a controlled external biliary fistula followed by referral to a center with an adequate infrastructure that can then perform the endoscopic procedure.

Routinely, simple cholecystectomies do not require the placement of drainages, but in the presence of a broad and bleeding gallbladder bed, a wide cystic duct, and a history of recent sphincterotomy, it is recommended to place a drainage that will prevent subhepatic collections and/or biliperitoneum.

This injury's prognosis is good since most leaks resolve with the described maneuvers. Close to 65% of all injuries are classified in this group.

Type B Injury

To generate this type of injury, a right biliary tract anatomical variant is required, whereby an accessory duct (that usually drains two segments of the right lobe) ends independently from the "main" right duct. In this condition, the confluence would be composed by the left and right ducts, with the accessory duct ending below the confluence (Figure 2). Some anatomists could argue that in this variant, the right duct ends in the left one and that the real confluence would be where the accessory duct drains. In this case, the cystic duct must drain into this accessory duct. It is an infrequent finding but not exceptional.

The result of this injury is complete occlusion of biliary drainage from part of the right hepatic lobe. Oftentimes, the injury is unnoticed or manifested as postoperative pain, or rarely as cholangitis.

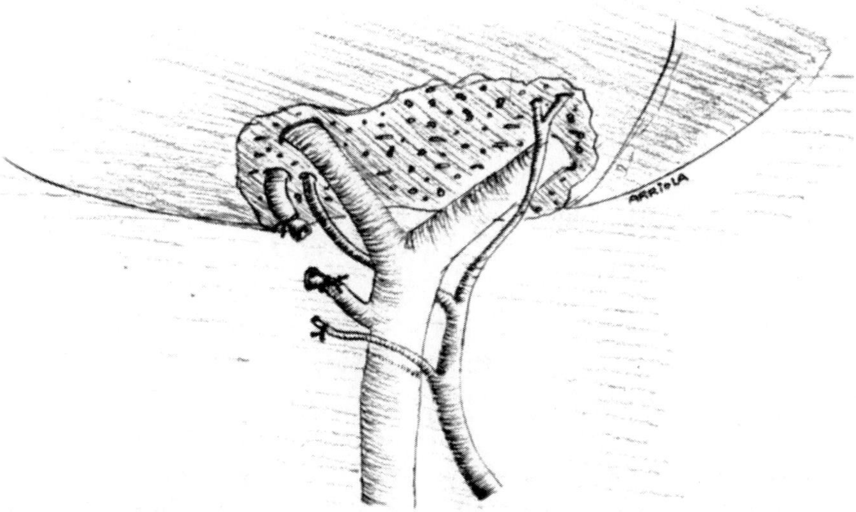

Figure 2. Anatomical variants may be present, and drainage of the accessory duct may be located below the confluence

If the patient is evaluated for postoperative pain, the segmental obstruction can be demonstrated by ultrasound if there is associated biliary dilation. Liver function tests show an increase in aminotransferases (4 to 8-fold), alkaline phosphatase and gamma glutamyl transferase while the rest are normal.

In general, no intervention is recommended, and only symptomatic management is required until the hepatic subsector becomes atrophic as a result of biliary cirrhosis secondary to the obstructive process.

This lesion is often unnoticed but may occasionally manifest as pain that may become incapacitating. In case of cholangitis, biliary drainage (percutaneous) becomes necessary. If cholangitis becomes refractory to medical treatment while the subsector atrophies, surgical resection of the affected segment is feasible.

Biliary derivation of a duct with this type of injury is difficult and there are only anecdotal cases reporting successful derivation. A Roux-en-Y hepatojejunoanastomosis may be attempted if an appropriate duct can be identified, along with the use of a transhepatic transanastomotic stent.

In the long term, these types of derivations do not have a good prognosis. The possibility of late obstruction and subsequent development of secondary biliary cirrhosis due to the obstructed segment is high. Under these circumstances, the probability of bile colonization and cholangitis is increased and the referred ablative measures should be suggested.

This type of injury is also difficult to prevent because the accessory duct is easily mistaken with the cystic duct in spite of complete dissection of Calot's triangle. Transoperative cholangiography reveals the right and left ducts with no gross evidence of injury, but a careful observer can detect that the entire right lobe is not completely opacified.

This variant can be detected by preoperative cholangiography (and, with less sensitivity, also with magnetic resonance cholangiography) and improve the transoperative efforts to avoid sectioning the accessory duct.

Strasberg designed a strategy mainly used in reconstruction cases, in which the two common ducts are separated (loss of confluence), but it can also be applied in cases of right accessory ducts.The hilar plate dissection is extended to the gallbladder bed, where the plate itself is projected. In this coronal plane, the right duct(s) is (are) identified, dissected and opened longitudinally in the anterior portion in order to create a wider anastomosis.

Strasberg's reported in his case series that 2 out of 23 patients with an accessory or common right duct with loss of confluence had a type B injury. In these cases, therapeutic endoscopy offers no possible solutions since there is loss of continuity of the biliary tract and the sectioned duct. [3]

Type C Injury

The mechanism of injury is very similar to that of type B and requires the same anatomical variant, the presence of a right accessory duct. In this situation, the proximal end of the accessory duct is not identified and a biliary fistula develops (Figure 3).

The proximal end is unnoticed by the surgeon since it is hidden in the infundibular portion of the gallbladder bed, perhaps even electrofulgurated and partially occluded by a staple after erroneously mistaking the duct with, for instance, an accessory artery.

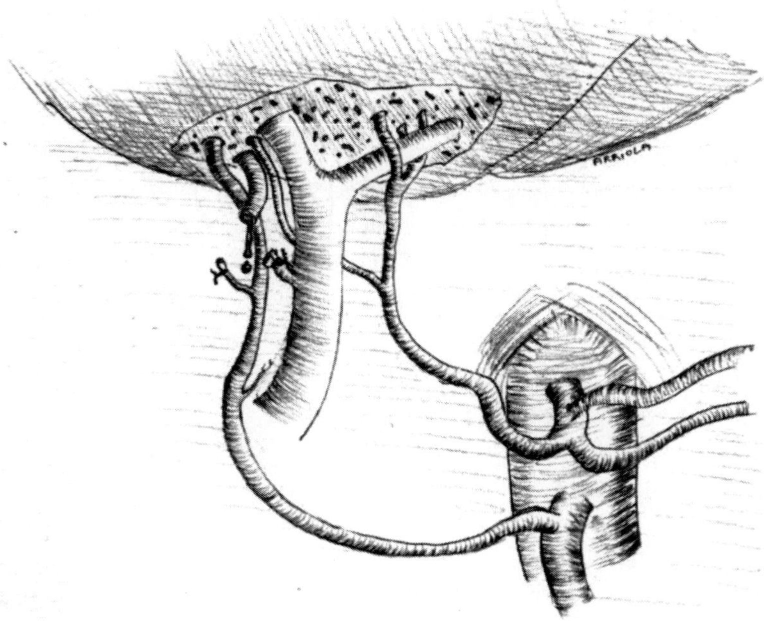

Figure 3. Biliary fistula in the presence of Type C injury.

It is manifested as a subhepatic collection with the same clinical features as type A injuries and since its output is considerable (approx. 200 - 300 mL bile per day produced by the segments it drains), the probability of developing biloperitoneum is increased.

The transoperative cholangiography shows filling of both lobes, but to the surgeon that is unfamiliar with this variant, the injury is unnoticed because, in general, what he identifies are the right and left ducts without observing full opacification of the right lobe.

When drainage is left after cholecystectomy, it manifests as a persistent external biliary fistula. Endoscopic cholangiography does not identify the absence of filling of the entire lobe, so endoscopic maneuvers are useless.

Performing a fistulography through the drain will reveal partial filling of the intrahepatic biliary tract but with no communication with the major ducts.

Appropriate subhepatic drainage, either by placing the drain percutaneously or surgically, will prevent the formation of collections.

It is occasionally possible to maintain the drain for several days or weeks (taking into account the possibility of adjacent visceral perforation, i.e. duodenum, colon) and the duct spontaneously occludes, leading to secondary biliary cirrhosis of the sector and subsequent atrophy.

Lillemoe et al. [4] has reported his experience in the management of these exceptional cases (11 cases, 5 less than Strasberg), and he treated them with a Roux-en-Y hepatojejunal biliary derivation, with good results (no symptoms and/or cholangitis, and normalization of liver function tests).

In our experience, these cases require a complex management. Identifying the duct is a demanding situation. Hidden in the vortex of the gallbladder bed, one can, at best, identify the bile leak but not an appropriate duct to create an anastomosis. If the duct is identified, it usually has poor quality so a transanastomotic stent must be placed. Its long-term prognosis is also uncertain since these anastomoses can be easily occluded.

We have found six cases of this type of injury in which the drainage in three of them was kept in place but it spontaneously occluded.

In a case in which a large collection was drained, the gallbladder was sutured and drained. In two others, one with associated refractory cholangitis, the hepatic segments drained by the duct were resected.

Hepatic resection must be carefully considered in these patients because, although capable of regeneration, it is recommended to maintain the hepatic mass. Extensive incision and dissection is required, so it must be noted that the surgical procedure also adds a risk factor to the patient's morbidity and mortality.

Type D Injury

This injury is basically exclusive of laparoscopic cholecystectomy [2, 5].This type of injury occurs after the common bile duct is dissected. The surgeon proceeds to dissect what he thinks is Calot's triangle, not realizing the real triangle is in the opposite side, thus the common hepatic duct is injured. A medial injury to the duct is generally present. This lesion varies in magnitude, maintaining partial integrity of the duct's circumference (Figure 4)

If the injury is minimal, it may be sutured with fine absorbable monofilaments (5 -0). It is highly recommended that the suture should be tension-free, otherwise subsequent necrosis (i.e. due to an overly generous cross-stitch) will develop.

If the injury is lineal and measures 25% less than the circumference, fine suture approximation stitches are appropriate, and the placement of a T-tube should be considered in order to decrease ductal pressure and bile leak. In extreme cases, the immediate postoperative placement of a stent with the same purpose may also be considered.

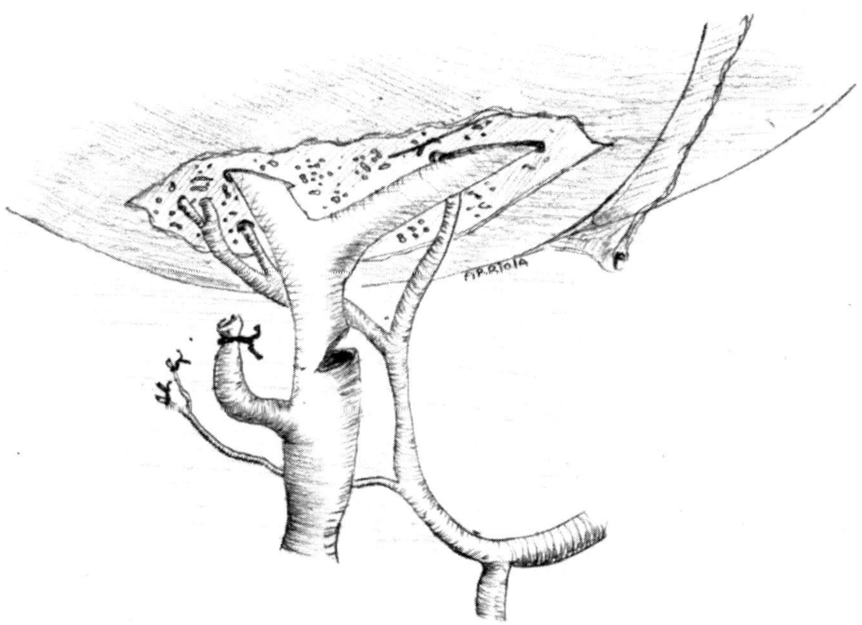

Figure 4. Type D lesions compromise the medial portion of the duct.

The duct's perfusion must be carefully evaluated, considering factors such as previous duct electrofulguration or devascularization, in order to guarantee a high quality and succesful repair.

A biliodigestive derivation is recommended in the following scenarios: a lesion that encompasses over 25% of the circumference, the repair decreases the duct's lumen, or it is concluded that the duct is devascularized.

Since the confluence is preserved in this type of injuries, a broad anastomosis is feasible, specially if the surgeon decides to open the anterior portion of the left duct longitudinally in order to to create a low-risk anastomosis; this procedure carries good long-term results.

Hepatojejunal derivation should be the first treatment option. In exceptional cases, hepaticoduodenal derivation may be performed according to some evidence. In our experience, this last option is not recommended when repairing iatrogenic biliary tract injuries.

The decision to perform a biliodigestive derivation may be threatened by the sugeon's tendency to conduct a less demanding repair by performing a choledoco-choledocal anastomosis. If such a scenario is presented, the inexpert surgeon must seek advice from personel trained in biliary injuries in order to obtain better long-term results.

If the injury is not identified during surgery, it will manifest as a biliary fistula with the previously described characteristics.

In type D injuries, the drainage of collections and/or biliperitoneum is no different to those described in the previous types. Endoscopic cholangiography can reveal the leak and/or lack of continuity. A long stent can be placed above the leak in order to subsequently control the fistula; the defect will heal through a second attempt and a stenotic area will develop in most cases. The partial stenosis may be endoscopically dilated and, if refractory, will require an elective biliodigestive derivation. The decision between endoscopic or surgical management should be taken through a multi-disciplinary group consensus.

In cases in which an endoscopic approach is possible, a transhepatic approach may be attempted in order to place a stent that will fulfill the same purpose and function as one placed endoscopically. [1, 7]

Another issue regarding this type of injury is an associated vascular injury. During the cephalic dissection of the misidintified duct, hemostasis is achieved by either electrofulguration of the duct's vessels or the placement of staples. The duct is completely separated from the hepatic hilum by placing a dissection forceps behind it. As the cephalic dissection progresses, an injury to the right hepatic artery may occur since it is usually located behind the main duct. During surgery, the spectrum of injury to the right hepatic artery ranges from occlusion by staples, occlusion by staples with section of the structure, or uncontrollable massive hemorrhage solved by indiscriminate placement of staples that can further injure the bile duct. This problem may also occur in open procedures after conversion. Strasberg and col. have described the consequences of ligating of the right hepatic artery. Segmental intrahepatic biliary tract stenoses may develop, and even intrahepatic abscesses may appear.

On cephalic dissection, the common duct is completely freed until the surgeon reaches the confluence (that may also present anatomical variants). The confluence offers resistance since it is located in the natural trajectory of the left duct, fixed to the hilar plate. In these conditions, the dissecting forceps may create an orifice on its medial and lateral portions. This is identified during surgery by a bile leak (usually different to gallbladder bile). Due to this erroneous dissection (Calot's triangle remains intact), only the distal end of the duct is opacified during cholangiography, and it may or may not be associated to extravasation with no proximal biliary filling. When fresh bile emerges with no stones or sludge, this kind of injury must be suspected. Bile's quality, continuous flow and the fact that the gallbladder is not completely emptied after continuous aspiration suggest this type of injury.

Within the spectrum of lesions to the common hepatic duct, we have observed a sub-group of three more injuries. Based on these findings, we he have proposed the expansion of the D classification as follows:

- Injury to the ductus hepatocholedochus: D1
- Injury at the confluence level: D2
- Injury to the left duct: D3
- Occlusion of the left duct: D4

The expansion of the classification is a minor variant within the spectrum of type D injuries, and it does have therapeutic implications. Injury to the left duct may occur when the confluence is low or the dissection is too high and medial to the hilum (a rare situation due to complete misunderstanding of the extrahepatic anatomy). In our series, we have found two cases: one in which a staple had been placed, and it was treated by selective derivation to the jejunum, and the second case, an injury during an anti-reflux procedure (Nissen fundoplication) associated with the left hepatic artery emerging from the left gastric artery; this required conversion to an open procedure due to hemorrhage and was solved with broad and deep transfictive suturing that obstructed the duct and, partially, the portal vein. The patient was referred to our center due to a large abscess that required left lateral hepatectomy.

Most type D injuries are identified during surgery. A small injury without significant devascularization of the duct may be treated with a small suture even during laparoscopy. In these rare cases, a drain should be placed and the patient should be referred for endoscopic assessment and sphincterotomy and/ or stent placement in order to decrease ductal pressure. If no leak is evident, the patient can be managed conservatively.

In other cases, when the duct is devascularized, the patient develops biliary leakage during the first days postoperatively, in spite of having placed small sutures; there is bile collection of various dimensions and different clinical manifestations. Some of these cases may be treated by percutaneous drainage and stent placement. However, many cases require a multi-disciplinary approach (radiologist, endoscopist and surgeon). If a large leak is detected, surgical treatment is necessary (evolves into a type E injury).

Biliary fistulas must close quickly. Maintaining drains for long time periods is not recommended since thay may perforate and/or penetrate adjacent viscera.

Once the fistula closes, the patient requires endoscopic follow-up to prevent the probable development of strictures where the injury healed. In these cases, ischemia also affects the long-term outcome. Ischemia during the immediate postoperative period may widen a small orifice in the biliary tract. After identifying the biliary leak, some surgeons tend to convert the procedure and place a T-tube after repair (some even do it laparoscopically). In these cases, the surgeon finds thin ducts and places a T-tube of an inappropriate caliber and also, inadequately closes the choledocotomy. The erroneous placement of T-tubes can injure the biliary tract. Placement of a T-tube in a devascularized duct may also evolve to a complete injury (Strasberg type E).

An intrahepatic anastomosis guarantees an appropriate anastomosis that, under favorable conditions, has a 95% succes rate. [5, 6]

It has been suggested that, if the injury encompasses less than 25% of the circumference, a primary repair is possible. Our group would suggest this therapeutic option only if the duct's circulation is adequate since, as previously mentioned, the duct's perfusion is always threatened in extensive dissections. If there is good circulation and the repair is performed with the appropriate material (absorbable monofilament 5-0), a primary repair can be attempted. In the remainig cases (8% in our series), we recommend bilioenteric anastomosis.

It is very difficult to obtain information on the accident during the index surgery. Many surgeons tend to minimize the type of injury and do not provide complete information on the event. In most cases, when attempting repair, reconstruction is possible depending on the type of accident and injury class.

Type E Injury [7-9]

This type of injury refers to the complete section of the biliary duct at different levels[24] and it is included among the injuries described in Bismuth's classification. According to Strasberg's classification, they are sub-divided according to the length of the main duct (E1>2 cm, E2<2 cm) (Figure 5), injury at the confluence , preserving the confluence (E3) (Figure 6), injury at the confluence without preserving it (E4) (Figure 7) and injury with a preserved confluence and accessory duct injury (E5) (Figure 8).

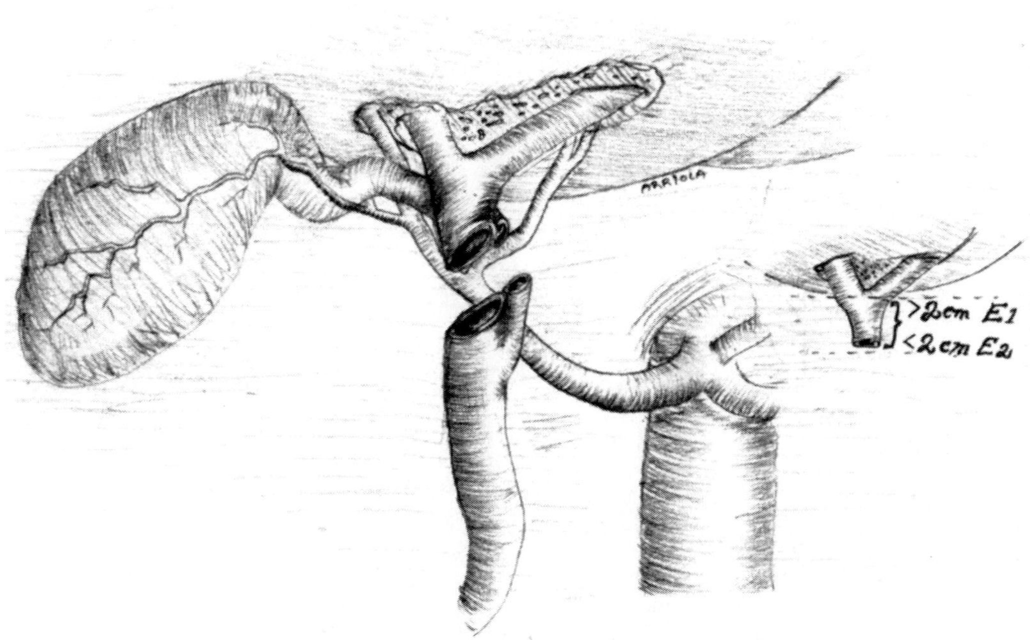

Figure 5. Type E injuries are further subdivided depending on its position in relation with the biliary confluence.

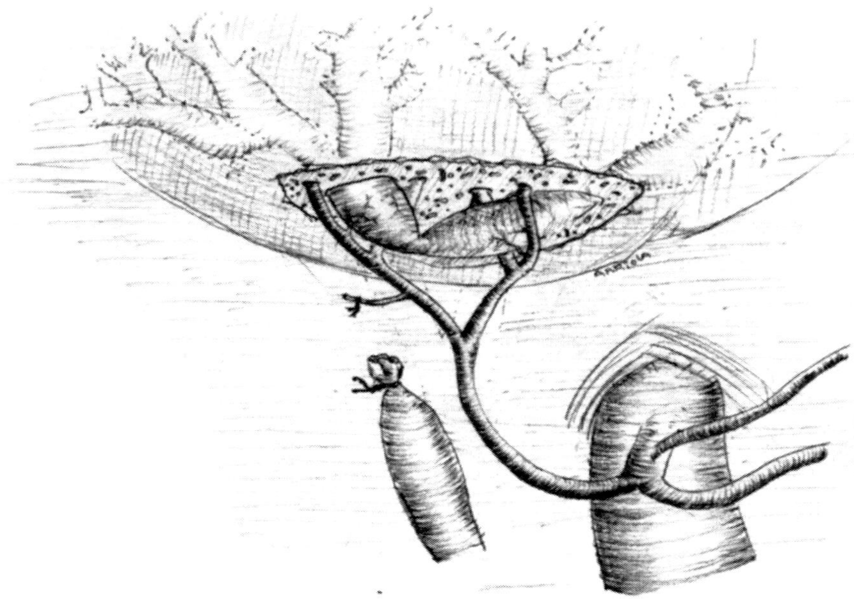

Figure 6. Type E3 lesions preserve the confluence.

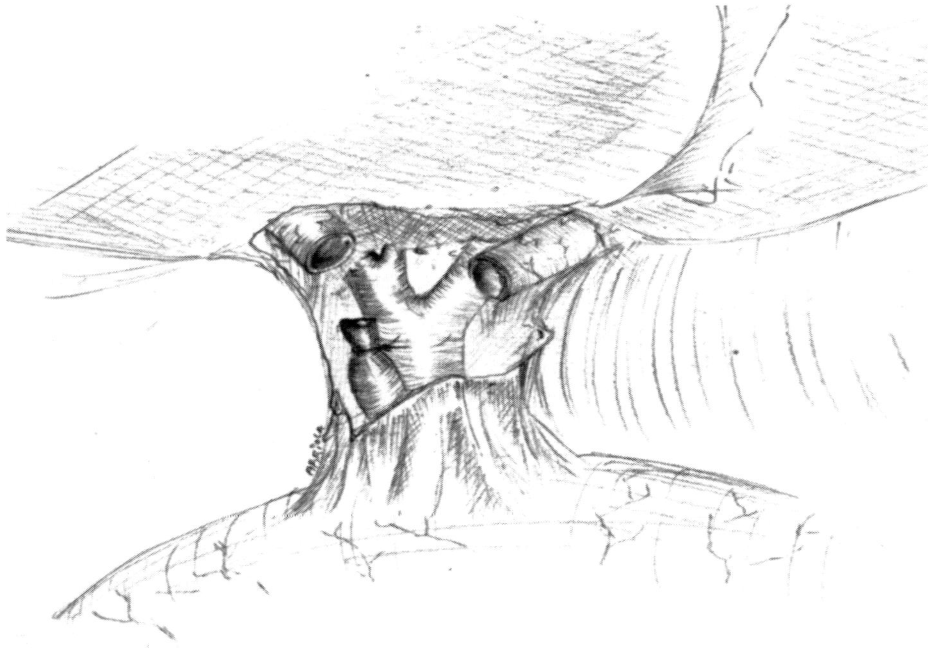

Figure 7. Type E4 lesions compromise the confluence.

These injuries are due to various causes but the most common mistakes are: misidentifying the common bile duct with the cystic duct, excessive traction of the hepatocystic union and staple occlusion, necrosis and subsequent dehiscence; other cases are due to the double section of the main duct (at the choledochal level and the hepatic level) with resulting tissue loss.

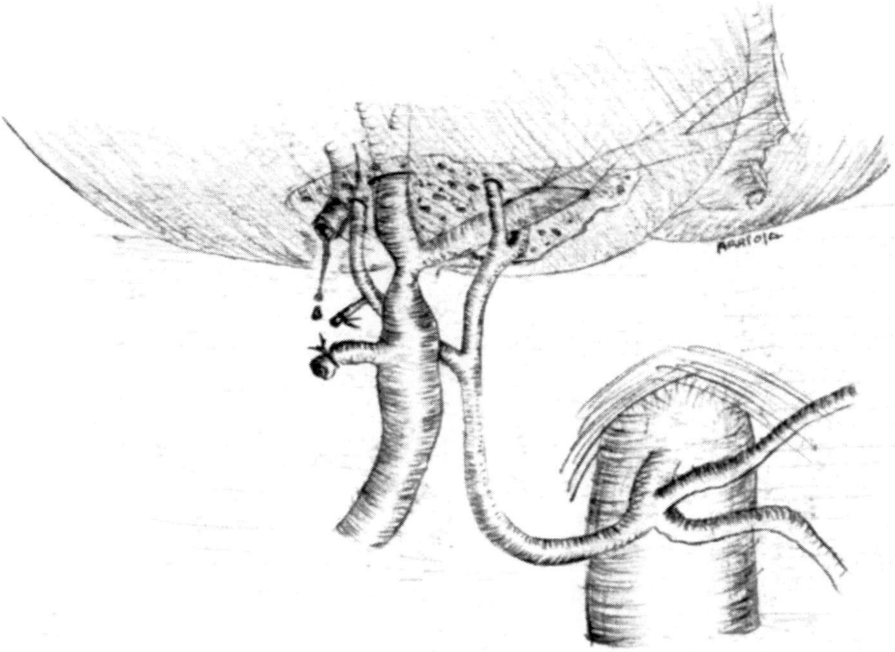

Figure 8. Type E5 injuries compromise both the main biliary ducts as well as the accessory duct.

Other injuries, such as thermal lesions, are manifested later in time as extreme duct stricture and, although its continuity is preserved, its physiopathological behavior is that of a complete section.

The incorrect placement of a T-tube (inappropriate caliber, inadequate suture) manifested as choledochorrhaphy dehiscence and T-tube dislocation, also leads to the loss of biliary tract tissue and behaves as a type E injury.

This type of injury is the most common after type A, accounting for 20 or 30% of all injuries. Retrograde cholangiography reveals complete duct obstruction or non-continuous extravasation of the contrast medium toward the intrahepatic ducts. This study is only indicated to corroborate the injury, sometimes even finding a type A injury amenable to endoscopic treatment. Unfortunately, this is occasionally used as a medico-legal argument, so many surgeons do not acknowledge it and prefer to reoperate.

Low complete sections of the biliary tract (E1 and E2) are by far the most attractive choice for the surgeon to perform a quick and low quality repair since they offer the possibility of performing duct termino-terminal anastomoses and hepatoduodenal derivations. [10] This leads to tense, high-risk anastomoses in spite of performing broad maneuvers to avoid tension, such as an extensive Kocher maneuver that allows access to the duodenum or the distal duct. The duodenum's caudal direction causes a high-tension anastomosis in addition to the probably associated duct ischemia. Injuries leading to complete section of the duct have two main issues to consider: duct devascularization and loss of tissue. This is why, no matter how low, complete duct sections must be managed with biliodigestive derivation without the aforementioned risks (tension and/or ischemia) such as a Roux-en-Y hepaticojejunal anastomosis. [11, 12]

Low biliary tract sections are technically the least demanding sub-group and they include all cases in which the confluence is preserved. In our experience, the best repair results are obtained when the confluence is *ad integrum* and allows a high quality and low risk anastomosis, such as that described in the "Reconstruction Technique" chapter. Partial resection of segments IV and V allows duct identification and execution of the anastomosis.

In contrast, separated ducts represent a greater technical challenge and may lead to a worse outcome. In these cases, the maneuvers described to repair type B injuries are necessary and oftentimes stents are required in order to guarantee the anastomosis' permeability. In the long-term follow-up, these cases have to be considered liver transplant recipients.

References

[1] Strasberg S. M., Hertl M., Soper N. J. An analysis of the problem of biliary injury during laparoscopic cholecystectomy. *J. Am. Coll. Surg.,* 1995; 180: 101- 25.

[2] Ahrendt S. A., Pitt H. A. Surgical therapy of iatrogenic lesions of biliary tract. *World J. Surg.,* 2001; 25: 1360-65.

[3] Strasberg S. M., Picus D. D., Drebin J. A. Results of a new strategy for reconstruction of biliary injuries having an isolated right-sided component. *J. Gastrointest. Surg.,* 2001; 5: 266-74.

[4] Lillemoe K. D., Petrofski J. A., Choti M. A., Venbrux A. C., Cameron J. L. Isolated right segmental hepatic injury: a diagnostic and therapeutic challenge. *J. Gastrointest. Surg.*, 2000; 2: 168-77.

[5] Mercado M. A., Chan C., Orozco H., Tielve M., Hinojosa C. A. Acute bile duct injury. *Surg. Endosc.*, 2003; 17: 1351-55.

[6] Mercado M. A., Orozco H., De la Garza L., López-Martínez L. M., Contreras A., Guillén-Navarro E. Biliary duct injury: partial segment IV resection for intrahepatic reconstruction of biliary lesions. *Arch. Surg.*, 1999; 134: 1008-1010.

[7] Lillemoe K. D., Pitt H. A., Cameron J. L. Current management of benign bile duct strictures. *Adv. Surg.*, 1992; 25: 119-74.

[8] Lillemoe K. D. Benign postoperative bile duct strictures. *Baillers Clin. Gastroenterol.,* 1997; 11: 749-79.

[9] Lillemoe K. D. To err is human, but should we expect more from a surgeon? *Ann. Surg.*, 2003; 237: 470-71.

[10] Moraca R. J., Lee F. t., Ryan J. A. Jr., Traverso L. W. Long term biliary function after reconstruction of major bile duct injuries with hepaticoduodenostomy or hepaticojejunostomy. *Arch. Surg.*, 2002; 137: 889-93.

[11] Melton G. B., Lillemoe K. D. The current management of postoperative bile duct strictures. *Adv. Surg.*, 2002; 36: 193-221.

[12] Lillemoe K. D. Current management of bile duct injury. *Br. J. Surg.*, 2008; 95: 403-5.

In: Bile Duct
Editor: Miguel Ángel Mercado

ISBN: 978-1-63321-771-3

Chapter 6

Reconstruction Techniques

Miguel Ángel Mercado, MD[1], Mario Vilatoba, MD[2], Fernando Ramírez del Val, MD[2], Daniel Zamora, MD[2], Santiago Mier-y-Teran, MD[2] and Bruno A. González-Nolasco, MD[2]

[1]Department of Surgery, National Institute of Medical Sciences and Nutrition "Salvador Zubiran", Mexico

[2]National Institute of Medical Sciences and Nutrition "Salvador Zubiran", Mexico

Abstract

When biliary tract injury is detected during surgery, conversion is necessary. Adequate exposure and dissection is critical. In patients with previous surgery, various kinds of anastomosis may be found. After obtaining a defunctionalized loop and mapping the biliary tract through thin dilators, the loop is anastomosed in a non-tense fashion to ensure a high quality derivation. The suture material used is important.

The hepaticoduodenal anastomosis, from our point of view, has the disadvantage of exposing the anastomosis to acidic content and food residues that hinder its function. Hepatocholedochal anastomosis and choledo-choledocal anastomosis, even though they are comfortable procedures, have high failure rates. Stents can be placed during surgery or transendoscopically, and they are used by our group in complex cases. Neoformation of gallstones after biliodigestive derivation or prosthesis placement is due to the presence of inadequate biliary drainage and/or bile colonization.

Technical Aspects of Reconstruction

Conversion is necessary when biliary tract injury is detected during surgery [1, 3, 4, 6, 15]. A subcostal incision provides adequate exposure of the right upper quadrant, although a median or paramedian incision may also provide good exposure with the use of mechanical retractors fixed to the table. In patients with previous surgery, access can be gained through the previous scar with the same recommendations.

In the case of patients with a history of median secondary wound closure, it is possible to make an alternate incision in the right upper quadrant.

Some may have post-incisional hernias, so the hernial sac should be carefully dissected to avoid injury to the viscera. Contiguous fistulous tracts (where drains are/were placed) are difficult to dissect due to firm adherences to intra-abdominal organs, and may occasionally penetrate into adjacent organs [14].

All organs should be freed and, in patients that have previously undergone biliodigestive derivation, it is essential to perform the lysis of adhesions of the small intestine in order to determine various factors: whether the anastomosed loop is not obstructed or defunctionalized, if there is an enteral anastomotic variant (Omega loop with Braun anastomosis, Nakayama Beta-anastomosis), or if there is an abnormal positioning of the loop compromising its appropriate function. In our case series (over 250 patients), we have found eight cases of loop dysfunction due to such variants. We have found rotated entero-entero anastomoses beyond the transmesenteric loop. Upon repositioning the intestine, loop emptying is compromised because it is anastomosed to the loop's contralateral portion, creating an angle that hinders emptying.

We have also found cases where termino-lateral anastomosis of an ileal loop with no defunctionalization was performed. In other cases, an unsuccesful attempt to defunctionalize the intestine due to the placement of an isoperistaltic loop in the direction of the hilum while performing an Omega loop and Braun anastomosis cannot prevent the ascent of intestinal content.

On many occasions, food residues such as fiber are deposited at the anastomotic level and lead to abnormal biliary drainage, particularly in non-dilated ducts.

It is therefore recommended to free the entire intestine and perform the necessary resections in order to obtain a defunctionalized loop measuring 40 to 50 cm that is then anastomosed to the proximal jejunum (termino-lateral) 20 to 30 cm from the angle of Treitz.

This last point is not essential and, in some cases, the anastomosis is done practically at the level of the ligament of Treitz. This is more risky due to the lack of mobility of one of its components.

The same condition of reflux and obstruction can be an argument for a hepaticoduodenal anastomosis, since it is further complicated by acid reflux. Although there is sufficient evidence to justify hepaticoduodenal anastomoses, in some cases the tension is so great due to caudal migration of the duodenum that we do not support this type of derivation.

It is important to carefully dissect the hepatic hilum. With the help of optical magnification, this is a safe and effective procedure that prevents injury of the biliary ducts and/or vessels.

In acute conditions, the bile leak may lead the surgeon to the detection of the injured duct or ducts. If such ducts are occluded, the staples are removed after verifying they are not vascular structures, and the bile source is confirmed (Figure 2).

Once identified, very thin dilators are introduced and directed towards the different ducts. In case of previous surgery, the site where the loop presents adherences guides the surgeon to identify the ducts once fibrous, scar and/or inflammatory tissue has been removed. After bile drainage, exploration of the ducts using dilators is performed.

We prefer to section the anterior aspect of the duct longitudinally (circulation is located on the lateral aspects) and continue this dissection towards the left duct without moving its posterior aspect. Bleeding is controlled through transfictive sutures using absorbable monofilament (5-0). Every section on the anterior aspect measures approximately 2 to 3 mm having thoroughly verified and certified the direction of the ducts.

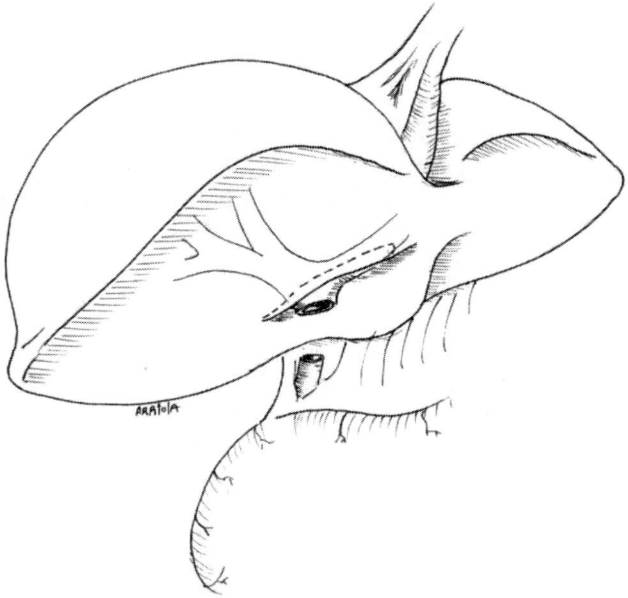

Figure 1. Sectional plane of biliary tract exposing the confluence.

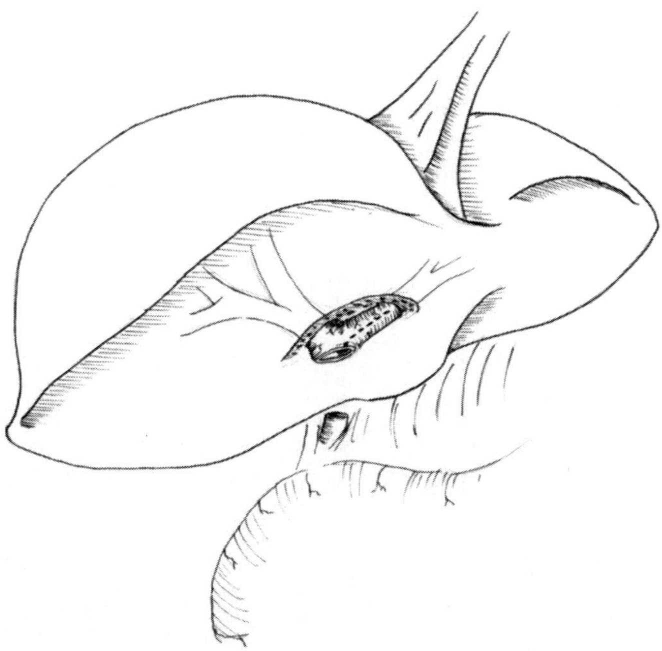

Figure 2. Section line for biliary tract opening.

In certain cases, the hilar plate is covered by the base of segment IV. The hilum is caudally tractioned and the transition between the liver parenchyma, its capsule and the hilar elements becomes evident. This line is sectioned in its entire extension, allowing the hilum to descend.

In order to facilitate exposure, the base of segment IV is removed with a 3x3x3 cm wedge. The small parenchymal bleeding is controlled with compression and, in some cases, with transfictive sutures. This maneuver adequately exposes the left duct, which follows an extrahepatic trajectory from the confluence to the round ligament's end. If the confluence is preserved, it is easy to see the right duct after the incision has been extended toward the left duct. If the confluence is not preserved, the right duct will be on the same plane as the left hepatic duct (antero-posteriorly). Scar fibrous tissue must be removed in order to identify its lumen. If the confluence is preserved, the jejunal loop is anastomosed with separate stitches that should be inverted in a latero-lateral manner where one angle is placed at the vertex of the left duct's longitudinal section and the other in the most distal portion of the main duct remnant. Sutures are placed in an outside-in fashion on the duct and inside-out on the edge of the loop in order to tie the knots on the outside. After completion of the posterior aspect, the ducts and the loop permeability are verified with dilators before placing separate stitches on the anterior aspect, with the same material (Figure 3).

Blumgart recommends placing the stitches on the biliary side of the anterior aspect before stitching the posterior aspect in order to make exposure easy. We keep the stitches placed for hemostasis of the anterior aspect in order to adequately expose the biliary tract's lumen.

After completing the anastomosis, the loop is fixed to the hepatic capsule far from the anastomosis in order to prevent loop rotation and dysfunctional positioning, as well as to decrease tension at the level of the anastomosis.

If the confluence is preserved, a double anastomosis must be attempted. In some cases in which the ducts are adequately preserved and close together, they may be joined with single stitches of the same material used in the anastomosis, making a single anastomosis possible.

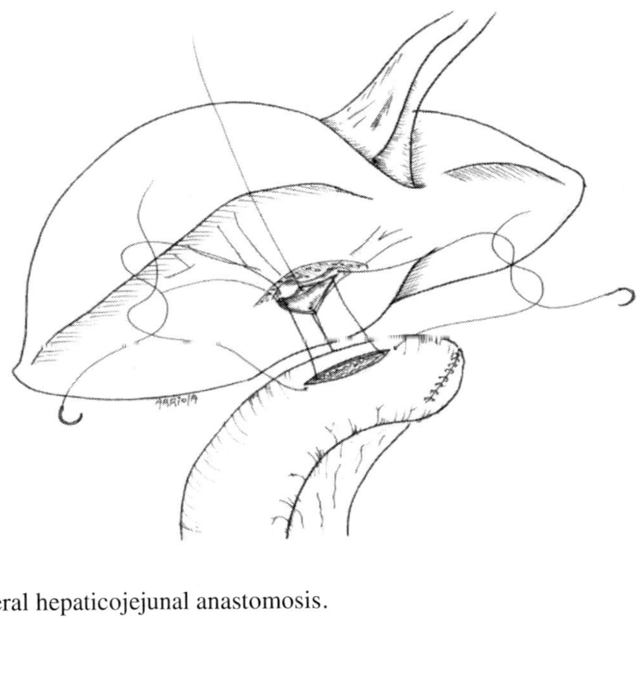

Figure 3. Latero-lateral hepaticojejunal anastomosis.

In case the ducts are separated, small and/or fibrous, it is preferred to place a transhepatic and transanastomotic stent since the anastomosis' permeability will depend on it.

There are unfortunate isolated cases in which an appropriate anastomosis is impossible to perform. The anastomosis of the jejunal opening to the hepatic parenchyma, and the need for stents in every duct included in the anastomosis, technically lead to a portoenterostomy, similar to Kasai's procedure [13].

In our experience and in that of other groups, these are very infrequent cases that often require prolonged permanence of the stents, they develop acute cholangitis, and should be considered for liver transplant.

The type of suture used is important. If there is no polydioxanone monofilament available, polyglycolic acid polyfilament or polypropylene monofilament may be used. This would imply the need for several knots but, if they are inverted, this is not a problem. Leaving an excessive number of intraluminal knots leads to biliary sludge and/or stone formation that prevent adequate function of the anastomosis.

Other suture materials such as silk or catgut should be avoided due to the foreign body granulomatous reaction caused by the first and the inflammatory process triggered by the second.

As previously mentioned, the anastomosis should be performed with optical magnification in order to correctly position the biliary epithelium and the jejunal mucosa.

The mucosal approximation with no sutures, such as the Rodney Smith patch, is a procedure that works well in only some cases and only with the previously described techniques. There is practically no justification not to perform a low risk anastomosis following the previously mentioned guidelines [5].

Some groups have developed techniques in which the proximal end of the defunctionalized loop is not exteriorized or is placed sub-cutaneously; this makes the intestine accessible using local anesthesia for endoscopic and, occasionally, radiological evaluation of the anastomosis. The anastomosis is performed 15 to 20 cm from the main stump of the defunctionalized loop. Some groups do this routinely. Endoscopic access is not easy because it is difficult to insufflate the loop. If this is feasible, there is also the problem of identifying the anastomosis that oftentimes is punctiform and/or obstructed. Some groups place a sub-cutaneous metallic ring that is easily detected radiologically. Our group has no experience with this variant. In a couple of cases, the loop has been placed sub-cutaneously but its use has not been necessary. When a high quality anastomosis is obtained with the mentioned techniques, the possibilities of success are close to 90%; thus, in our judgment, that variant should not be frequently used [9, 10].

Other groups anastomose the loop with the duodenum in order to have access to the anastomosis. This variant has been used and reported even less frequently than that previously described.

Hepaticoduodenal Anastomosis

In general, biliary tract injuries [11] develop at a certain level and under certain conditions that preclude the possibility of using the duodenum for derivation. There are numerous reports that have discussed the use of this derivation to successfully repair the biliary tract, such as Traverso's and Stewart-Way's groups; Stewart-Way recommends it for injuries in which the ductus choledochus has an acceptable length and there is no tissue loss.

From our viewpoint, it has the disadvantage of exposing the anastomosis to acidic content and food residues that may compromise the function of the anastomosis.

Moreover, even if an extensive Kocher maneuver is performed to obtain appropriate exposure of the structures, the duodenum and the pancreatic head tend to return to their anatomical position (as a result of the fixation provided by anatomical structures i.e. celiac trunk and gravity), creating tension on the anastomosis and consequently its avulsion.

There are no controlled prospective studies that prove the superiority of the Roux-en-Y hepaticojejunal anastomosis over hepatoduodenostomy, but dysfunction of the latter requiring reoperation is certainly a fact.

Close to 60 cases in our series comprise failed hepatoduodenostomies.

Another disadvantage of this type of derivation is the presence of a concomitant duodenal fistula when early dehiscence develops. This type of fistula implies disastrous short and long-term consequences, leading to septic complications and severe hydroelectrolytic imbalance as well as negative nutritional repercussions. The biliary fistula associated to hepaticojejunal anastomosis avoids this type of complications and, in most cases, it does not preclude the PO route, its output is low, and it generally closes with no repercussions.

Therefore, hepaticojejunal anastomosis appears to be a better option in all conditions.

Hepatocholedochal Anastomosis, Choledo-Choledochal Anastomosis

This type of repair is one of the most frequently used by the surgeons that caused the injury, in an acute setting. This procedure is comfortable for the surgeon, it is quick, it does not require anastomoses or intestinal mobilization and, somehow, during the first days or weeks, it minimizes the injury in the eyes of everybody involved.

Termino-terminal anastomosis is performed on a stent, usually a T-tube. It requires the cephalic mobilization of the duodenum since this type of injury leads to duct tissue loss and is, by definition, tense.

Another problem is that this procedure is often performed on ischemic ducts (proximal and distal), preparing the anastomosis for failure such as early dehiscence and/or late stenosis. It is not possible to visualize the ducts in the immediate period after the injury. This situation is opposite to that which occurs with duct anastomoses in liver transplants, where circulation is optimal and there is no tension.

Moreover, inappropriate material such as silk is often used, leading to a foreign body inflammatory reaction that contributes to the anastomosis' stenosis.

Again, a judicious and multidisciplinary approach (surgical and endoscopic) will establish the best course of action for each individual patient.

There are no published prospective results on this type of repair and, aside from the fact that there are very few case candidates for this reconstruction, the consensus is that most, probably over 70 to 80%, tend to become stenotic over time.

Transhepatic and/or Transanastomotic Stents (Figure 4)

Stents can be placed percutaneously, during surgery or transendoscopically. The latter require integrity of the biliary tract in order to be successfully placed.

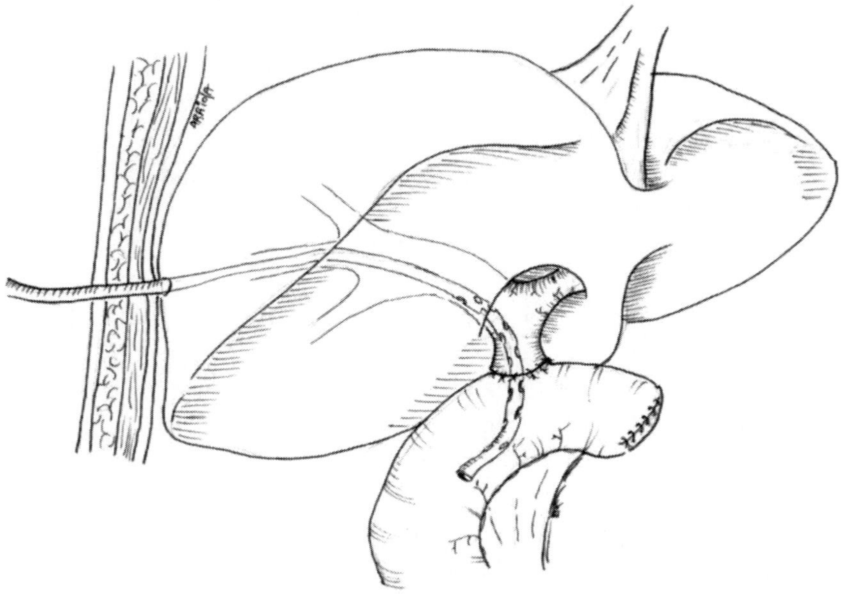

Figure 4. Transhepatic stent. Hepaticojejunal anastomosis with transhepatic tuve.

Percutaneous stents are placed under fluoroscopic visualization; once the biliary tract has been opacified, metal guide-wires are inserted, afterwards dilators are introduced and the stent is placed. Its final position is decided fluoroscopically.

Stents are placed during surgery in different ways. Usually, a perforating dilator is advanced through the biliary tract. The dilator is then used to perforate the parenchyma, making an exit through the hepatic dome. The parenchyma is perforated again and once the surgeon detects resistance, he carefully diverts the perforator. This step must not be difficult and, in general, it is smooth and presents only mild resistance upon exiting the duct [8].

The reason why the dilator must be diverted is that vascular structures offer more resistance. A variant of the dilator is a small Randall forceps with a hole at its end, through which the stent can be sutured. Once the stent is fixed, the dilator is removed through the biliary tract lumen.

One of the most discussed issues in biliary tract reconstruction is the use of transhepatic and/or transanastomotic stents. There are groups that use them routinely, but others suggest that their use increases morbidity without other advantages. Stents can be placed in various ways:

a) Transhepatic stent: it is usually placed percutaneously and occasionally during surgery. The stent is placed through the surface of the liver, into a biliary duct but without reaching the anastomosis.

b) Transhepatic transanastomotic stent: it is placed during surgery and it is passed through the anastomosis into the intestinal loop.
c) Transanastomotic stent: it is placed during surgery when performing the anastomosis. It does not go through the parenchyma and only remains in the duct's lumen. The distal end may be left in the intestinal lumen and fixed with absorbable sutures, or it may emerge like a jejunostomy to the exterior by extracting it at a variable distance from the anastomosis.
d) Endless transhepatic transanastomotic stents: they are placed through the liver surface, moving through the anastomosis and the intestinal lumen, and exiting to the exterior. Both the proximal and distal ends are outside the skin.

Transhepatic and/or transanastomotic stents have several functions:

a) Control ductal pressure; the intestinal loop allows for external drainage and it can avoid dehiscences.
b) Promote epithelio-mucosal healing over the stent, thus maintaining the anastomosis' diameter.
c) Postoperative port for instrumentation with or without radiological guidance in order to maintain the anastomosis open.
d) Easy access for radiological controls of the anastomosis.

They do have some disadvantages or negative issues:

a) No one has proven that they are essential.
b) The duration they remain in place is practically random and biased by the surgeon's experience.
c) Their permanence and placement increases morbidity.
d) They occasionally behave like foreign bodies and are a potential nidus for calculus formation.
e) Most surgeons keep them in place for 6 to 9 months with no real justification; they argue that it is the necessary time period for anastomosis epithelization.
f) The stents' material (Teflon, Silastic, vulcanized rubber) is also a matter of controversy.

In our judgment, a selective use of stents is the best option. An electively performed anastomosis without associated cholangitis results in a biliary tract of a good caliber (not necessarily requiring dilation). Performing a low-risk and high quality anastomosis is feasible if it fulfills all the requirements described in the technique and this case is unlikely to need a stent. Otherwise, an anastomosis with separated, retracted, inflamed and scarred ducts, in which placing sutures is impossible and the intestine is adhered to the parenchyma and/or hepatic capsule, requires the placement of a transhepatic transanastomotic stent.

In many centers, non-transanastomotic transhepatic stents are placed by radiologists before surgery. This controls biliary fistulae and outlines the anatomy allowing for careful planning of the procedure. During surgery, they serve as a guide to find the ducts, and after the anastomosis, they maintain the duct pressure low and prevent leaks that may appear in a newly created, edematous anastomoses. They also allow postoperative radiological control of the anastomosis and it can be removed later with full knowledge of the anastomosis' function.

Aside from the mentioned purposes, transanastomotic stents also maintain the anastomosis mechanically permeable. In extraordinarily complex cases with injured biliary ducts and all possible negative associated factors, stents act as an internal and external fistula, both controlled and amenable to manipulation.

Silastic stents cause a minimal inflammatory reaction and oftentimes upon removal, there may be bile accumulations since an adequate trajectory is not formed. Therefore, if the postoperative plan includes repeated procedures, leaving a vulcanized rubber or latex stent is preferable since they do create an appropriate trajectory, ideal for radiological instrumentation.

Our group uses stents in complex cases, particularly latex stents, to ensure safe access to the anastomosis.

In a comparative study conducted by our group, in which similarly complex cases were managed with or without transhepatic transanastomotic stents, we found similar long-term results in both groups (adequate anastomosis function, no cholangitis, normal liver function tests) in almost 80% of cases. Stents led to higher long-term morbidity manifested as the neoformation of gallstones and complex fistulae such as arterio-biliary (due to selective transfemoral embolization) or bilio-pleural (as a result of decortication) fistula.

Subhepatic fluid accumulations were more common in the group with no stent and the frequency of secondary surgeries was similar in both groups (under 10%).

In many cases, the placement and use of stents is biased by the surgeon's experience and training. Again, the judicious balance of the risks and benefits of stent placement must be established before deciding to place one. If it is placed, they should be washed after surgery in saline solution following an aseptic technique; this requires training the patient and his relatives.

The stent must be periodically changed by an expert radiologist. Its removal should be a consensus between the surgeon and the radiologist.

Gallstones After Biliary Tract Reconstruction [16, 17]

Gallstone neoformation after biliodigestive derivation or endoprosthesis placement is due to two problems (either alone or combined): the presence of biliary stricture due to inadequate bile drainage and/or, more importantly, bile colonization.

Between the three type of calculi described in the literature (cholesterol, black pigmented, brown pigmented), the most common ones are those due to the hydrolysis of conjugated bilirubin to unconjugated bilirubin by bacterial beta glucuronidase and/or phospholipase. Bile colonization develops due to the communication of the biliary tree with the digestive tract as well as to the presence of foreign bodies (transhepatic stents, endoprosthesis, etc.).

Since microorganisms synthesize beta glucuronidase and phospholipase, palmitate is released; this is why the stones have calcium along with unconjugated bilirubin. Stones are formed by nucleation due to the binding of calcium bilirubinate to a glycoprotein.

Therefore, patients with transhepatic stents and/or biliodigestive derivations develop pigmented biliary calculi that manifest as obstructive jaundice and even right upper quadrant pain.

It is not unusual for a patient with a biliodigestive derivation, particularly regarding a high-risk anastomosis, to develop small calculi due to the above-mentioned mechanisms or as a result of the shedding of sutures into the lumen of the anastomosis. In this sense, it is recommended to perform the anastomosis procedure using disposable hydrolysable sutures that cannot act as a nidus for calculi formation and bile accumulation.

When the anastomosis is sufficiently ample, stones can spontaneously pass and more often than not, they do not produce symptoms. If the anastomosis has flow problems, the stone may become impacted and lead to fever, jaundice, choluria and right upper quadrant pain that disappear once the stone passes. Occasionally, cholangitis develops, requiring antibiotic therapy and even percutaneous and/or surgical drainage.

Patients with a closed transhepatic stent have a higher risk of developing these symptoms more often. That is why the stent should be periodically changed since biliary sludge forms around the stent and within its lumen.

A comparative study conducted by our group [7], analyzed the value of oral biliary acids in the prevention of cholangitis and/or stent obstruction. Ursodeoxycholic acid administration was not found to be useful in the prevention of stent obstruction or in decreasing the frequency of gallstones. Patients with recurrent cholangitis after derivation should be reevaluated, and reintervention should be considered; this procedure should be a low-risk anastomosis wide enough to prevent obstruction by gallstones.

Occasionally, when a thin caliber biliary tract is found through imaging studies, a poor long-term prognosis is expected since it is impossible to perform another anastomosis with better functional characteristics.

These patients develop hepatocellular injury and must eventually be considered liver transplant recipients.

References

[1] Asbun, H. J., Rossi, R. L., Lowell, J. A., Munson, J. L. Bile duct injury during laparoscopic cholecystectomy: mechanism of injury, prevention and management. *World J. Surg*. 993; 547-54.

[2] Al-Ghnaniem, R., Benjamin, I. S. Long-term outcome of hepatico-jejunostomy with routine access loop formation following iatrogenic bile duct injury. *Br. J. Surg*. 2002; 89: 1118-24.

[3] Bingener-Casy, J., Richardo, M. L., Strodel, W. E., Schwesinger, W. A., Sirinek, K. R. Reasons for conversion from laparoscopic to open cholecystectomy: a 10-year review. *J. Gastrointest. Surg*. 2002; 6: 200-5.

[4] Fruhauf, N. R., Malago, M., Broelsch, C. E. Management of iatrogenic lesions of the biliary tract. *Med. SC: Monit*. 2001; 7: 60-3.

[5] Jarnagin, W. R., Blumgart, L. H. Operative repair of bile duct injuries involving the hepatic duct confluence. *Arch. Surg*. 1999; 134: 769-75.

[6] Ludwig, K., Bernhardt, J., Steffen, H., Lornz, D. Contribution of intraoperative cholangiography to incidence and outcome of common bile duct injuries during laparoscopic cholecystectomy. *Surg. Endosc.* 2002; 16: 1098-1104.

[7] Mercado, M. A., Chan, C., Orozco, H., Cano-Gutierrez, G., Galindo, E., Chaparro, J. M., Lozano-Salazar, R. R., Lopez-Loredo, A. Biliary stents for reconstruction in bile duct injuries. The role of bile acids. *Rev. Gastroenterol. Mex.* 2002; 67: 82-6.

[8] Mercado, M. A., Chan, C., Orozco, H., Cano-Gutierrez, G., Chaparro, J. M., Galindo, E., Vilatoba, M., Samaniego-Arrizu, G. To stent or not to stent bilioenteric anastomosis alter iatrogenic injury: a dilemma not answered? *Arch. Surg.* 2002; 137: 60-3.

[9] Mercado, M. A., Chan, C., Tielve, M., Contreras, A., Galvez-Treviño, R., Ramos-Gallardo, G., Orozco, H. Lesión yatrogénica de la vía biliar. Experiencia de 180 casos. *Rev. Gastroenterol. Mex.* 2002; 67: 245-9.

[10] Melton, G. B., Lillemoe, K. D. The current management of postoperative bile duct strictures. *Adv. Surg.* 2002; 36: 193-221.

[11] Moraca, R., Lee, F. T., Ryan, J. A. Jr, Traverso, L. W. Long term biliary function after reconstruction of mayor bile duct injuries with hepaticoduodenostomy or hepaticojejunostomy. *Arch. Surg.* 2002; 137: 889-93.

[12] Nordin, A., Halme, L., Maksalo, H., Isoniem, H., Hockerstedt, K. Management and outcome of major bile duct injuries after laparoscopic cholecystectomy: form therapeutic endoscopy to liver transplantation. *Liver Transpl.* 2002; 8: 1036-43.

[13] Pickleman, J., Marsan, R., Borge, M. Portoenterostomy: an old treatment for a new disease. *Arch. Surg.* 2000; 135: 811-17.

[14] Rossi, R. L., Tsao, J. L. Biliary reconstruction. *Surg. Clin. North Am.* 1994; 74: 825-41.

[15] Strasberg, S. M. Avoidance of biliary injury during laparoscopic cholecystectomy. *J. Hepatobiliary Pancreat. Surg.* 2002; 9: 543-7.

[16] Stewart, L., Ponce, R., Oesterle, A. L., Griffiss, J. M., Way, L. W. Pigment gallstone pathogenesis: slime production by biliary bacteria is more important than beta-glucuronidase production. *J. Gastrointest. Surg.* 2000; 4: 547-53.

[17] Stewart, L., Smith, A. L., Pellegrini, C. A., Moston, R. W., Way, L. W. Pigment gallstones form as a composite of bacterial microcolonies and pigment solids. *Ann. Surg.* 1987; 206: 242-50.

In: Bile Duct
Editor: Miguel Ángel Mercado

ISBN: 978-1-63321-771-3

Chapter 7

Perioperative Complications of Hepatoduodenostomy and Choledoco-Choledocal Anastomosis in Bile Duct Injuries

Miguel Ángel Mercado, MD[1], Alan Contreras, MD[2], Lizeth Luna, MD[2], Mariana Morales, MD[2], Leticia Carrete, MD[2], Santiago Mier-y-Teran, MD[2] and Bruno A. González-Nolasco, MD[2]

[1]Department of Surgery, National Institute of Medical Sciences and Nutrition "Salvador Zubiran", Mexico

[2]National Institute of Medical Sciences and Nutrition "Salvador Zubiran", Mexico

Abstract

Introduction: This survey analyzes the correlation between perioperative complications in patients who underwent hepatojejunostomy after a primary surgery (hepatoduodenostomy or choledoco-choledocal anastomosis), and those whom the first intervention was hepatojejunostomy.

Methods: A quantitative and retrospective analysis was done, including patients in which hepatojejunostomy was performed at the "National Institute of Medical Sciences and Nutrition" from 1990 to 2010. The confidence interval was set at 95% and the statistical analysis was performed using Chi-squared test.

Results: 116 patients were included; group 1 ($n=39$) was constituted by patients with previous repairs and group 2 ($n=77$) with patients without previous repair. Preoperative complications were found in *76% (30)* in group 1, whereas in the group 2 these complications were present in *54% (42)* ($p<.005$). Laparoscopic cholecystectomy was the most frequent type of surgery from the total number of patients, *66% (26)* in the group 1 and *44% (34)* in the group 2. Cholangitis was the most frequent complication found preoperatively; *66% (26)* in group 1 and *44% (34)* in group 2 ($p=.04$). We compared the proportion of postoperative complications in both groups, along with segment IV resection, and whether the confluence was preserved or not. In this regard, *30% (12)* of patients assigned to group 1 suffered this type of complications, while the group 2, *23% (29).*

Conclusion: In this study, patients with primary repairs had more preoperative complications than patients with no previous repairs prior to hepatojejunostomy.

Introduction

During the last years, laparoscopic cholecystectomy has become the primary treatment for diverse gallbladder diseases. The reported incidence of iatrogenic injuries secondary to these procedures has been constant (0.4-0.6%) [1-3]. Although bile duct injuries are not considered a public health problem, the potential consequences for the patient should always be taken into consideration. These injuries are associated with high perioperative morbidity and mortality, consequently carrying an impact in postoperative quality of life and survival [4, 5]. Some authors have stated that 75%-98% of these cases could experience a total recovery after surgical repair [6, 7]. The Roux-en-Y Hepatojejunostomy is currently considered by many groups, as the best option when it comes to a bile duct injury repair [12].

However, other groups are still using different surgical techniques and procedures as primary interventions; the hepatoduodenostomy and choledoco-choledocal anastomosis are the most frequently performed. As the main reference center specialized in the treatment of bile duct injuries in Mexico, near half the patients who attend have already had a primary intervention. Therefore, it is necessary to determine the potential differences regarding perioperative complications between the patients who underwent primary repair and those who were primarily repaired in our institute.

Methods

A retrospective database was created including all patients treated for bile duct injury in the National Institute of Medical Sciences and Nutrition "Salvador Zubirán" from January 1990 to December 2010. Data collection and patient follow-up was approved by the medical ethics committee of the institute. Data collected included gender, age, comorbidities, previous repairs, type of cholecystectomy, date of the hepatojejunostomy, preoperative complications, postoperative complications, resection of segment IV, biliary confluence preservation, anastomosis stenosis, cholangitis and abscesses.

The variables were categorized as qualitative data.

Patients

The sample selection included 116 patients, from which *33.6%* (39) were assigned to group 1; this group includes patients with previous repairs such as hepatoduodenostomy and choledoco-choledocal anastomosis.

Table 1. Group distribution. Group 1 conformed by patients with previous repair. Group 2 for patients whom the first repair was the index hepatojejunostomy

	Group 1	Group 2	Total
Frequency	39	77	116
Percentage	33.6	66.4	100
Valid Percentage	33.6	66.4	100

On the other hand, *66.4%* (77) were allocated in group 2, regarding patients in which hepatojejunostomy was the first approach to repair the bile duct injury (Table 1).

The following inclusion criteria were implemented:

- Patients with hepatojejunostomy performed in this institute during 1990-2010
- Iatrogenic bile duct injury as the cause of repair
- Patients for whom radiologic and/or endoscopic treatment had been ruled out
- Previous primary bile duct injury repair.

Statistical Analysis

In order to execute the statistical analysis, we considered qualitative variables only. Hence, the survey would be able to establish meaningful associations or independence between the events. The analysis was carried out using the statistical software SPSS v.19 and the Chi-squared test. The accepted confidence interval was set at 95% *($p<.05$).*

Results

From the total number of patients included, *36.2% (42)* were men, whereas *63.8% (74)* were women. The age frequency analysis revealed that *85%* were under 65 years and the rest were over that age. The mean age between patients was 45.6 years old (Graphic 1).

The sample distribution analysis revealed a non-Gaussian distribution. The difference between preoperative complications and postoperative complications was obtained considering the index hepatojejunostomy as a reference in time.

The primary intervention type depended entirely on the surgeon's decision. However, the classification of the injury was not considered since in many cases the data was unknown. The respective contingency tables were built based on the groups and the event compared.

Tables 2 and 3 illustrate the results for each analyzed variable including the proportion of patients who presented the studied event and the corresponding p values.

The proportion of preoperative complications found in group 1 was *76% (30),* whereas in group 2 these types of complications were present in *54% (42)*. When we applied the statistical test, they appeared to be related significantly ($p<0.05$).

The variables considered as preoperative complications were the following: type of cholecystectomy, biliary fistula, sepsis, biloma, pericholangitic abscesses and cholangitis.

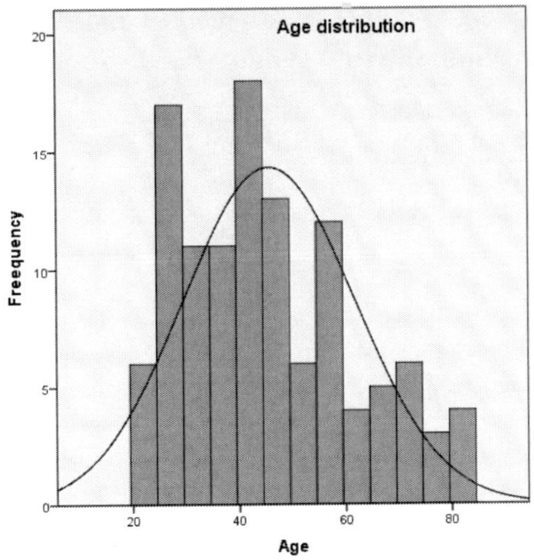

Mean age = 45.6.
SD = 16.1.
N = 116.

Graphic 1. Age Frequency Analysis.

From the total number of patients, laparoscopic cholecystectomy was the most frequent type of surgery performed, *66% (26)* in group 1 and *44% (34)* in group 2. Nevertheless, this association was not statistically significant.

As mentioned above, preoperative complications were analyzed individually. Thereby, as shown in table 2, biliary fistula was present in *15% (6)* of patients in group 1 while in group 2 the proportion was *27% (21) (p=.15)*. The percentage of patients who presented sepsis was *2% (1)* for group 1 and *7% (6)* for group 2 *(p=.26)*.

On the other hand, the proportion of patients in whom biloma was diagnosed preoperatively was *5% (2)* in group 1 and *9% (7)* in group 2 *(p=.45)*. Abscesses were found in *12% (5)* of patients in the first group and in *3% (3)* of patients in the second group. Cholangitis was the most frequent complication found preoperatively with *66% (26)* in group 1 and *44% (34)* in group 2, being statistically significant (p=.04).

We compared the proportion of postoperative complications in both groups, along with IV segment resection, and whether the confluence was preserved or not. In this regard, *30% (12)* of patients assigned to group 1 suffered this type of complications, while in group 2, *23% (29)*.

During the follow up, stenosis was diagnosed in *5% (2)* of patients in group 1 *and 5% (4)* of patients in group 2 with no statistical significance between them *(p=.98)*. Abscesses in the postoperative period were found in *5% (2)* of group 1, whereas in *7% (6)* of group 2 *(p=.59)*.

Bile duct fistula was documented in *2% (1)* of patients in group 1 and 5% (4) of patients in group 2 *(p=.5)*, while cholangitis proportion was *20% (8)* in group 1 and *21% (16)* in group 2, this was not of statistical significance *(p=.7)*.

When analyzing the relation between surgical procedures and preservation of the confluence, our results show that there is no association considering that *71% (28)* and *74% (57)* of patients who belong to group 1 and 2, respectively, the confluence could be preserved *(p=.79)*.

In the same way, resection of the fourth liver segment did not show any correlation neither with group 1 nor group 2; *46% (18) and 40% (31)*, respectively, the difference was not statistically significant *(p=.54)*.

Odds ratio was calculated. Statistical significance was found in the case of preoperative complications and particularly, cholangitis. Table 4 shows the odds ratio value as well as the respective confidence intervals (95%).

Table 2. Ratio of preoperative complications

Variable	Group 1 (n=39)	Group 2 (n=77)	P (<.05)
Preoperative complications	30/39 *(76%)*	42/77 *(54%)*	.01
Cholecystectomy*	26/39 *(66%)*	34/77 *(44%)*	.36
Biliary fistula	6/39 *(15%)*	21/77 *(27%)*	.15
Sepsis	1/39 *(2%)*	6/77 *(7%)*	.26
Biloma	2/39 *(5%)*	7/77 *(9%)*	.45
Pericholangitic abscesses	5/39 *(12%)*	3/77 *(3%)*	.07
Cholangitis	26/39 (66%)	34/77 (44%)	.02

Table 3. Ratio of postoperative complications

Variable	Grupo 1 (n=39)	Grupo 2 (n=77)	P (<.05)
Postoperative complications	12/39 *(30%)*	23/77 *(29%)*	.92
Confluence	28/39 *(71%)*	57/77 *(74%)*	.79
Resection fourth segment	18/39 *(46%)*	31/77 *(40%)*	.54
Stenosis	2/39 *(5%)*	4/77 *(5%)*	.98
Abscesses	2/39 *(5%)*	6/77 *(7%)*	.59
Fistula	1/39 *(2%)*	4/77 *(5%)*	.50
Cholangitis	8/39 *(20%)*	18/77 *(23%)*	.70

Table 4. Odds ratio of the association between preoperative complications and cholangitis

Variable	Odds ratio	Confidence Intervals
Preoperative Complications	2.77	1.1-6.2
Cholangitis	2.59	1.1-5.6
Pericholangitic abscesses	3.6	.81-16.6

Discussion

Reuver et al. [13] considered 151 cases of iatrogenic bile duct injuries, showing that 26.4% of patients with secondary repairs suffered perioperative complications.

On the contrary, these complications were present in only 7.9% of patients referred to perform a primary repair *(p=0.04)*. Moreover, postoperative complications rose up in patients with secondary repairs *(p=0.04)*.

Melton et al. [8] carried out a survey analyzing patient's quality of life who underwent a bile duct repair was performed. They selected a sample of 89 patients from which *24% (21)* were secondary repairs, while *42% (35)* were primary repairs; the rest of injuries were diagnosed during the surgery. It was documented that, as a consequence of the procedure´s high mortality, the long term quality of life decreases dramatically in patients who have undergone a secondary repair [4, 8].

End-to-end choledocal anastomosis, which is also known as choledoco-choledocal anastomosis with T-tube, is technically suitable when the injury is diagnosed during cholecystectomy. However, because of its multiple complications, the results tend to be poo [14].

Whenever tension exists on the anastomosis, it is not indicated to perform a primary repair. Even though, Kocher maneuver would help the surgeon gain intestinal length on the duodenum´s side, this approach is not sufficiently effective to create a low-tension anastomosis.

Therefore, we have demonstrated that there is a higher degree of preoperative complications than expected, as well as septic complications such as cholangitis and pericholangitic abscesses. After the index hepatojejunostomy, the outcome is actually similar to the results obtained with the primary intervention. Hence, it is apparent that there is no increased risk of postoperative issues.

According to a survey concerning end-to-end choledocal anastomosis, which was carried out by DeReuver et al. [14], this procedure might be performed as primary treatment when the injury does not bear a significant loss of tissue, resulting in low postoperative mortality and morbidity. In contrast, it has been documented a broad stenosis ratio (70%-80%) after the aforementioned surgery. Nonetheless, the stenosis ratio is even higher after a secondary repair with previous end-to-end choledocal anastomosis [15-17].

The hepatoduodenostomy is chosen by some surgical groups since it is more physiological and, technically, less complicated.

Moreover, this procedure bears the possibility to carry out postoperative cholangiographies and radiological interventions, if necessary [18].

Nonetheless, in this surgery, manipulating and stretching the duodenum in order to perform the anastomosis may cause the intestine to return to its original position later on. Constant tension in the anastomosis site is present and it might lead to dehiscence of the anastomosis, which is a critical event in these patients.

Duodenum fistulas may appear in the postoperative period, increasing the morbidity. Significant hydroelectrolytic losses and high flow pancreatic and gastric secretion, as well as biliary fluid, are capable of eroding the surrounding structures. Furthermore, this type of anastomosis could be blocked by intestinal content deposits over time. The mortality of this complication is considerably high and often requires gastric drain. Even percutaneous biliary intervention and necrotic tissue removals may be necessary.

The definitive procedure may have to be postponed due to this complication, with the resultant consequences regarding time and quality of the recovery. However, it is impossible to determine accurately the exact number of failed hepatoduodenostomies that end up in fistulization.

This situation contrasts with the setting found in pancreatic or distal biliary neoplasms, where the progressive rise of intraductal pressure produces dilation of biliary ducts, consequently, making the procedure technically easier.

The effectiveness of this type of anastomosis is limited. It might be noted that loss of tissue and devascularization are frequent drawbacks during surgery, while subsequent tension exerts its harmful effects upon the duodenal joint. Thereby, the ideal conditions would have been set for dehiscence. In this sense, there are not sufficient reports to objectively assess the hepatoduodenostomy and its effectiveness.

It is possible that primary repairs, either hepatoduodenostomy or choledoco-choledocal, do work well. Nonetheless, our center merely rescues those who have had a failed primary attempt elsewhere. Thereby, it is not possible to determine clearly what the proportion of failed primary interventions is. On the other hand, the consequences of dehiscence in end-to-end anastomosis are less catastrophic. Actually the results tend to be better than the ones obtained with hepatoduodenostomy, and generally, the treatment of late stenosis is suitably performed through endoscopic procedures. Bile duct quality is different when bile duct injury anastomosis is compared to the anastomosis performed in liver transplants, where the surgeon has two well-vascularized ends without important tissue losses. In this case there should not be tension on the anastomosis.

Well-qualified surgeons must evaluate every type of repair. According to the author's experience, unless favorable conditions were present, the hepatojejunostomy should be considered as the first line of treatment.

Conclusion

End to end anastomosis possess the advantage that it might be performed in an acute setting, just after the surgeon identifies the injury. It has been documented that stenosis is a common complication in the long term. When permeability is lost, the patient's quality of life is harshly affected.

In selected patients, it is possible to perform a hepatoduodenostomy as a primary repair. Yet, this is not the case for most of the patients with bile duct injuries since the anastomosis will suffer from high tension. It is only suitable when the surgeon has two large and thick duct ends to perform the anastomosis.

In addition to its poor outcome, the hepatoduodenostomy is subject to irritation and erosion derived from pancreatic, gastric and biliary secretions.

The treatment of choice must be assessed by multiple areas and evaluated ideally by an expert surgeon in order to avoid posterior complications.

In conclusion, preoperative complications seem to be more frequent in patients with primary repairs prior to hepatojejunostomy and they are manifested particularly as cholangitis. However, there are no apparent differences in the postoperative span, once these patients are sent to a specialized center in order to be evaluated correctly for treatment. So, we strongly recommend adequate training of surgeons so that they may be able to identify bile duct injuries, treat them, or transfer these patients to more experienced centers.

References

[1] Deziel, D. J., Millikan, K. W., Economou, S. G., Doolas, A., Ko, S. T., Airan, M. C. Complications of laparoscopic cholecystectomy: a national survey of 4,292 hospitals and an analysis of 77,604 cases. *Am. J. Surg*. 1993; 165:9-14?

[2] Wherry, D. C., Marohn, M. R., Malanoski, M. P., Hetz, S. P., Rich, N. M. An external audit of laparoscopic cholecystectomy in the steady state performed in medical treatment facilities of the Department of Defense. *Ann. Surg*. 1996; 224:145-54.

[3] Orlando, R., 3rd, Russell, J. C., Lynch, J., Mattie, A. Laparoscopic cholecystectomy. A statewide experience. The Connecticut Laparoscopic Cholecystectomy Registry. *Arch. Surg*. 1993;128:494-8; discussion 8-9.

[4] Boerma, D., Rauws, E. A., Keulemans, Y. C., et al. Impaired quality of life 5 years after bile duct injury during laparoscopic cholecystectomy: a prospective analysis. *Ann. Surg*. 2001;234:750.

[5] Moore, D. E., Feurer, I. D., Holzman, M. D., et al. Long-term detrimental effect of bile duct injury on health-related quality of life. *Arch. Surg*. 2004;139:476-81; discussion 81-2.

[6] De Santibanes, E., Ardiles, V., Pekolj, J. Complex bile duct injuries: management. *HPB* (Oxford) 2008;10:4-12.

[7] Connor, S., Garden, O. J. Bile duct injury in the era of laparoscopic cholecystectomy. *Br. J. Surg*. 2006;93:158-68.

[8] Melton, G. B., Lillemoe, K. D., Cameron, J. L., Sauter, P. A., Coleman, J., Yeo, C. J. Major bile duct injuries associated with laparoscopic cholecystectomy: effect of surgical repair on quality of life. *Ann. Surg*. 2002;235:888-95.

[9] Lillemoe, K. D., Melton, G. B., Cameron, J. L., et al. Postoperative bile duct strictures: management and outcome in the 1990s. *Ann. Surg*. 2000;232:430-41.

[10] Flum, D. R., Cheadle, A., Prela, C., Dellinger, E. P., Chan, L. Bile duct injury during cholecystectomy and survival in medicare beneficiaries. *JAMA* 2003;290:2168-73.

[11] Walsh, R. M., Vogt, D. P., Ponsky, J. L., Brown, N., Mascha, E., Henderson, J. M. Management of failed biliary repairs for major bile duct injuries after laparoscopic cholecystectomy. *J. Am. Coll. Surg*. 2004;199:192-7.

[12] Lillemoe, K. D. Current management of bile duct injury. *Br. J. Surg*. 2008;95:403-5.

[13] De Reuver, P. R., Grossmann, I., Busch, O. R., Obertop, H., van Gulik, T. M., Gouma, D. J. Referral pattern and timing of repair are risk factors for complications after reconstructive surgery for bile duct injury. *Ann. Surg*. 2007;245:763-70.

[14] De Reuver, P. R., Busch, O. R., Rauws, E. A., Lameris, J. S., van Gulik, T. M., Gouma, D. J. Long-term results of a primary end-to-end anastomosis in peroperative detected bile duct injury. *J. Gastrointest. Surg*. 2007;11:296-302.

[15] Mercado, M. A., Borja-Cacho, D., Dominguez, I., et al. An unusual cause of bilioenteric anastomotic dysfunction after iatrogenic bile duct injury. *Ann. Hepatol*. 2006;5:120-2.

[16] Pellegrini, C. A., Thomas, M. J., Way, L. W. Recurrent biliary stricture. Patterns of recurrence and outcome of surgical therapy. *Am. J. Surg*. 1984;147:175-80.

[17] Stewart, L., Way, L. W. Bile duct injuries during laparoscopic cholecystectomy. Factors that influence the results of treatment. *Arch. Surg*. 1995;130:1123-8; discussion 92-3.

[18] Moraca, R. J., Lee, F. T., Ryan, J. A., Jr., Traverso, L. W. Long-term biliary function after reconstruction of major bile duct injuries with hepaticoduodenostomy or hepaticojejunostomy. *Arch. Surg*. 2002;137:889-93; discussion 93-4.

In: Bile Duct
Editor: Miguel Ángel Mercado

ISBN: 978-1-63321-771-3

Chapter 8

Iatrogenic Bile Duct Injury: Surgical Rescue of Endoscopic Treatment Failures

Miguel Ángel Mercado, MD[1], Lizeth Luna, MD[2], Daniel Zamora, MD[2], Ismael Domínguez, MD[2], Julio Alfaro, MD[2], Erick Misael-Saucedo, MD[2], Santiago Mier-y-Teran, MD[2] and Bruno A. González-Nolasco, MD[2]

[1]Department of Surgery, National Institute of Medical Sciences and Nutrition "Salvador Zubiran", Mexico

[2]National Institute of Medical Sciences and Nutrition "Salvador Zubiran", Mexico

Abstract

Introduction: This study evaluates the postoperative outcome of patients who had hepaticojejunostomy as treatment for iatrogenic bile duct injuries, with previous use of endoprosthesis.

Methods: A retrospective study was performed from 2005 to 2010. Patients who had endoscopic biliary stenting (minimum 6 months with 2 exchanges) previous to surgical reconstruction were included. Group 1 consisted of 25 patients repaired with endoscopic biliary endoprosthesis before surgical intervention and group 2 consisted of 75 patients who required surgical treatment as first approach.

Results: Preoperative sepsis ($p=0.012$), number of preoperative episodes of cholangitis ($p<0.001$), postoperative stenosis ($p<0.0001$) and radiological intervention ($p= 0.017$) had a statistically significant difference between the two groups.

A subanalysis of patients with criteria for endoscopic treatment failure (endoscopic treatment for minimum 1 year with 4 stent exchanges) was performed. Furthermore, the differences in the variables measured were statistically significant, and the stented group presented more complications.

Conclusion: Management of bile duct injury must be multidisciplinary. When continuity of the bile duct is preserved, endoscopic biliary stenting is the treatment of choice. However, if the stenosis cannot be solved in a short period of time, it is necessary to promote early surgery to prevent postoperative long-term stenosis or radiological intervention. Early intervention would facilitate surgical reconstruction and improve long-term outcome.

Introduction

Nowadays, 70–80% of all cholecystectomies are performed laparoscopically, although complex cases still require the open technique [1, 2]. In the era of open cholecystectomy, the incidence of bile duct injuries remained at the level of 0.1-0.2%.

After the introduction of laparoscopic cholecystectomy, this rate has doubled. If leakages from the cystic duct and the gallbladder bed are included, the reported incidence of bile duct injuries has varied between 0.8 and 2.8% [3].

Different treatment options exist including percutaneous biliary drainage, balloon dilation with stenting, and endoscopic biliary stenting. Although bile duct leaks can be managed successfully using these treatments, complete bile duct transection requires surgery.

For postoperative biliary strictures, hepaticojejunostomy is widely accepted as the treatment of choice because it is perceived that a good one-time fix by an experienced surgeon will provide an excellent outcome [4].

The aim of this study is to evaluate the postoperative outcome of patients who underwent hepaticojejunostomy as treatment for iatrogenic bile duct injuries, with previous use of stents.

Methods

Patients

From January 2005 to December 2010, a total of 339 patients were treated with hepaticojejunostomy in our center. From this total, 268 were treated for iatrogenic bile duct injury. Patients who underwent endoscopic biliary stenting previously (6 months at minimum with 2 exchanges) were included in this study. Group 1 consisted of 25 patients repaired with endoscopic biliary endoprosthesis before surgical intervention and group 2 consisted of 75 patients with complete section of the bile ducts, requiring surgical intervention as the first line approach (Roux-en-Y hepaticojejunostomy).

The groups were paired by age, gender, type of cholecystectomy (open or laparoscopic), type of injury (Type E4 and E5 according to Strasberg´s classification, were excluded from group 2) and comorbidities (Diabetes Mellitus, systemic arterial hypertension). There were 18 males and 57 females, with a mean age of 38.0 ±12 years (range 20-64 years).

Patients were evaluated at 3, 6 or 12 months according to their clinical course and laboratory test results. We used our institution normal values for liver function test as a reference to define enzymes elevation.

Statistical Analysis

Stata 12.0 software and Microsoft Excel were used for data collection and analysis. Comparison between groups was performed using the Mann–Whitney U-test, the T-test, and the $\chi 2$ test as appropriate. A p-value below 0.05 was considered statistically significant.

Results

Table 1 shows the baseline features of both groups. The mean age of patients in group 1, who were mainly female (25 % from the total number of patients), was 38 years (±11) and did not differ statistically from the mean age of group 2 (38 ± 12 years). No statistical difference was noted in terms of comorbidities between the two groups (p = 1.000).

75 cholecystectomies were performed, 17% were open in group 1 and 41% in group 2, whereas 15% laparoscopic approaches were performed in group 1 and 25% in group 2. Once established that there was no significant difference between groups, preoperative variables were evaluated (Table 2). A total of 3 patients in group 1 developed preoperatory sepsis (4%), while 0 patients developed preoperatory sepsis in group 2. Significant difference was obtained when bile fistulae were analyzed; 17% of patients in group 2 versus 1.3% in group 1. Patients with surgery as first line of approach had significantly higher AST levels than patients with previous endoscopic biliary stenting (p = .038).

As shown in Table 3 (operative variables), the analysis of patients with previous endoscopic biliary stenting showed a statistical significant value in bleeding (p <0.001), however, it did not represent a clinical difference in abdominal surgeries (difference between groups 31 ml).

Clinical Outcome

As we can observe in Table 4, levels of transaminases were significantly higher in group 1 (previous endoprosthesis), 12 months after the surgical intervention (ALT G1: 9.2, G2: 2.6 p=0.004; AST G1 6.6%, 2.6% p= 0.0035).

Table 1. Baseline characteristics of patients with Roux en Y anastomosis

	GROUP 1 With endoprosthesis	GROUP 2 Without endoprosthesis	p
	n (%)	n (%)	
N=75	25 (33)	50 (66)	
Male	6(8)	12(16)	
Female	19(25)	38(50)	0.823
Comorbidities (Hypertension, DM2)	2(2.6)	4(5.2)	1.000
Age (ED)	38 (11)	38 (12)	0.874
Open Cholecystectomy	13 (17)	31(41)	
Laparoscopic Cholecystectomy	12 (15)	19(25)	0.407

Also, previous endoscopic biliary stenting in patients with repeated episodes of cholangitis without early surgical treatment seems to be a relevant risk factor to develop postoperative stenosis (G1: 10.5%, G2: 1.3% p<0.0001). On the other hand, significant difference in terms of reoperation was not observed. The following variables did not show statistical difference: rate of cholangitis/5 years, reoperation and time to first episode of cholangitis.

Table 2. Preoperative Variables

	GROUP 1 With endoprosthesis	GROUP 2 Without endoprosthesis	p
	n (%)	n (%)	
N=75	25 (33)	50 (66)	
Number of previous stents (Mean, median, mode) (ED)	8, 4, 2 (8) Min, Max. 2-30	0	.
Preoperative complications			
Fistula	1(1.3)	13(17)	0.021*
Sepsis	3(4)	0(0)	0.012*
Biloma	3(4)	9(12)	0.504
Abscess	0(0)	5(0)	0.102
Preoperative Laboratories			
Total bilirubin >1.5	15(20)	36(47.5)	0.408
Direct bilirubin >0.2	18(23.8)	46(60.7)	0.052
ALT >59	13(17)	33(43.5)	0.429
AST >56	8(10.5)	29(38.2)	0.038*
ALP >153	19(25)	42(55.4)	0.609
Number of cholangitis episodes	6.36(1.4)	1 (.503)	<. 0001*
Number of cholangitis episodes/months (ED)	.22 (.28)	.20 (.34)	<. 0001*

*Significant values.
ALT: Alanine transaminase,
AST: Aspartate transaminase.
ALP: Alkaline phosphatase.

Table 3. Operative Variables

	GROUP 1 With endoprosthesis	GROUP 2 Without endoprosthesis	p
	n (%)	n (%)	
N=75	25 (33)	50(66)	
Segment IV resection	4(5.2)	46(60.7)	<0.0001*
Duration of operation Median (hours)	4.16 (ED 0.97)	4.20 (ED 0.87)	0.862
Operative bleeding ml	378.63 (ED 343.98)	347 (ED 294.25)	<. 0001*

*Significant Values.

A subanalysis (Table 5) of patients with criteria for endoscopic treatment failure (endoscopic treatment for 1 year with minimum 4 stent exchanges) was performed to avoid the selection bias caused by the authors preference to select all cases with previous endoscopic biliary stenting (with minimum 6 months of endoscopic treatment) as the main groups (Table 2, 3, 4); thereby, the main analysis was made to clear up if either immediate or mediate surgery treatment (<30 days, 1-12 months respectively after injury) influence clinical outcome in patients with hepaticojejunostomy.

Furthermore, the differences in the variables measured (preoperative sepsis, number of preoperative episodes of cholangitis, postoperative stenosis and radiological intervention) kept significantly higher on the stented group, as shown in table 5. Clinical outcome is the same as the ones showed with the main groups (N=75 G1: 25, G2: 50).

Table 4. Postoperative Variables

	GROUP 1 With endoprosthesis	GROUP 2 Without endoprosthesis	p
	n (%)	n(%)	
N=75	25 (33)	50(66)	
Laboratory Test (3 months)			
Total Bilirubin >1.5	6(8)	5(6.6)	0.102
Direct Bilirubin >0.2	0(0)	3(4)	0.152
ALT >59	5(6.6)	19(25)	0.090
AST >56	4(5.2)	19(25)	0.038*
ALP >153	12(16)	24(31.6)	0.922
Laboratory Test (12 months)			
Total Bilirubin >1.5	4(5.2)	3(4)	0.219
Direct Bilirubin >0.2	3(4)	2(2.6)	0.247
ALT >59	7(9.2)	2(2.6)	0.004*
AST >56	5(6.6)	2(2.6)	0.035*
ALP >153	7(9.2)	17(22.4)	0.349
Early Biliary Complications			
Early cholangitis	4(5.3)	3(4)	0.160
Abscess	1(1.3)	1(1.3)	0.612
Fistula	1(1.3)	1(1.3)	0.612
Biloma	1(1.3)	3(4)	0.716
Late Biliary Complications			
Stenosis	8(10.5)	1(1.3)	<. 0001*
Primary patency (Radiological Intervention)	5(6.6)	2(2.6)	0.017*
Secondary assisted patency (Reoperation)	4(5.3)	2(2.6)	0.071
Time to first episode of cholangitis (ED)	13.6 (22 months)	15.6 (15 months)	0.490
Rate of Cholangitis/5 years	1.25	1.20	0.095

*Significant values, ALT: Alanine transaminase, AST: Aspartate transaminase ALP: Alkaline phosphatase.

Discussion

Regarding the spectrum of postoperative bile duct injuries (BDI), the final result presents different outcomes.

It is possible to rehabilitate the bile duct completely using endoscopic treatment, in case of lateral injuries, but in other cases, patients might present late stenosis. These results are influenced by a myriad of factors, making it mostly unpredictable.

Factor that should be considered about these lesions are size, anatomical location, vascular involvement and the possibility of thermal injury, since they might play an important role on their evolution (incomplete or punctate lesions can be converted in complex injuries).

Table 5. Subanalysis of Preoperarive and Postoperative Variables in Patients with Endoscopic Treatment Failure

	GROUP 1 With endoprosthesis	GROUP 2 Without endoprosthesis	p
	n (%)	n (%)	
N=75	18 (33)	36(66)	
Preoperative Variables			
Bile Fistula	1 (2)	10 (18)	0.056
Sepsis	3 (6)	0	0.012*
Cholangitis episodes (DE)	2.38 (1.41)	0.5 (.5)	0.0007*
Cholangitis episodes/months (DE)	0.20 (.37)	0.17(.291)	0.0009*
Operative Variables Segment IV resection	2 (4)	34 (62)	<0.0001*
Postoperative Variables			
Laboratory Test (3 months)			
Total Bilirubin >1.5	4 (7)	4 (7)	0.228
Direct Bilirubin >0.2	6 (11)	6 (11)	0.215
ALT >59	3 (5)	12 (22)	0.204
AST >56	2 (4)	11(20)	0.118
ALP >153	7 (13)	18(33)	0.467
Laboratory Test (12 months)			
Total Bilirubin >1.5	3(6)	2(4)	0.343
Direct Bilirubin >0.2	3(6)	2(4)	0.343
ALT >59	7(13)	1(2)	0.003*
AST >56	5(9)	1(2)	0.021*
ALP >153	6(11)	12(22)	0.414
Early Biliary Complications			
Early cholangitis	3(5.5)	2(4)	0.183
Late Biliary Complications			
Stenosis	6(11)	1(2)	0.002*
Primary patency (Radiological Intervention)	4(7)	1(2)	0.020*
Secondary assisted patency (Reoperation)	4(7)	2(4)	0.066

*Significant values, ALT: Alanine transaminase, AST: Aspartate transaminase ALP: Alkaline phosphatase.

Endoscopic treatment is the mainstay of therapy for benign biliary strictures and surgery is reserved for selected patients in whom endoscopic treatment fails or is not feasible [5]. Complex lesions with complete section or obstruction of a main duct (Strasberg E) should receive surgical treatment through Roux-en-Y anastomosis as first line approach.

Minor bile duct injuries (Strasberg lesions from A to D, which are the most common, 68% of cases in our series) that preserve continuity are usually candidates for endoscopic treatment (endoprosthesis placement) and/or radiological intervention [6, 7].

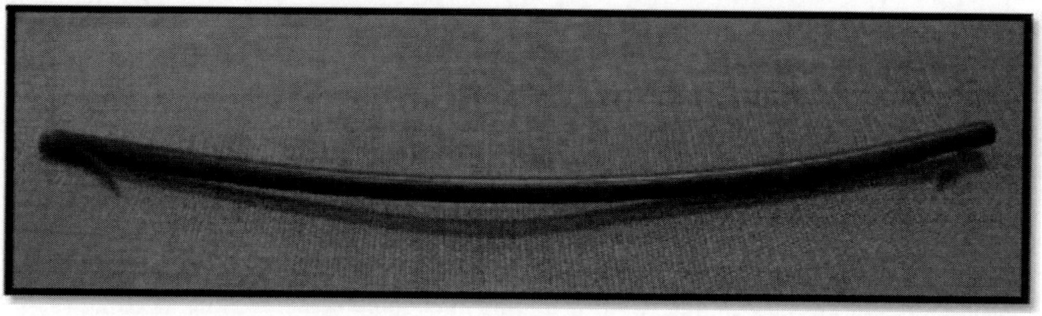

Figure 1. Endoprothesis used for small bile duct injuries.

The endoscopic insertion of plastic stents represents an effective system of biliary decompression, contributing to the improvement of the symptoms, determining a significant enhancement in quality of life in patients suffering from obstructive jaundice associated with benign strictures. However, the number of major limitations of this approach is mainly represented by stent occlusion, often followed by life-threatening cholangitis requiring repeated interventions and stent exchange [8]. Some papers have hypothesized about the mechanisms presumably involved in the clogging phenomenon of biliary endoprosthesis, for instance, deposition of biliary sludge and the presence of the multispecies nature of microbial biofilm, which progressively becomes thicker and contributes significantly to provoke occlusion of the endoprosthesis lumen [9-12].

Also, we report a greater number of preoperative sepsis in those patients with biliary endoprosthesis placement. Motte et al. mentioned risk factors for sepsis associated with this group of patients, including quality of drainage after the procedure, nature of the stricture, the type of drainage or prior cholangitis [13].

We reported a lower incidence of preoperative biliary fistula in group 1 (with endoprosthesis prior to surgical therapy). Weber et al. reported that endoscopic treatment of bile duct lesions was effective after cholecystectomy, particularly in patients with peripheral bile duct leakages and bile duct strictures [14].

After stenting the bile duct endoscopically and solving issues such as biliary compression, stenosis or bile duct leakages, it is necessary to evaluate weeks or months later the anatomic and functional conditions of the bile ducts, as well as those cases with duct-to-duct anastomosis (sometimes used to repair injuries with loss of continuity detected during the surgery). In our group no end-to-end anastomosis of the transected duct was performed in order to avoid tension and an undervascularized anastomosis, which, in consequence, might be associated with early dehiscence and/or fistulization of the anastomosis with late stenosis, making endoscopic treatment necessary [15]. However, in the case of liver transplants, the conditions and results of this therapy are opposite [16]. It is better to perform a high and wide hepaticojejunostomy at the outset due to the aforementioned reasons.

The endoscopic approach generally involves the placement of one or multiple plastic stents simultaneously with frequent replacements, dilation of the strictures or a combination of these approaches [5] (it requires a mean of four ERCPs over a 12 month period [4]). Both procedures require months of follow up. In consequence, it is not possible to determine when to consider an endoscopic treatment as a failure. Many times endoscopists face a stenotic area that is difficult to cross; in these cases it is necessary to perform immediate surgery, even though in other cases it is possible to maintain the patient without jaudince or cholangitis while the stent remains permeable. Therefore, this group of patients must be managed by a multidisciplinary team (surgeons, radiologists and gastroenterologist) to distribute the treatment options.

Our study confirms the long-term outcome of endoscopic treatment, taking into account the presence of a foreign body produces epithelial irritation, inflammatory reaction of the bile duct, and establishment of a biofilm; a key event in the formation of biliary sludge, pigment gallstones and the blockage of biliary stents [10-12, 17, 18].

Therefore, during surgical intervention all bile duct components are thickened.

Generally, circumferential stenotic injuries are classified as Strasberg E (with different distribution through the bile duct) and the advantage carried by this type of lesions, opposite to the 'classical' laparoscopic bile duct injury, is a longer proximal biliary tree in continuity with the gastrointestinal tract; this allows the opening of the bile duct proximal to the stenotic area and extension of the opening through the left bile duct, sometimes requiring partial resection of segment IV to find nonscarred and nonischemic ducts. This creates a safe and high quality anastomosis with significantly better results.

Our study shows long-term difference in relation to the anastomosis function. Patients in whom a stent was placed, inflammatory reaction of the bile duct secondary to foreign body and the newly formed stones causes long-term permeability problems requiring interventional radiology support to restore the proper function of the anastomosis.

For this reason, the communication between endoscopists and surgeons must be broad to decide the timing and fashion of the intervention.

We propose that if a long or difficult to cross stenotic area is found, this case must be referred to an advance surgery group to optimize the repair results.

It would be important to establish criteria to allow us to decide when should be the best time to perform surgical treatment and, thereby, avoid the preoperative and postoperative biliary complications.

Conclusion

Management of bile duct injuries must be multidisciplinary. When continuity of the bile duct is preserved, endoscopic biliary stenting is the treatment of choice. However, if a stenosis cannot be solved in a short period of time, it is necessary to promote early surgery (Roux-en-Y hepaticojejunostomy) to prevent postoperative long-term stenosis or radiological intervention. The presence of stents induces stone formation secondary to stasis, biliary colonization and foreign body reaction, provoking bile duct inflammation; surgery does not present such complications because the bile duct is complete and adequate for repair. Early intervention would decrease these three events, which would make surgical reconstruction easier and improve the long-term outcome.

References

[1] Fletcher, D. R., Hobbs, M. S., Tan, P., Valinsky, L. J., Hockey, R. L., Pikora, T. J., et al. Complications of cholecystectomy: risks of the laparoscopic approach and protective effects of operative cholangiography: a population-based study. *Ann. Surg*. 1999; 229: 449–457.

[2] Russell, J. C., Walsh, S. J., Mattie, A. S., Lynch, J. T. Bile duct injuries, 1989–1993. A statewide experience. Connecticut Laparoscopic Cholecystectomy Registry. *Arch. Surg*. 1996; 131: 382–388.

[3] Connor, C., Garden, O. J. Bile duct injury in the era of laparoscopic cholecystectomy. *British Journal of Surgery* 2006; 93: 158–168.

[4] Dumonceau, J. M., Tringali, A., Blero, D., Devière, J., Laugiers, R., Heresbach, D., Costamagna, G. *Biliary stenting: Indications, choice of stents and results: European Society of Gastrointestinal Endoscopy (ESGE) clinical guideline Endoscopy 2012*; 44: 277–298.

[5] Zepeda-Gómez, S., Baron, T. H. Benign biliary strictures: current endoscopic management. *Nat. Rev. Gastroenterol. Hepatol*. 2011 Sep. 6;8(10): 573-81.

[6] Mercado, M. A., Dominguez, I., Classification and management of bile duct injuries. *WJGS*. 2011; 3(4): 43.

[7] Lillemoe, K. D., Current management of bile duct injury. Department of Surgery, *British Journal of Surgery* 2008; 95: 403–405.

[8] Donielli, G., Di Rosa, R., Fiocca, F., Plastic Biliary Stent Occlusion: Factors Involved and Possible Preventive Approaches, *Clinical Medicine and Research* 2007; 5, (1): 53-60.

[9] Guaglianone, E., Cardines, R., Vuotto, C., Di Rosa, R., Babini, V., Mastrantonio, P., et al., Microbial biofilms associated with biliary stent clogging. *FEMS Immunol. Med. Microbiol*. 2010 Aug.; 59(3): 410–20.

[10] Speer, A. G., Cotton, P. B., Rode, J., Sedan, A. M., Neal, C. R., Holton, J., Costerton, J. W. Biliary stent blockage with bacterial biofilm. A light and electron microscopy study. *Ann. Intern. Med*. 1988; 108:546-553.

[11] Leung, J. W., Ling, T. K., Kung, J. L., Vallance-Owen, J. The role of bacteria in the blockage of biliary stents. *Gastrointest. Endosc*. 1988; 34:19-22.

[12] Leung, J. W., Liu, Y. L., Desta, T., Libby, E., Inciardi, J. F., Lam, K. Is there a synergistic effect between mixed bacterial infection in biofilm formation on biliary stents? *Gastrointest. Endosc*. 1998; 48:250-257.

[13] Motte, S., Deviere, J., Dumonceau, J. M., Serruys, E., Thys, J. P., Cremer, M. Risk factors for septicemia following endoscopic biliary stenting. *Gastroenterology*. 1991; 101(5): 1374-81.

[14] Weber, A., Feussner, H., Winkelmann, F., Siewert, J. R., Schmid, R. M., Prinz, C. Long-term outcome of endoscopic therapy in patients with bile duct injury after cholecystectomy. *J. Gastroenterol. Hepatol.* 2009 May; 24(5): 762–9.

[15] Mercado, M. A., Vilatobá, M., Chan, C., Domínguez, I. Intrahepatic Bilioenteric Anastomosis After Biliary Complications of Liver Transplantation: Operative Rescue of Surgical Failures.

[16] Mercado, M. A., Chan, C., Long-term Evaluation of Biliary Reconstruction After Partial Resection of Segments IV and V in Iatrogenic Injuries, *J. gastrointest. Surg.* 2006; 10:77–82.

[17] Sung, J. Y., Leung, J. W., Shaffer, E. A., Lam, K., Costerton, J. W. Bacterial biofilm, brown pigment stone and blockage of biliary stents. *J. Gastroenterol. Hepatol.* 1993; 8: 28-34.

[18] Van Berkel, J., van Marle, A., Groen, M. J., Mechanisms of Biliary Stent Clogging: Confocal Laser Scanning and Scanning Electron Microscopy, *Endoscopy* 2005; 37: 729-734.

In: Bile Duct
Editor: Miguel Ángel Mercado
ISBN: 978-1-63321-771-3

Chapter 9

Bile Duct Injury in the Elderly: A Single Center 20 Year Experience in Reconstruction

Miguel Ángel Mercado, MD[1], Alan Contreras, MD[2], Julio Alfaro Varela, MD[2], Ana Leticia Carrete, MD[2], Gerardo Tena, MD[2], Santiago Mier-y-Teran, MD[2] and Bruno A. González-Nolasco, MD[2]

[1]Professor, Chairman of the Department of Surgery,
National Institute of Medical Sciences and Nutrition "Salvador Zubiran"
[2]National Institute of Medical Sciences and Nutrition "Salvador Zubiran"

Abstract

Background: Hepatobiliary disease, especially issues concerning the gallbladder, is the most common indication for abdominal surgery in the elderly; therefore, cholecystectomies and bile duct injuries are expected to increase as the population ages. The aim of the study was to analyze the characteristics, management and outcome of bile duct injury repair in the elderly population through a 20-year period.

Methods: A retrospective analysis of the institutional database identified all patients that underwent surgical repair of the biliary tract secondary to bile duct injury from July 1992 to July 2012.

Results: A total of 486 patients were identified; 53 patients were identified as elderly population. They were allocated into two groups; Group 1 included 38 patients between 60 and 74 years of age and Group 2 included 15 patients with >75 years of age. The median age was 70 years. We found a direct correlation between the age of the patient and the amount of comorbidities associated; 64% of all patients had comorbidities, 58% in Group 1 and 80% in Group 2. Primary surgical repair was the most frequent procedure (51%) and the Hepp-Couinaud technique was performed in 70% of the cases. Postoperative complications were observed in 53% of the patients. Partial resection of segment IV-V was used in 51% of the patients and hepatectomy was necessary in 3

(5.6%) of the patients. Vasculobiliary injuries were found in 4 (7%) patients. Excellent outcome was achieved in 74% of the patients, successful outcome in 89% and poor outcome in 11% of the patients. Death occurred in 4 (7.5%) patients.

Conclusions: The present study's outcomes confirm that bilioenteric anastomoses in the elderly is a safe procedure with acceptable morbidity and mortality, and that using different techniques in order to achieve an adequate anastomosis does not increase morbidity. Excellent outcomes are expected in specialized centers and poor results occur in older patients with co-existing morbidities.

Keywords: Bile duct injury, bilioenteric anastomoses, elderly

Introduction

Life expectancy worldwide has increased. By the year 2025, the world will host 1.2 billion people aged 60 and over. This number will rise up to 1.9 billion in 2050 [1]. The incidence of diseases tends to increase with age [2] as well as the need for surgical procedures. Hepatobiliary disease, especially issues concerning the gallbladder, is the most common indication for abdominal surgery in the elderly; [3-7] therefore, cholecystectomies and bile duct injuries are expected to increase too.

Age is one of the critical factors that affect the mortality and morbidity rates after open or laparoscopic cholecystectomy [8, 9, 10]. Elderly patients who underwent surgery have more postoperative complications and prolonged hospital stay [2]. Macintyre et al. [11] described death as a complication after open cholecystectomy occurring almost exclusively in patients over 60 years. Although age has been identified as a risk factor for postoperative complications and poor outcome in hepatobiliary disease, there is scarce information in the medical literature regarding bile duct injury and its management in the elderly. The aim of the study is to describe bile duct injury in the elderly and provide an analysis of the surgical management and outcome in this age group.

Materials and Methods

Literature Search Strategy

Searches were conducted in PubMed and MEDLINE database using the MESH/Em Tree heading "bile duct injury in the elderly". We were only able to retrieve two articles, one published by Li Yan-xu et al. [12] published in the Chinese literature in 2009 with 38 cases and the second by Mercado et al. [13] published in 2004 with 20 cases.

Patients

The study was performed in a third level reference center specialized in bile duct injuries. During a 20 year period from July 1992 to July 2012, a total of 486 patients underwent surgical treatment for bile duct injury. We defined the elderly population according to the

World Health Organization as above 60 years of age for developing countries [14]. 53 patients were included in the study as part of the elderly population. These patients were allocated into two groups; Group 1 included patients between 60 to 74 years of age and Group 2 included patients >75 years.

All patients underwent a standard pretreatment evaluation that required a cholangioresonance or endoscopic retrograde cholangiopancreatography performed in our institution to diagnose the bile duct injury. Patients underwent either a primary repair surgery or surgical remodeling of a dysfunctional bilioenteric anastomosis. All surgeries were performed by the same surgeon. Patients referred to our institution with bile duct injury that didn't required surgical treatment were excluded from the study.

Complications

Complications were analyzed using the Clavien-Dindo Classification of Surgical Complications [15, 16] and Accordion Severity Grading System [17] during the first 30 postoperative days.

Follow-Up

Patients were followed-up at 3 month intervals during the first year, at 6 month interval during the second year and at 1 year interval after the second year from the surgery. Routine follow-up included physical examination and biochemical blood tests (liver function tests and complete blood count). Imaging studies were only indicated when dysfunction of the anastomosis was suspected. The bilioenteric anastomosis patency was assessed through the Terblanche Scale [18]. Patients that did not assist to their follow-up at least at 3 months after surgery were excluded from the follow-up analysis (Terblanche Scale) and those that didn't show up to their last scheduled check-up were considered lost; not being able to determine if they were alive or dead.

Statistical Analysis

Statistical analyses were performed using SPSS Version 20.0 (SPSS, Inc., Chicago, IL, USA). P-values ≤ 0.05 were deemed to indicate statistical significance.

Results

From a database of 486 cases of bilioenteric anastomosis due to bile duct injury performed through a 20 year period, 53 patients were considered elderly and thus selected for the study. Surgical repair was performed during the first decade of the study (July 1992 -July 2002) in 8 patients and during the second decade (July 2002 - July 2012) in 45 patients. This represents 29 (54%) more cases than those expected for the same time period. The elderly patients represented 11% of all the bilioenteric anastomosis performed during the study period. (Figure 1) The data was subdivided into two groups; Group 1 included patients between 60-74 years and Group 2 patients >75 years.

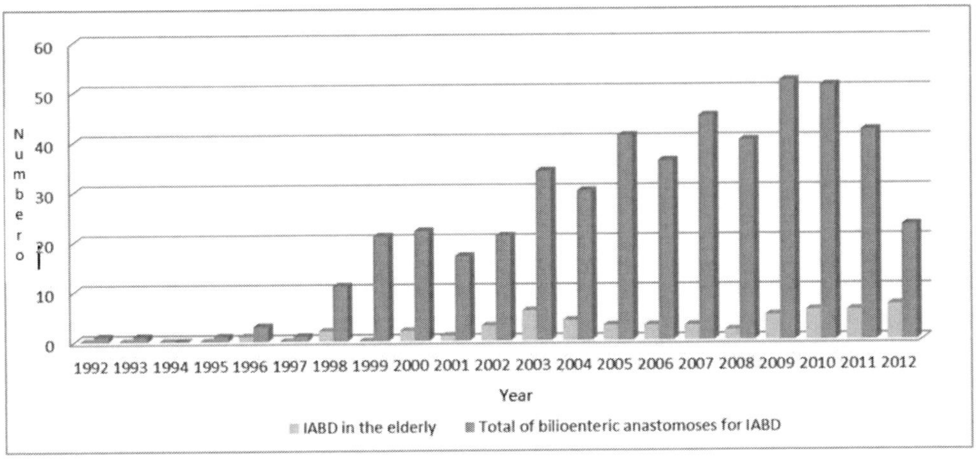

IBDI, Iatrogenic bile duct injury.

Figure 1. Bilioenteric anastomoses performed in 20 years.

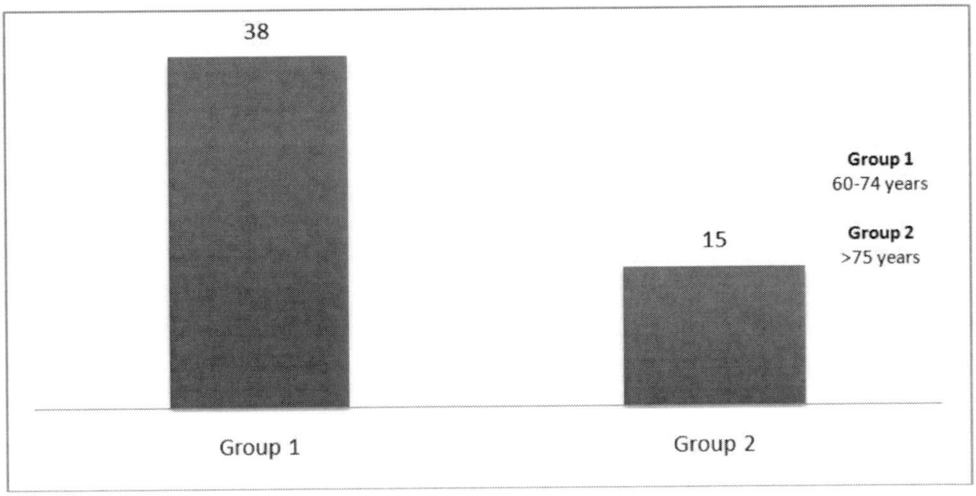

Figure 2. Group distribution.

General characteristics of both groups are described in Table 1. 23 patients (43%) were female and 30 (57%) were male (p= 0.35). Patients were divided as follows: 38 (72%) belonged to Group 1 and 15 (28%) to Group 2. (Figure 2) The median age of the population was 70 years (range 60 – 85 years); Group 1 had a median age of 66.8 $\pm$ 3.9 years and Group 2 had a median of 79 $\pm$ 3.5 years ($p < 0.05$).

Comorbidities were observed in 34 (n=53; 64%) patients from the whole population. 22 patients from Group 1 presented comorbidities (n=38; 58%) compared with 12 (n=15; 80%) patients (p=0.13) in Group 2. As expected, the older the patient, the more frequent the presence of comorbidities. The referral time from the patient´s original surgery place to our institution ranged from 7 days to 14 years (median 21.7 months). Group 1 had a referral time median of 23.6 months and Group 2 had a median of 19.9 months. The interval was less than 1 month in 11 patients (n=53; 22%), between 1 to 12 months in 21 patients (n=53; 39%) and more than 12 months in 21 patients (n=53%; 39%).

Postoperative complications were observed in 28 patients (n=53; 53%) (p=0.53). Group 1 had 20 observed complications (n=38; 53%) compared with Group 2 that had 8 observed complications (n=15; 53%) (p=1.0). Seventeen patients (32%) were considered lost and 32 (60.5%) were alive. There were 4 deaths (n=53) in the postoperative period, accounting for a perioperative mortality rate of 7.5%. Group 1 had 2 deaths (n=38; 5%); the cause of dead in the first case was septic complications during the placement of percutaneous pacemaker leading to piercing of the cardiac wall, and the second case was caused by mesenteric thrombosis. Group 2 had two deaths (n=15; 13%); the first death was due to septic shock secondary to cholangitis, and the second was caused by abdominal sepsis after right hepatectomy and primary repair.

Operating time, estimated blood loss, number of blood transfusions, partial resection of segment IV-V, the need of hepatectomy and vasculobiliary injuries were compared between Group 1 and Group 2 (Table 2).

Table 1. General characteristics of the study Groups

	Group 1	Group 2	TOTAL	P
Number of patients	38 (72%)	15 (28%)	53	
Age (median)	66.8 ±3.9	79 ±3.5	70	P<0.05
Gender				P=0.35
Male	15 (39.5%)	8 (53%)	23 (43%)	
Female	23 (60.5%)	7 (47%)	30 (57%)	
Comorbidities				P=0.13
Yes	22 (58%)	12 (80%)	34 (64%)	
No	16 (42%)	3 (20%)	19 (36%)	
Bilioenteric Anastomoses				P=0.15
Primary	17 (45%)	10 (67%)	27 (51%)	
Remodeling	21 (55%)	5 (33%)	26 (49%)	
Postoperative Complications				P=1.0
Yes	20 (53%)	8 (53%)	28 (53%)	
No	18 (47%)	7 (47%)	25 (47%)	
Interval time to referral	23.6 m	19.9 m	21.7 m	
< 1 month	8 (21%)	3 (20%)	11 (22%)	
1-12 months	14 (37%)	7 (47%)	21 (39%)	
>12 months	16 (42%)	5 (33%)	21 (39%)	
Deaths	2 (5%)	2 (13%)	4 (7.5%)	P=0.31
Lost	13	4	17 (32%)	
Alive	23	9	32 (60.5%)	

Table 2. Surgical characteristics of the study groups

	Group 1 N=38	Group 2 N=15	TOTAL N=53	P
Operating Time (Mean) Range	183 min (180-720)	169 min (180-330)	244 min (180-720)	
Blood loss	615 ml	482 ml	581 ml	*P*=0.47
Partial resection of segment IV - V	22 (58%)	5 (33%)	27 (51%)	*P*=0.1
Hospital stay (mean) Range	12 días (5-69)	10 días (6-29)	11 días (5-69)	
Blood transfussions	250 ml	250 ml	250 ml	
Type of bilioenteric anastomoses (Primary) Hepp-Couinaud Portoenterostomy HJ + neo-formation of confluence	17/38 (45%) 12/17 (70%) 3/17 (18%) 2/17 (12%)	10/15 (67%) 7/9 (67%) 1/9 (11%) 2/9 (22%)	27/53 (51%) 18/26 (70%) 4 (15%) 4 (15%)	
Remodeling Hepp-Couinaud Portoenterostomy HJ + neo-formation of confluence	21/38 (55%) 12/21(57%) 1/21 (5%) 8/21 (38%)	5/15 (33%) 5/5 (100%) 0 0	26/53 (49%) 17/26 (65%) 1/26 (4%) 8/26 (31%)	
Hepatectomy Right Left	 2 (5%) 0	 1 (6%) 0	 3/53 (5.6%) 0	*P*=0.84
Vasculobiliary injuries	3 (8%)	1 (6%)	4/53 (7%)	*P*=0.88

HJ, hepaticojejunostomy.

Group 1 showed a longer operative time, with a median of 183 minutes (range=180-720 minutes). Group 2 had a median operative time of 169 minutes (range=180-330 minutes). Operative blood loss median was 581 ml for the whole population; 615 ml for Group 1 and 482 ml for Group 2 (p=0.47).

Partial resection of segment IV-V was more frequently done in Group 1, accounting for twenty-one (n=38; 55%) patients compared to 6 patients of Group 2 (n=15; 40%), with no statistical difference (p=0.1). Group 1 showed an Odds ratio of 2.75 (95% CI 0.78-9.61) for partial liver segment resection and a longer operative time, suggesting that this group required more technically challenging procedures, with more remodeling surgeries than primary repairs when compared to Group 2. In the whole population, 27 patients (51%) had primary repair surgery and 26 (49%) had remodeling of a previous bilioenteric anastomoses. Group 1 had primary repair performed in 17 cases (n=38; 45%) and remodeling in 21 (n=53; 55%). Group 2 patients underwent primary repair in 10 cases (n=15; 67%) and remodeling in 5 (n=15; 33%). Older patients showed more primary reconstructions.

The average hospital stay was 12 days (range=5-69 days) for Group 1 and 10 days (range=6-29 days) for Group 2.

Three type of reconstruction techniques were performed by the same surgeon: hepaticojejunostomy (Hepp-Couinaud), portoenterostomy and hepaticojejunsotomy with neo-formation of the confluence. All procedures had a Roux-en-Y intestinal loop. Surgical techniques in Group 1 distributed as follows: Hepp-Couinaud in 12 cases (n=17; 70%), portoenterostomy in 3 patients (n=17; 18%) and hepaticojejunostomy with neo-formation of the confluence in 2 patients (n=17; 12%). In Group 2, seven patients (n=9; 67%) underwent a Hepp-Couinaud, 1 patient (n=9; 11%) went through a portoenterostomy and 2 patients (n=9; 22%) had a hepaticojejunostomy with neo-formation of the confluence.

Group 1 had the following remodeling surgical procedures: 12 Hepp-Couinaud (n=21; 57%), 1 portoenterostomy (n=21; 5%) and 8 hepaticojejunostomy with neo-formation of the confluence (n=21; 38%). In Group 2 the only remodeling technique used was the Hepp-Couinaud in 5 patients (n=5; 100%).

Nineteen patients (n=21; 90%) in Group 1 that underwent a remodeling of the anastomosis had only one previous surgery, 1 patient (n=21; 5%) had two previous surgeries and 1 other (n=21; 5%) had 3 previous surgeries. In Group 2, all 5 patients (n=5; 100%) that required remodeling of the anastomosis had only one previous surgery.

Two right hepatectomies (n=38; 5%) were performed in Group 1, and only one (n=15; 6%) in Group 2 (p=0.84). Vasculobiliary injuries were found in 4 patients (n=53; 7%); 3 of them (n=38; 8%) in Group 1 and one (n=15; 6%) in Group 2 (p=0.88). The mortality rate for hepatectomies in the elderly with bile duct injury was 33%.

It is expected that older patients will have more associated comorbidities. Indeed, patients in Group 2 had more comorbidities as shown in table 3. Two concomitant comorbidities co-existed in 6 patients of Group 1 (n=38; 28%).

Three concomitant comorbidities were presented in 5 patients (n=38; 23%). In group 2, four patients (n=15; 33%) had two co-existing comorbidities and 3 patients (n=15; 33%) had three combined comorbidities.

The most frequent form of clinical presentation of the bile duct injury was cholangitis, reported in 31 patients (n=53, 58%) (p=0.16), followed by jaundice in 11 patients (N=53; 21%) (p=0.5). In Group 1, cholangitis was observed in 20 patients (n=38; 53%), jaundice in 7 of them (n=7; 18%), and biliary fistula in 6 (n=38; 16%). In Group 2, cholangitis was reported in 11 patients (n=15; 73%), and jaundice in 4 (n=38; 27%). Older patients are more likely to present with cholangitis (73% vs. 53%) according to our data (Figure 3).

Table 3. Associated comorbidities

	Group 1 (n=38)	Group 2 (n=15)	TOTAL (n=53)
High blood pressure	5	1	6/53 (11%)
Diabetes Mellitus 2	2	1	3/53 (6%)
Hyperuricemia	1		1/53 (2%)
Dyslipidemia	1		1/53 (2%)
Heart disease		1	1/53 (2%)
Obesity	1		1/53 (2%)
Liver cirrhosis		1	1/53 (2%)
2 Comorbidities	6 (28%)	4 (33%)	10 (19%)
3 Comorbidities	5 (23%)	3 (25%)	8 (15%)
> 3 Comorbidities	1 (4%)	1 (8%)	2 (4%)
TOTAL	22/38 (58%)	12/15 (80%)	34 (64%)

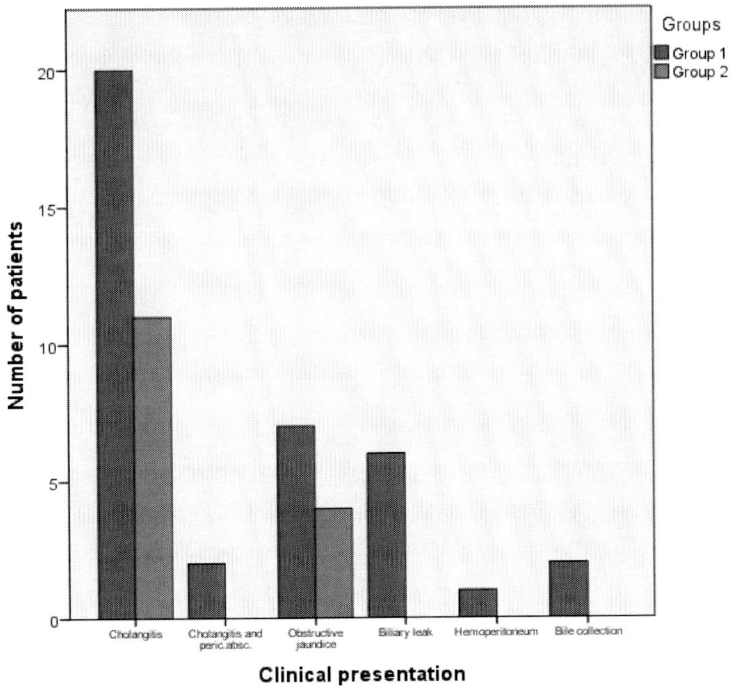

Figure 3. Clinical presentation of bile duct injuries.

Table 4. Postoperative complications

	Group 1 N=20	Group 2 N=8	TOTAL N=28	p
Intraabdominal fluid collection	5/20 (25%)	3/8 (37.5%)	8/28 (28%)	*P*=0.33
Cholangitis	9/20 (45%)	2/8 (25%)	11/28 (36%)	*P*=0.50
Biliary fistula	2/20 (10%)	1/8 (12.5%)	3/28 (11%)	*P*=0.72
Pericholangitic abscess	3/20 (15%)	0	3/28(11%)	
Wound infection	3/20 (15%)	0	3/28 (11%)	
Wound hematoma	1/20 (5%)	2/8 (25%)	3/28 (11%)	*P*=0.07
Pneumonia	1/20 (5%)	2/8 (25%)	3/28 (11%)	*P*=0.07
Acute renal failure	1/20 (5%)	0	1/28 (4%)	
Urinary tract infection	1/20 (5%)	0	1/28 (4%)	
Mesenteric thrombosis	1/20 (5%)	0	1/28 (4%)	
Bactcricmia	2/20 (10%)	0	2/28 (8%)	
Sepsis	3/20 (15%)	0	3/28 (11%)	
Septic shock	0	1/8 (12.5%)	1/28 (4%)	
Hypovolemic shock	1/20 (5%)	1/8 (12.5%)	2/28 (8%)	*P*=0.39
TOTAL	21/38 (50%)	7/15 (47%)	28/53 (53%)	*P*=0.57

In the present study, 28 (n=53; 53%) patients had postoperative complications. Group 1 had 20 postoperative complications (n=38; 53%), and Group 2 had 8 postoperative complication cases (n=15; 53%).

The most common complication was cholangitis (11/28; 36%) and intrabdominal fluid collection (8/28; 28%). It is important to notice that in most cases complications were not unique, and were usually combined with more than one concomitant complication. Younger patients were more likely to present cholangitis (45% vs. 25%) and older patients were more likely to present intraabdominal fluid collections (37.5% vs. 25%) (Table 4).

The Clavien-Dindo and Accordion classifications were used to standardize our results (Table 5). According to the classification of Clavien-Dindo, in Group 1 there was no complication Grade 1; 9 patients (n=20; 45%) had Grade 2 complications; 4 patients (n=20; 20%) had Grade 3a; 1 (n=20; 5%) had Grade 3b; 3 patients (n=20; 15%) had Grade 4a, 1 patient (n=20; 5%) had Grade 4b and 2 patients (n=20, 10%) had Grade 5 complications. Patients in Group 2 had no complications considered Grade 1; 2 patients (n=8; 25%) had Grade 2; 3 (n=8; 37.5%) patients presented Grade 3a; 1 patient (n=8; 12.5%) had Grade 3b, and 2 patients (n=8; 25%) had Grade 5.

We also used the Accordion classification. Group 1 had no complications Grade 1; 9 patients (n=20; 45%) had Grade 2; 4 patients (n=20; 20%) had Grade 3; 5 (n=20; 25%) had Grade 5; 2 patients (n=20; 10%) had Grade 6 complications. Group 2 had 1 patient (n=8; 12.5%) with Grade 1; 1 (n=8; 12.5%) with Grade 2; 3 patients (n=8; 37.5%) with Grade 3; 1 patient (n=8; 12.5%) with Grade 4; and 2 patients (n=8; 25%) with Grade 6 complications.

The indications for surgery in the elderly are summarized in Table 6. Cholecystolithiasis was the main surgical indication in our series with 33 patients (n=53; 62%). In Group 1, cholecystolithiasis presented in 26 patients (n=38; 68%), acute cholecystitis in 10 (n=38; 26%), acalculous cholecystitis in 1 patient (n=38; 3%) and chronic colecystitis in 1 other patient (n=38; 3%). In Group 2, acute cholecystitis presented in 7 patients (n=15; 47%), cholecystolithiasis in 7 patients (n=15; 47%) and chronic cholecystitis in 1 (n=15; 6%) (Figure 4). Younger patients are more likely to suffer bile duct injury during elective surgery for cholecystolithiasis than older patients (68% vs. 47%), with no statistical significance (p=0.14). Older patients are more likely to suffer bile duct injury during emergency surgery for acute cholecystitis than younger patients (47% vs. 26%), with no statistical significance (p=0.15).

Table 5. Postoperative complications (Clavien-Dindo and Accordion)

CLASIFICATION OF COMPLICATIONS	Group 1 N=20 (%)	Group 2 N=8 (%)
Clavien-Dindo		
1	0	0
2	9 (45%)	2(25%)
3ª	4 (20%)	3 (37.5%)
3b	1 (5%)	1 (12.5%)
4ª	3 (15%)	0
4b	1 (5%)	0
5	2 (10%)	2 (25%)
ACCORDION		
1	0	1 (12.5%)
2	9 (45%)	1 (12.5%)
3	4 (20%)	3 (37.5%)
4	0	1 (12.5%)
5	5 (25%)	0
6	2 (10%)	2 (25%)

Table 6. Etiology of the injury

Etiology	Group 1 N=38 (%)	Group 2 N=15 (%)	TOTAL N=53 (%)	P
Acute cholecytitis	10 (26%)	7 (47%)	17/53 (32%)	p=0.15
Chronic cholecystitis	1 (3%)	1 (6%)	2/53 (4%)	P=0.48
Cholecystolithiasis	26 (68%)	7 (47%)	33/53 (62%)	P=0.14
Acalculous cholecystitis	1 (3%)	0	1/53 (2%)	

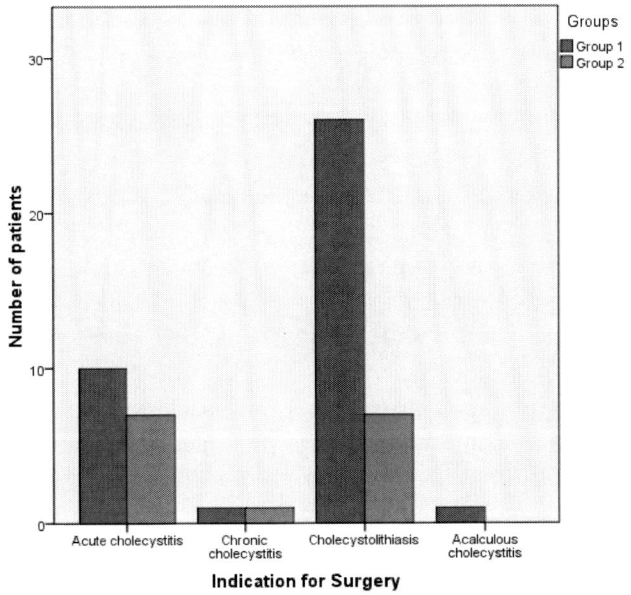

Figure 4. Etiology of the injury.

Table 7. Type of surgery in which the injury occurred

Type of surgery	Group 1 (%)	Group 2 (%)	TOTAL	OR
Open Cholecystectomy	27 (71%)	10 (67%)	37 (70%)	OR 1.22 95%CI 0.34-4.43
Laparoscopic Cholecystectomy	11 (29%)	5 (33%)	16 (30%)	OR 0.81 95% CI 0.23-2.93

Bile duct injury occurred in patients who underwent either open or laparoscopic cholecystectomy. Among all 53 patients, injury occurred during open cholecystectomy in 37 patients (70%) and during laparoscopic cholecystectomy in 16 patients (30%). Injury during open cholecystectomy had an Odds ratio of 1.22 (95% CI 0.34-4.43) (Table 7). In Group 1, injury occurred during open cholecystectomy in 27 cases (n=38; 71%) and during laparoscopic cholecystectomy in 11 patients (n=38; 29%). Among Group 2, injury occurred during open cholecystectomy in 10 patients (n=15; 67%) and during laparoscopic cholecystectomy in 5 patients (n=15; 33%) (Figure 5). Injury is more likely to occur in the elderly during open cholecystectomy than laparoscopic (70% vs. 30%).

Outcome of the anastomosis was evaluated according to the Terblanche scale (Table 8). It is important to consider that in this analysis we excluded 7 patients that did not assist to their follow-up consult in at least the first 3 months.

Table 8. Outcome of definitive surgical treatment

Terblanche scale	Group 1 N=36 (%)	Group 2 N=10 (%)	Total N= 46	Odds Ratio CI 95%
I Excellent results	29 (80%)	5 (50%)	34 (74%)	OR 4.14 95%CI 0.93-18.36
II Good results	2 (6%)	1 (10%)	3 (6%)	
III Satisfactory results	3 (8%)	1 (10%)	4 (9%)	
IV Poor results	2 (6%)	3 (30%)	5 (11%)	

Table 9. Factors associated to predicting outcome after surgical repair

Factors predicting outcome	Failure/Total (%)	*P* value
Total	5/46 (11%)	
No previous repair Hepaticojejunostomy Portoenterostomy HJ + neo-confluence	2/21 (9.5%) 1/15 (6.6%) 1/4 (25%) 0/2 (0%)	P=0.8
Previous repair Hepaticojejunostomy Portoenterostomy HJ + neo-confluence	3/25 (12%) 2/17 (11.7%) 0/1 (0%) 1/7 (14.2%)	P=0.8
Partial resection of segment IV-V	2/26 (7.6%)	P=0.43
Vasculobiliary injury	1/4 (25%)	P=0.44
Hepatectomy	0/2 (0.0%)	
Comorbidities 1 2 3 >3	4/30 (13%) 1/12 (8%) 2/10 (20%) 0/5 (0.0%) 1/3 (33%)	P=0.93
No comorbidities	1/16 (6%)	P=0.79
Interval to reference <1 month 1-12 months >12 months	 1/11 (9%) 1/16 (6.25%) 3/19 (15.7%)	P=0.59
Age 60-74 years >75 years	 2/36 (6%) 3/10 (30%)	P=0.02

HJ, hepaticojejunostomy.

Patient follow-up in Group 1 showed the following: 29 patients (n=36; 80%) had excellent results (Grade I), 2 patients (n=36; 6%) had good results (Grade II), 3 patients (n=36; 8%) had satisfactory results (Grade III) and 2 patients (n=36; 6%) had poor results (Grade IV). Patients in Group 2 showed the following pattern: excellent results were achieved in 5 patients (Grade I) (n=10; 50%), good results (Grade II) in 1 patient (n=10; 10%), satisfactory results (Grade III) in 1 patient (n=10; 10%) and poor results (Grade IV) in 3 patients (n=10; 30%). Younger patients are more likely to have an excellent outcome than older patients (80% vs. 50%) Older patients are more likely to have poor outcome when compared to younger patients (6% vs. 30%). Factors predicting possible outcome failure are listed in Table 9.

Discussion

In the present study we show the results of our experience as a tertiary level reference center for biliary duct reconstruction after bile duct injury, having performed more than 486 bilioenteric derivations in over 20 years (1992-2012). Of all the surgical reconstructions performed, 53 of them were done in elderly patients, representing 11% of all the surgeries. During the second decade (2002-2012) we experienced an increase of 54% of elderly patient cases in this study group, and as shown in other studies, this aging group will continue to increase [1].

Cholecystolithiasis is the most common abdominal surgical disease in the elderly, considering 50% of women and 15% of men aged ≥60 years are estimated to have gallstones. [19] It has a prevalence of 21.4% in people aged 60 to 69 years and 27.5% in individuals aged over 70 years [20]. Therefore, surgical treatment of different biliary tract diseases has increased in the elderly, and iatrogenic bile duct injuries may be expected to increase as well. There is scarce information regarding bile duct injury reconstruction or repair reported in the medical literature, which makes the need for information in this growing population more evident. Mercado et al., [13] published a 10 year experience with bile duct reconstruction after iatrogenic bile duct injury in the elderly, which is one of the few studies available that addresses this group of patients.

As age increases, comorbidities are expected to appear more frequently. In our study, we found that 64% of all the patients had associated comorbidities, generally more than one of them. The older the patient, the more comorbidities associated at the time of the study. 58% of the patients presented comorbidities when they were <74 years of age. This proportion increases to 80% in patients >75 years.

Although the elderly are at increased risk for surgery because of associated comorbidities [21], this study shows that post-operative complications in patients <74 years and older than 75 years were similar (53% vs. 53% respectively), without statistical significance p=1.0, and it was not associated with the presence of comorbidities. Old age is one of the critical factors affecting the morbidity and mortality rates after biliary surgery [8,9], but based on our results, bilioenteric anastomoses are a safe procedure and should not have worse outcome when performed in elderly people; less invasive procedures should not be attempted based solely on age, but definitive surgical resolution of the injury. Promptly referrering patients to centers specialized in bile duct injuries is essential for the achievement of excellent results. The low complication rates between young and elderly may be associated with an improvement in surgical and anesthetic techniques, as well as with better management in the post-operative period in highly specialized centers.

Laparoscopic cholecystectomy is now accepted by most surgeons as the "gold standard" procedure for biliary diseases, even for acute cholecystitis [22] and it is the treatment of choice in elderly patients [23]. It is important to remember that age has never been a contraindication for laparoscopic cholecystectomy [24], but most authors advise maintaining a low threshold for conversion to an open procedure in such patients [25, 26]. Bile duct injuries are more frequent during laparoscopic cholecystectomy (3 to 6 in 1000 cases) compared with an open approach [27]. Flum et al. [28] described that the incidence of bile duct injuries in the elderly patient is completely comparable to that of the younger population. During our 20 year study period, most of the injuries in elderly patients referred to our institution occurred during open cholecystectomy compared to laparoscopic cholecystectomy (70% vs. 30% respectively); this finding does not correlate with data previously published. Interestingly, most bile duct injuries occurred while performing surgery indicated for cholecystolithiasis (62%) and not for acute cholecystitis (32%). In patients older than 75 years, injuries occurred with the same frequency while performing surgery for cholecystolithiasis (47%) and acute cholecystitis (47%). This is probably explained by the need of more emergency surgery in older patients.

Different types of surgical techniques have been described to repair bile duct injuries; including end-to-end anastomosis [29], choledochoduodenostomy, [30] and hepaticojejunostomy [31]. The Roux-en-Y hepaticojejunostomy offers the best results, and is the authors´ preferred approach [32]. Lillemoe et al. [33 described that surgical Roux-en-Y hepaticojejunostomy reconstruction is associated to an overall success rate of 90%. Portoenterostomy is a technique used when the injury does not allow adequate anastomosis to the biliary ducts and in the authors experience, a third of these cases require radiological o surgical reintervention [32, 34]. When the injury is near the confluence and when a simple anastomosis is difficult, the "bile duct growing factor" is an excellent alternative for repair [35]. Our results demonstrate that in patients below 74 years, most of the anastomoses (55%) had previous repair attempts and patients above 75 years, most of them (67%) had no previous repair attempts. The Hepp-Couinaud technique was the most frequent surgical repair performed in our study group. Patients who had poor outcome according to the Terblanche scale had previous repair attempts in 60% of the cases. The repair technique that was associated to worst complications; according to Clavien (Grade 5) and Accordion (Grade 6) was portoenterostomy (100%) for Group 1 and for Group 2 was portoenterostomy (50%) and Hepp-Couinaud (50%), all of them had previous repair attempt. The mortality for our study group was higher in patients who underwent portoenterostomy, with 75% of the deaths occurring in this group. Our mortality rate for portoenterostomy in the elderly was of 60% and should be considered as a high risk factor for death in this group of age. To achieve the best surgical results, patients should be promptly referred to specialized centers.

Achieving a high quality anastomosis; defined as a tension-free, wide, done with the adequate suture material, and performed on healthy bile ducts, offers the best results [35]. Additional maneuvers may be needed in order to complete such an anastomosis. These techniques include partial resection of segment IV and V [36, 37, 38], these are especially useful in complex injuries with loss of the biliary confluence or in patients with multiple repair attempts, allowing adequate exposition of the ducts and a high quality anastomosis.

Our study demonstrated that 49% of our patients required partial resection of segment IV or V; this was more frequent in Group 1, which was also the group with higher number of remodeling procedures (55%). Therefore, partial resection of liver segments is more frequent in patients with previous reconstruction attempts and is not associated with increased complication rates in the elderly. Mercado et al., [37] demonstrated that partial liver resection improves the probability of achieving a high quality bilioenteric anastomosis, without increasing morbidity or mortality rates.

Biliary injuries are commonly associated with vascular injuries, especially arterial injuries [39]. Deziel et al. found that 12% of bile duct injuries were associated with right hepatic artery injury [40]; two centers reported an incidence of right hepatic artery injury in 41% of the patients in one study [41] and 61% of the patients in the another [42, 43]. In our study we found 4 vasculobiliary injuries, which represented 7% of all cases, requiring right hepatectomy in two cases (50%). Seventy five percent of the vasculobiliary injuries occurred in patients between 60 and 74 years. It is important to emphasize that most of the patients in the former group had had at least one previous repair attempt. Strassberg et al. [43] recommends the image assessment of the hepatic arteries as part of the work up in all major biliary injuries. This also indirectly indicates that liver blood flow is compensated through collaterals that during complex biliary injury are interrupted and cause liver ischemia. We consider that it is important to assess the vascular status of the patients because atherosclerotic changes may affect the formation of collateral shunts; this would explain the high incidence of vasculobiliary injuries and the need for hepatectomy in the elderly. Strassberg et al. [43] estimates that the incidence of right liver infarction in right hepatic artery vasculobiliary injuries is about 10%. Nevertheless, a 50% incidence of hepatectomy in confirmed vasculobiliary injuries is very high; suggesting that probably in the elderly the incidence of liver infarction is much higher. Our mortality rate of vasculobiliary injuries and right hepatectomy in the elderly was 25%, similar to that described by Li et al. [44] It has been reported that biliary-enteric anastomosis for bile duct injury is potentially lethal if associated with vascular injury, leading to a high rate of morbidity with reduced long-term survival [41, 45, 46]. Buell et al. [47] found that an associated arterial injury is an independent predictor of mortality (38% with arterial injury versus 3% without it $p<0.001$). The physiopathology of vasculobiliary injuries in the elderly should be explored more thoroughly in future studies.

The objective of bilioenteric anastomosis in bile duct injury is to reconstruct the biliary tract allowing bile to flow into the gastrointestinal tract, preventing cholestasis, cholangitis, recurrent strictures and, ultimately, secondary biliary cirrhosis and death. There are several grading systems to evaluate the outcome of bilioenteric anastomosis based in clinical and biochemical parameters, including the scales of Terblanche, Mcdonald and Lillemoe, among others. Obtaining a bilioenteric anastomosis, in which no clinical or biochemical parameters of cholestasis are detected, may be considered a successful anastomosis. In our study, we used the Terblanche [18] grading system. A successful outcome after surgical repair of bile duct injury was observed in 70-90% of patients in referral centers. [18, 48, 49] Lillemoe et al. [33] described in a series of cases from John Hopkins, an excellent result in 71.1% of the cases, successful outcome in 90.8% of the cases and failure in 9.2% of their cases. Our results are similar, with an excellent outcome in 74% of our cases, a successful outcome in 89% of our patients and failure or poor results in 11% of our cases. Terblanche classification Grade 1-3 was considered a successful treatment. It is important to consider that patients with more than 75 years had worse outcome than the younger ones, obtaining excellent results only in 50% of these cases and failure in 30%, compared to the younger patients that obtained excellent results in 80% of the cases and failure only in 6% of the patients. Age should be considered as a poor prognosis factor in the follow-up after bile duct injury reconstruction.

The mortality rates for emergency cholecystectomy among the elderly have been reported to range from 6 to 15 % [50]. In general, these results are similar to the outcomes when gastrointestinal surgery is performed on the elderly [51]. Previous studies in open cholecystectomy in elderly patients have found mortality rates of 0.6–7.5% [52-56] and in the elderly patients who have undergone laparoscopic cholecystectomy, an overall mortality rate of 0.7% has been shown [22, 25, 57-60]. Savassi-Rocha et al. [61] published their results regarding 167 patients with bile duct injury, in which a mortality rate of 4.2% was found. Our mortality rate for bilioenteric derivations secondary to bile duct injuries was 7.5 % with no difference with respect between age groups. Therefore, bilioenteric derivations do not confer a higher risk of mortality in the elderly. It is important to report that the death events in our study were associated to postoperative complications, and many patients were lost to follow-up, not being able to determine if they were alive or deceased.

Conclusion

Surgical procedures in patients > 60 years of age are increasing steadily, including bilioenteric anastomosis secondary to bile duct injury. In the present study, we provide evidence that bilioenteric anastomosis in the elderly can be performed safely after bile duct injury with a high likelihood of long-term patency. Age is a poor prognostic factor for dysfunction of the anastomosis in the long-term, but not for postoperative complications. The portoenterostomy procedure is a risk factor for complications and death in the elderly, and vasculobiliary injuries are associated to more frequent liver infarction and the need for hepatectomy.

References

[1] World Population Prospects: The 2002 Revision, Highlights. New York: Unite Nations Population Division; 2003. (ESA/P/WP. 180).

[2] Joshi K, Kumar R, Avasthi A. Morbidity profile and its relationship with disability and psychological distress among elderly people in Northern India. *International Journal of Epidemiology, 2003*; 32:978-987.

[3] Bennion LJ, Grundy SM. Risk factors for the development of cholelithiasis in man. *N. Engl. J. Med.,* 1979;299:1221–1227.

[4] Brunt LM, Quasebarth DL, Dunnegan DL, et al. Outcomes analysis of laparoscopic cholecystectomy in the extremely elderly. *Surg. Endosc.,* 2001;15:700–705.

[5] Shamburek RD, Farrar JT. Disorders of the digestive system in the elderly. *N. Engl. J. Med.,* 1990;322:438–443.

[6] Kahng KU, Roslyn JJ. Surgical issues for the elderly patient with hepatobiliary disease. *Surg. Clin. North Am.,* 1994;74:345–373.

[7] Rege RV. 1998 Asymptomatic gallstones. In: Cameron JL (editor). Current Surgical Therapy, 6th edition. Mosby–Year Book, St. Louis, 403–405.
[8] Deziel DJ. Complications of cholecystectomy. *Surg. Clin. N Am.,* 1994; 74: 809-23.
[9] McSherry CK, Glenn F. The Incidence and causes of death following surgery for non-malignant biliary tract disease. *Ann. Surg.,* l98O; 191:271-5.
[10] Jatzko GR, Lisborg PH, Pert! AM, Stettner HM. Multivariate comparison of complications after laparoscopic cholecystectomy and open cholecystectomy. *Ann. Surg.,* 1995; 221: 381-6.
[11] Macintyre IMC, Wilson RG. Laparoscopic cholecystectomy. *Br. J. Surg.,* 1993; 80: 552-9.
[12] LI Yan-xu,CHAI Xin-qun,FENG Xian-song,et al. Bile duct reoperations in elderly patients: An analysis of 38 cases. *Journal of Abdominal Surgery,* 2009-03.
[13] Mercado MA, Chan C, Hinojosa C, et al. Bile Duct Reconstruction after Iatrogenic Injury in the Elderly. *Annals of Hepatology,* 2004; 3(4): 160-162.
[14] World Health Organization. 2012. "Definition of an Older or Elderly Person." Retrieved January 28, 2012 (http://www.who.int/healthinfo/survey/ageingdefnolder /en/index.html).
[15] Clavien PA. Sanabria JR. Strasberg SM. Proposed classification of complications of surgery with examples of utility in cholecystectomy. *Surgery,* 1992;111(5):518 –526.
[16] Dindo D, Demartines N, Clavien PA. Classification of surgical complications. A new proposal with evaluation in a cohort of 6336 patients and results of a survey. *Ann. Surg.,* 2004;240:205–213.
[17] Strasberg SM, Linehan DC, Hawkins WG. The accordion severity grading system of surgical complications. *Ann. Surg.,* 2009; 250:177–186.
[18] Terblanche J, Worthley CS, Spence RAJ, Krige JAJ. High or low Hepaticojejunostomy in Biliary Stricture 167 hepaticojejunostomy for bile duct strictures. *Surgery,* 1990; 108: 828-834.
[19] A-Hon Kwon, Matsui Y. Laparoscopic Cholecystectomy in Patients Aged 80 Years and Over. *World J. Surg.,* (2006) 30: 1204–1210.
[20] Régo RE, de Campos T, de Moricz A, Silva RA, Pacheco Júnior AM. Cholecystectomy in the elderly: early results of open versus laparoscopic approach. *Rev. Assoc. Med. Bras.,* 2003; 49(3):293-9.
[21] Escarce JJ, Shea JA, Chen W, Qian Z, Schwartz JS. Outcomes of open cholecystectomy in the elderly: a longitudinal analysis of 21,000 cases in the prelaparoscopic era. Surgery 1995; 117: 156-164.
[22] Lujan JA, Sanchez-Bueno F, Parrilla P, Robles R, Torralba JA,Gonzalez-Costea R. Laparoscopic vs. open cholecystectomy in patients aged 65 and older. *Surg. Laparosc. Endosc.,* 1998; 8: 208-210.
[23] Polychronidis A, Botaitis S, Tsaroucha A, Tripsianis G, Bounovas A, Pitiakoudis M, et al. Laparoscopic cholecystectomy in elderly patients. *J. Gastrointest. Liver Dis.,* 2008; 17(3):309-13.
[24] Reddick EJ, Olsen DO. Laparoscopic laser cholecystectomy. *Surg. Endosc.,* 1989; 3: 131-3.
[25] Behrman SW, Melvin WS, Babb ME, Johnson J, Ellison EC. Laparoscopic cholecystectomy in the geriatric population. *Am. Surg.,* 1996; 2001: 15: 700-705.

[26] Pessaus P, Tuech JJ, Derouet N, Rouge C, Regenet N, Arnaud JP. Laparoscopic cholecystectomy in the elderly: a prospective study. *Surg. Endosc.,* 2000; 14: 1067-1069.

[27] Strasberg SM, Hertl M, Soper NJ. An analysis of the problem of biliary injury during laparoscopic cholecystectomy. *J. Am. Coll. Surg.,* 1995; 180: 101-125.

[28] Flum DR, Cheadle A, Prela C, Dellinger EP, Chan L. Bile duct injury during cholecystectomy and survival in medicare beneficiaries. *JAMA,* 2003; 290: 2168-2173.

[29] Cattel RB, Braasch JW. Two stage repairs of benign strictures of the bile duct. *Surg. Gynecol. Obstet.,* 1959; 109:691-696.

[30] Aust JB, Root HD, Urdaneta L, Varco RL. Biliary stricture. Surgery1967; 62:601-608.

[31] Bismuth H, Franco D, Corlette MB, Hepp J. Long term results of Roux-en-Y hepaticojejunostomy. *Surg. Gynecol. Obstet.,* 1978; 146:161-167.

[32] Mercado MA et al. Intrahepatic reapir of bile duct injuries. A comparative study. *J. Gastroinest. Surg.,* 2008, 12 :364-368.

[33] Lillemoe K, Melton G, Cameron JL, Pitt HA, Campbell KA, Talamani MA, et al. Postoperative bile duct strictures:management and outcome in the 1990s. *Annals of Surgery,* 232 (3):430-441.

[34] Pickelman J, Marsan R, Borge M. Portoenterostomy: An old treatment for a new disease. *Arch. Surg.,* 2000; 135: 644-648.

[35] Mercado MA, Orozco H, Chan C, Quezada C, Barajas-Olivas A, Borja-Cacho D, et al. Bile duct growing factor: an alternate technique for reconstruction of thin bile ducts after iatrogenic injury. *J. Gastrointest. Surg.,* 2006;10:1164-1169.

[36] Strasberg SM, Picus DD, Drebin JA. Results of a new strategy for reconstruction of biliary injuries having an isolated right-sided component. *J. Gastrointest. Surg.,* 2001;5: 266-274.

[37] Mercado MA, Chan C, Orozco H, Villalta JM, Barajas-Olivas A, Eraña J, et al. Long term evaluation of biliary reconstruction after partial resection of segments IV and V in iatrogenic injuries. *J. Gastrointest. Surg.,* 2006;10 :77-82.

[38] Mercado MA, Chan C, Orozco H, de la Garza L, et al. Biliary duct injury: Partial segment IV resection for intrahepatic reconstruction of biliary lesions. *Arch. Surg.,* 1999; 134: 1008-1010.

[39] Davidoff AM, Pappas TN, Murray EA, Hillern DJ, Johnson RD, Baker ME, et al. Mechanisms of major biliary injury during laparoscopic cholecystectomy. *Ann. Surg.,* 1992;215:196–202.

[40] Deziel DJ, Millikan KW, Economou SG, Doolas A, Ko ST, Airan MC. Complications of laparoscopic cholecystectomy: a national survey of 4292 hospitals and an analysis of 77 604 cases. *Am. J. Surg.,* 1993;165:9–14

[41] Alves A, Farges O, Nicolet J, Watrin T, Sauvanet A, Belghiti J, et al. Incidence and consequence of an hepatic artery injury in patients with postcholecystectomy bile duct strictures. *Ann. Surg.,* 2003;238:93–96.

[42] Koffron A, Ferrario M, Parsons W, Nemcek A, Saker M, Abecassis M. Failed primary management of iatrogenic biliary injury: incidence and significance of concomitant hepatic arterial disruption. *Surgery,* 2001;130:722–728.

[43] Strasberg SM, Helton SW .An analytical review of vasculobiliary injury in laparoscopic and open cholecystectomy. HPB (Oxford). 2011 January; 13(1): 1–14.

[44] Li J, Frilling A, Nadalin S, Paul A, Malagò M, Broelsch CE. Management of concomitant hepatic artery injury in patients with iatrogenic major bile duct injury after laparoscopic cholecystectomy. *Br. J. Surg.,* 2008 Apr;95(4):460-5.

[45] Seeliger H, Furst A, Zulke C, et al. Surgical management of bile duct injuries following laparoscopic cholecystectomy: analysis and follow-up of 28 cases. *Langenbecks Arch. Surg.,* 2002;387:286 –293.

[46] Chijiiwa K, Yamashita H, Yoshida J, et al. Current management and long-term prognosis of hepatolithiasis. *Arch. Surg.,* 1995;130:194 –197.

[47] Buell JF, Cronin DC, Funaki B, Koffron A, Yoshida A, Lo A, et al. Devastating and fatal complications associated with combined vascular and bile duct injuries during cholecystectomy. *Arch. Surg.,* 2002;137:703–10.

[48] Pellegrini CA, Thomas MJ, Way LW. Recurrent biliary stricture. Patterns of recurrence and outcome of surgical therapy .*Am. J. Surg.,* 1984; 147: 175-180.

[49] Davids PH, Tanka AK, Rauws EA, van Gulik TM, van Leeuwen DJ, de Wit LT, Verbeek PC, Huibregtse K, van der Heyde MN, Tytgat GN. Benign biliary strictures. Surgery or endoscopy? *Ann. Surg.,* 1993; 217: 237-243.

[50] Glenn F, Hays DM. The age factor in the mortality rate of patients undergoing surgery of the biliary tract. *Surg. Gynecol. Obstet.,* 1955; 100: 11.

[51] Siegel K. Biliary tract diseases in the elderly: management and outcomes. *Gut,* 1997; 41: 433–435

[52] Tagle FM, Lavergne J, Barkin JS, Unger SW. Laparoscopic cholecystectomy in the elderly. *Surg. Endosc.,* 1997; 11: 636-638.

[53] Houghton PW, Jenkinson LR, Donaldson LA. Cholecystectomy in the elderly: a prospective study. *Br. J. Surg.,* 1985; 72: 220-222.

[54] Margiotta SJ Jr, Horwitz JR, Willis IH, Wallack MK. Cholecystectomy in the elderly. *Am. J. Surg.,* 1988; 156: 509-512.

[55] Pigott JP, Williams GB. Cholecystectomy in the elderly. *Am. J. Surg.,* 1988; 155: 408-410.

[56] Smith N, Max MH. Gallbladder surgery in patients over 60: is there an increased risk? *South Med. J.,* 1987; 80: 472-474.

[57] Askew AR. Surgery for gallstones in the elderly. *Aust. N Z J. Surg.,* 1995; 65: 312-315.

[58] Magnuson TH, Ratner LE, Zenilman ME, Bender JS. Laparoscopic cholecystectomy: applicability in the geriatric population. *Am. Surg.,* 1997; 63: 91-96.

[59] Mayol J, Martinez-Sarmiento J, Tamayo FJ, Fernandez-Represa JA. Complications of laparoscopic cholecystectomy in the ageing patient. *Age Ageing,* 1997; 26: 77-81.

[60] Nenner RP, Imperato PJ, Alcorn CM. Complications of laparoscopic cholecystectomy in a geriatric population group. *NY State J. Med.,* 1992; 92: 518-520.

[61] Savassi Rocha PR, Almeida SR, Sanches MD, Andrade MA, Ferreira JT, Diniz MT, et al. Iatrogenic Bile duct injuries. *Surg. Endosc.,* 2003; 17: 1356-61. 265-69.

In: Bile Duct
Editor: Miguel Ángel Mercado
ISBN: 978-1-63321-771-3

Chapter 10

Vasculobiliary Injuries Associated to Laparoscopic Cholecystectomy

Miguel Ángel Mercado, MD[1,*], Bernardo Franssen, MD[2], Alejandro Elnecavé, MD[2], Santiago Mier-y-Teran, MD[2], Christopher Kauffman, MD[2] and Bruno A. González-Nolasco, MD[2]
[1]Professor, Chairman of the Department of Surgery,
National Institute of Medical Sciences and Nutrition "Salvador Zubiran"
[2]National Institute of Medical Sciences and Nutrition "Salvador Zubiran"

Abstract

Introduction: Injury of major vessels associated to bile duct injury in laparoscopic cholecystectomy has been reported with variable frequency. There is no consensus of what a surgeon has to do in this setting, although most of the reports show that there is no negative effect on long term results of reconstruction.

Methods: The files of patients repaired at our hospital in the last three years in which hepatic arterial injury was specifically searched for at the operation were reviewed. In all cases an intrahepatic hepatojejunostomy was done.

Results: A total of 195 cases were repaired, and the frequency of right arterial injury was 22% (43 cases). In 4 cases, the injury was identified at the index operation and in 25 cases within 36 hours. In the remaining 14 cases the repair was performed later.

Postoperative cholangitis was found in 8% of the cases, with 4% requiring radiological and/or surgical reintervention to dilate the anastomosis.

Of the patients that were repaired at the index operation or hours later, we observed that in 80% of the cases, retrograde flow of the injured hepatic artery was present.

---

* Correspondence: Miguel Ángel Mercado, Chairman of the Department of Surgery, National Institute of Medical Sciences and Nutrition "Salvador Zubirán".Vasco de Quiroga 15, Colonia Seccion XVI, Tlalpan C.P.14000, Mexico D.F. miguel.mercadod@quetzal.innsz.mx, 5487 0900 ext. 2130.

Conclusion: Almost one third of complex bile duct injuries have some type of arterial involvement. They are produced mainly laparoscopically. Moreover, most of the injured arteries have retrograde flow and do not need reconstruction.

Keywords: Vasculobiliary, bile duct injuries, hepatic injuries, cholecystectomy, hepatic infarction.

Introduction

Bile duct injury associated to cholecystectomy, mainly laparoscopic, has been extensively studied [1]. Causes, mechanisms, scenarios of presentation, as well as short and long term results have been reviewed and reported [2]. Several of these reports have stressed about injury to major hilar vessels, mainly the right hepatic artery (Figures 1A and 1B), and its consequences [3, 4, 5].

A number of reports of the operative results of biliary reconstruction in this setting have been done [6, 7, 8]. Nevertheless, there is no consensus about what a surgeon has to do when he or she finds an injury to the artery. Some authors tend to repair the bile duct without repairing the artery, while others advice to attempt the repair every time, [9] or according to the time of evolution of the injury [10].

Herein, we report our experience and results of repair in cases in which the right hepatic artery was injured. A review of the literature was also done, as well as a report of our strategy for repair in this type of injury.

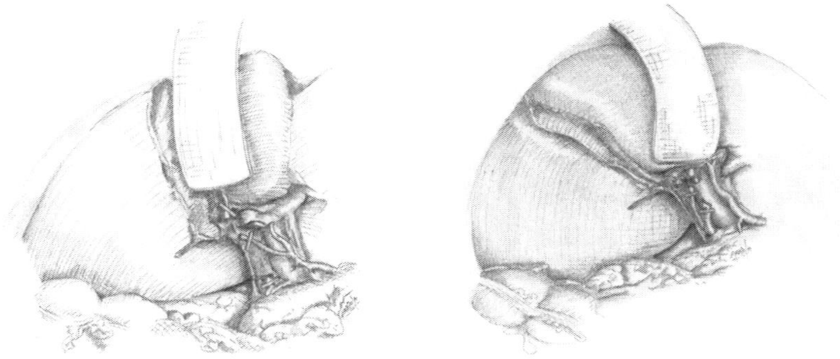

(a) (b)

Figure 1. *A.* The right hepatic duct has been severed and clips are placed in the distal and proximal stumps. Loss of substance is evident. *B.* Section of the right hepatic artery, a branch of the mesenteric artery. Loss of substance is observed as well.

Methods

The clinical history of patients repaired in the last three years at our hospital was reviewed. In this period of time we routinely performed an operative search for the right hepatic artery.

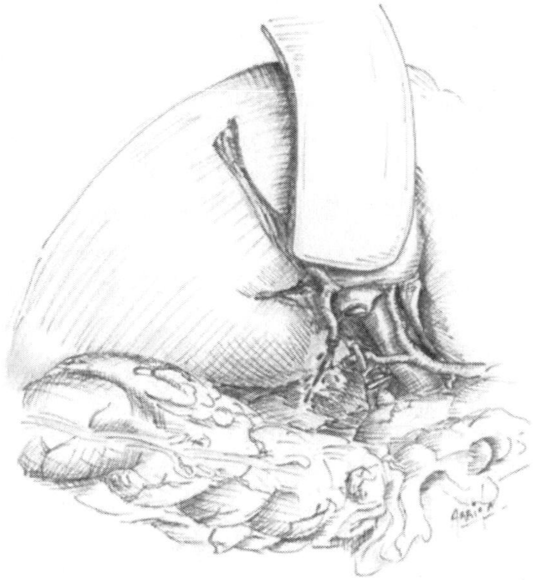

Figure 2. After removal of the distal clip at the proximal stump, retrograde flow is observed. This is a common scenario according to our experience, and requires reconstruction.

All cases were treated with a Roux-en-Y hepatojejunostomy, done after partial removal of the base of segments IV and V. Anterior opening of the left duct was done, taking care not to damage the branches to segment IV. A wide side-to-side anastomosis with isolated hydrolizable 5-0 stitches was done, obtaining a tension free, wide, and non ischemic anastomosis. In cases in which the confluence was lost, a neo-confluence was built with isolated stitches. If the distance between the two ducts was larger than 1 cm, a double barrel anastomosis was done, and for cases in which only secondary ducts were identified, a portoenterostomy was performed. In all cases, we attempted to identify the right hepatic artery. This was achieved by visualization and palpation. No attempt was done to free the artery by dissection, in order to avoid injury. Ligations and/or sutures were removed from the stumps of the injured arteries, in order to observe retrograde flow from the distal artery (Figure 2). Postoperatively, cholangitis and liver function tests were recorded. Cholangitis was diagnosed when fever and abnormal liver function tests were observed. We also recorded the need of reintervention, either surgical or radiological.

Results

In the last 3 years, our surgical team repaired a total of 195 cases. The estimated frequency for arterial injury was *22% (43 cases)*. In patients treated at the index operation *(4 cases)*, or within the next hours of injury *(<24 hours, 25 cases)*, all clips and/or sutures were removed in order to identify retrograde flow of the artery. This was observed in *25* of these *29 cases*. In the four patients without retrograde flow, no attempt was done to reconstruct the artery.

In the remaining *14* cases, the repair was done weeks, months or years after the injury *(average 247 days)*. Most of them had failed bilioenteric anastomosis *(8 cases)* and in *6* cases, a large and hard stenosis, consequence of an end-to-end repair, was observed.

All cases were treated with an intrahepatic bilioenteric anastomosis (Roux-en-Y hepatojejunostomy). Postoperative cholangitis was found in *8%* of the cases with *4%* requiring radiological dilation of the anastomosis. In the last 3 years no major hepatectomy has been done. We have not observed a single case of hemobilia related to right hepatic arterial injury.

Discussion

Vasculobiliary lesions are commonly associated to bile duct injury [11]. Most of the injuries to the bile duct have concomitant damage of the microcirculation of said structure. Misidentification of the common duct promotes devascularization, by means of electrofulguration and/or clips placement that interrupt the lateral arterial circulation of the duct. The dissection necessary to place a clip also promotes some type of devascularization. Damage to the small vessels produces ischemia of the stump of the transected bile duct. This is why several authors have advised to defer the repair until the complete establishment of the ischemic injury [10]. If an anastomosis is done to ischemic ducts, dehiscence and/or stenosis of the anastomosis can be observed in the early or late postoperative period.

There are some anecdotic cases in which the hilium has been completely injured, with complete damage to the porta hepatis. Zaydfudim et al. reported on a case treated by means of a portocaval shunt and subsequent liver transplantation [13]. In our hospital we observed a case that was transferred immediately, and arterial liberation (the artery was actually only tied without loss of substance) with an end-to-end porto-portal anastomosis was done. A Roux-en-Y bilioenteric anastomosis was performed.

Injury to the right hepatic artery is also observed associated to the bile duct injury, in direct relation to its height. Therefore, the higher the injury, the probability of right hepatic compromise is higher [14].

The reported frequency of right hepatic injury varies greatly. Koffron et al. reported an incidence of 61%, suggesting that arterial disruption may affect the outcome [15]. Buell et al. analyzed 27 complex injuries with a frequency of 26%. They found arterial compromise irrespective of the injury level. The presence of arterial injury was a predictor of mortality [16]. Alves et al. found an incidence of 47% and stated that if a Hepp-Couinaud repair is done, the arterial injury does not affect the results of reconstruction [17]. Shmidt et al. found 11 injuries in 54 patients. They concluded that the outcome of patients with arterial injury is worse than those without it [18].

Stewart et al. made an extensive investigation of the subject [14]. In their series of 261 cases, 84 (32%) had an arterial injury. Correlation between injury and the level of the bile duct involvement was observed (64% in class IV of the Stewart-Way classification). The consequences of the ligature were abscesses, bleeding, hemobilia, and right lobe ischemia. They found that the right hepatic arterial injury had no influence on the success of repair or mortality rate, but was associated with an increased morbidity.

They observed that 54% of their documented right hepatic arterial injuries had intrahepatic repercussion. In our whole experience, along 20 years, these events (cholangitic abscesses, right lobe ischemia) surfaced in 11 cases, which required hepatectomy.

In the last three years, however, we did not observe these events and we have not done hepatectomies. This is perhaps the consequence of a more conservative approach, waiting for response to medical treatment, percutaneous drainage and subsequent atrophy of the right liver. In a retrospective analysis we found that, of the cases treated by means of hepatectomy, not all of them had a right arterial injury. Thus, the decision to remove the right liver has to be individualized. In our experience, this is an uncommon approach (less than 3% of the total cases). The most relevant conclusion of this paper is that the result of reconstruction is related to the experience and surgical background of the surgeon, obtaining comparable results in patients presented with and without right hepatic arterial injury. It is important to stress that we have not found hemobilia and/or hemorrhage as a consequence of right hepatic arterial injury, in opposition to the cases described by Stewart et al.

Intraoperative bleeding (found in 69% of 38 patients with right hepatic arterial injury) and postoperative bleeding (including hemobilia) was not observed in our series. In our whole experience we have only seen two cases of postoperative hemobilia. One case presented with severe bleeding and the other with bleeding at the anastomosis level. These bleedings were the consequence of non coagulated vessels near the anastomosis, but in no case came from the intrahepatic biliary tree. Postoperative hemoblia can be the result of bleeding at the edge of the mucosa of the jejunum, at the edge of the bile duct or both. Intrahepatic biliary tree hemorrhage has been observed by our group after instrumentation of the biliary tract with Bakes dilators, when forced dilation is done, and/or when an inadequate placement of the dilator is performed with disruption of the bile duct and parenchymal injury. In all cases the hemorrhage was not significant, and stopped spontaneously.

Tzovaras et al. [19] showed in their study that interruption of hepatic arterial flow is usually well tolerated and that there is strong evidence that concomitant vascular injuries do not have any impact on mortality. The frequency of long-term stenosis in these cases, however, is increased.

Khanmorali et al. [20] reported that the injury of the artery was not only an interruption of flow, but also loss of substance. In the cases in which intraoperative diagnosis was possible or repair was done within 24 hours, an attempt of reconstruction was done: end-to-end anastomosis repair using an autologous venous graft, and in other cases using the gastroduodenal artery.

Li et al. [21] documented a frequency of 10 arterial injuries in their series of 60 cases. Rearterialization was done in 5 cases and hepatectomy in 2, with a mortality of 30%.

Laurent et al. [22], reviewing the indication of hepatectomy in bile duct injury, showed 11 arterial injuries in 18 cases, all of which required major hepatectomy. The morbidity was increased, mainly by biliary fistula and ascites.

Winslow et al. [10], in their review of biliary repair, state that the presence of a major arterial injury for ore than 24 hours was an indication for delayed repair, and that early detection would be an indication to attempt arterial reconstruction. Nevertheless, they remark that they had no opportunity to treat such a patient. In the cases with evident liver infarction (4 cases) resection was done.

An unanswered question in relation to the arterial anatomy of each individual patient remains. As it is well known, the fetal liver has three main arteries (right, a branch of the mesenteric artery; medial, a branch of the celiac trunk; and left, a branch of the left gastric artery). In most cases, the right and left ones obliterate, remaining only the medial artery that derives in the right and left hepatic arteries. These two vessels have a better interconnection than the two arising from the mesenteric and gastric arteries. It has been shown that the ligature of the branch arising from the mesenteric artery can promote liver abscesses on the right lobe, as has been observed in Whipple procedures. Perhaps the injury to this artery, associated to a complex injury of the bile duct, evolves into the cases that are more prone to the development of complications related to the interruption of said vessel, such as liver infection, abscesses, hemobilia, etc.

According to our experience, we can point the following observations:

a) Not all arterial injuries occur at the index operation.
b) Some of them occur in the first attempt of repair, usually done by the primary surgeon.
c) Most of the arterial injuries are evident lately in the patients evolution.

In all cases, our advice is to do a high repair, at the confluence level, whenever possible. We have observed better long term results, with fewer cases of postoperative stenosis and lesser need of reoperation [7].

We do not advice to do routine angiography. It is time consuming, expensive, and with radiation exposure. Furthermore, the probability or rehabilitating the artery is extremely low. The repair of right hepatic arterial injuries is anecdotic, and long term patency of the repair has not been documented (or even reported).

As with the cases repaired at the index operation or hours lately, for elective repair and/or correction of failed repairs, we advocate the high hilar repair. Partial removal of segments IV and V as a maneuver to lower the plate is routinely performed in our hospital. The advantage of this maneuver is that no injury to the duct vasculature is presented.

The classic hilar plate descent achieved with the Hepp Couinaud approach jeopardizes the circulation of the ducts. The probability of injury to the communicating artery between the vasculature of the left and right duct is higher. Lowering the plate after partial removal of segments IV and V does not jeopardize the circulation of the duct at the confluence level. After lowering the plate, a large anterior opening of the left duct allows a wide, tension free, non ischemic anastomosis (Strasberg's sideways technique).

We always start the dissection of the hilus after resection of the small wedge of segments IV and V. A complete dissection of the hilus is not usually performed, in order to prevent damage to small arterial collaterals that can compromise the circulation that develops after the interruption of the right hepatic artery flow. The dissection of the left duct, close to the insertion of the round ligament, exposes the vascularity of segment IV. An attempt to avoid interruption of these vessels should be done. The anterior opening of the duct is carried out at this level.

This approach warrants better results of the anastomosis, even when a right arterial injury is present.

In the cases repaired at the index operation or hours later we had the opportunity to remove clips and/or sutures (placed by the primary surgeon after converting the laparoscopic surgery to an open operation). Most of these cases show retrograde flow of the artery. If such condition is found, no attempt to repair should be done. In the cases with no retrograde flow (less than 5 in our series) an attempt for revascularization should be considered. Nevertheless, these arteries are usually very small, the repair is time consuming, and no long term patency can be warranted.

There is no strong evidence published stating that this approach promotes better results. On the contrary, reconstructions performed in experienced centers, without attempt of arterial repair, have a better impact [14].

Conclusion

We conclude that almost one third of complex injuries have some type of major arterial involvement. They are produced in the laparoscopic approach as well as after conversion to an open procedure. By means of MRI angiography, nowadays it is easier to identify them, but very few cases can be reconstructed. A large number of repairs and experienced surgeons minimize the impact of arterial injury on long-term outcome.

We found cases with refractory segmental cholangitis and/or liver infraction that need major liver resection. These situations are now anecdotic.

In cases evaluated days or weeks after the injury, there is no need to investigate arterial injury. These patients have done a self selection, and either present the less common consequences of arterial injury (such as abscess, hemobilia, or segmentary stenosis of the intrahepatic ducts along with liver atrophy), or have already developed compensatory flow through hilar and intrahepatic collaterals. We recommend a high repair for these cases.

References

[1] Connor S, Garden OJ. Bile duct injury in the era of laparoscopicholecystectomy. *Br. J. Surg.,* 2006; 93:158-68.

[2] Stewart L, Way LW. Laparoscopic bile duct injuries: timing of surgical repair does not influence success rate. A multivariate analysis of factors influencing surgical outcomes. *HPB,* (Oxford). 2009; 11:516-22.

[3] Bachellier P, Nakano H, Weber JC, Lemarque P, Oussoultzoglou E, Candau C, Wolf P, et al. Surgical repair after bile duct and vascular injuries during laparoscopic cholecystectomy: When and how?. *World J. Surg.,* 2001; 25:1335-45.

[4] Schmidt SC, Langrehr JM, Hintze RE, Neuhaus P. Long-term results and risk factors influencing outcome of major bile duct injuries following cholecystectomy. *Br. J. Surg.*, 2005; 92:76-82.

[5] Schmidt SC, Langrehr JM, Settmacher U, Neuhaus P. Surgical treatment of bile duct injuries following laparoscopic cholecystectomy. Does the concomitant hepatic arterial injury influence the long term outcome? *Zentralbl. Chir.*, 2004; 129:487-92.

[6] Fischer CP, Fahy BN, Aloia TA, Bass BL, Gaber AO, Ghobrial RM. Timing of referral impacts surgical outcomes in patients undergoing repair of bile duct injuries. *HPB,* (Oxford). 2009; 11:22-27.

[7] Mercado MA, Chan C, Orozco H, Tielve M, Hinojosa CA. Acute bile duct injury. The need for a high repair. *Surg. Endosc.*, 2003; 17:1351-55.

[8] Bektas H, Schrem H, Winny M, Klempnauer J. Surgical treatment and outcome of iatrogenic bile duct lesions after cholecystectomy and the impact of different clinical classification systems. *Br. J. Surg.*, 2007; 94:1119-27.

[9] Mathisen O, Soreide O, Bergan A: Laparoscopic cholecystectomy: bile duct and vascular injuries: management and outcome. *Scand J. Gastroenterol.*, 2002; 37: 476-81.

[10] Winslow ER, Fialkowski EA, Linehan DC, Hawking WG, Picus DD, Strasberg SM. "Sideways": Results of repair of biliary injuries using a policy of side to side hepaticojejunostomy. *Ann. Surg.*, 2009; 249:426-34.

[11] Mercado MA. Early vs late repair of bile duct injuries. *Surg. Endosc.*, 2006; 20:1644-47.

[12] Strasberg SM. Error traps and vasculo-biliary injury in laparoscopic and open cholecystectomy. *J. Hepatobiliary Pancreat Surg.*, 2008; 15(3):284-92.

[13] Zaydfudim V, Wright JK, Pinson CW. Liver transplantation for iatrogenic porta hepatic transaction. *Am. Surg.*, 2009; 75:313-16.

[14] Stewart L, Robinson TN, Lee CM, Liuk, Whang K, Way LW. Right hepatic artery injury associated with laparoscopic bile duct injury: incidence, mechanism and consequences. *J. Gastrointest Surg.*, 2004; 8:523-30.

[15] Koffron, Ferrario M, Parsons W, Nemcek A, Saker M, Abecassis M. Failed primary management of iatrogenic biliary injury: incidence and significance of concomitant hepatic arterial disruption. *Surgery*, 2001; 130:722-28.

[16] Buell JF, Cronin DC, Funaki B, Koffron A, Yoshida A, Lo A, Leef J, et al. Devastating and fatal complications associated with combined vascular and bile duct injuries during cholecystectomy. *Arch. Surg.*, 2002; 137:708-10.

[17] Alves A, Farges O, Nicolet J, Watrin T, Sauvanet A, Belghiti J. Incidence and consequence of an hepatic artery injury in patients with postcholacystectomy bile duct strictures. *Ann. Surg.*, 2003; 238:93-6.

[18] Schmidt SC, Settmachor U, Langrehr JM, Neuhaus P. Management and outcome of patients with combined bile duct and hepatic arterial injuries after laparoscopic cholecystectomy. *Surgery,* 2004; 135:613-18.

[19] Tzovaras G, Dervenis C. Vascular injuries in laparoscopic cholecystectomy: an underestimated problem. *Dig Surg.*, 2006; 23:370-74.

[20] Khanmorali K, Defaria W, Moore RE, Guarneri R, Tzakis AG. Gastroduodenal artery as the inflow tract to repair the right hepatic artery in a combined vasculobiliary injury after laparoscopic cholecystectomy. *Am. Surg.*, 2007; 73:888-9.

[21] Li J, Frilling A, Nadalin S, Paul A, Malago M, Broelsch CE. Management of concomitant hepatic artery injury in patients with iatrogenic major bile duct injury after laparoscopic cholecystectomy. *Br. J. Surg.*, 2008; 95:460-5.

[22] Laurent A, Sauranet A, Farges O, Watrin T, Riukins E, Belghiti J. Major hepatectomy for the treatment of complex bile duct injury. *Ann. Surg.*, 2008; 248:77-83.

[23] Mercado MA, Chan C, Salgado-Nesme N, López-Rosales F. Intrahepatic repair of bile duct injuries. A comparative study. *J. Gastrointest Surg.,* 2008; 12:364-368.

In: Bile Duct
Editor: Miguel Ángel Mercado

ISBN: 978-1-63321-771-3

Chapter 11

Avoidance, Prevention and Recognition of Bile Duct Injury

Adnan Alseidi, MD, EdM*, Farzad Alemi and W. Scott Helton
Virginia Mason Medical Center, Department of General,
Thoracic and Vascular Surgery, Seattle, Washington

Abstract

Iatrogenic injury through operative trauma is the main cause of bile duct injury (BDI), accounting for 96% of all BDIs. The incidence of BDI has dramatically increased with the adoption of laparoscopy as the method of choice for gallbladder removal. Recent data suggests that incidence resulting from laparoscopic cholecystectomy is 0.3-0.7%, compared to 0.16-0.2% for the traditional open approach. Morbidity and mortality is reported to be as high as 47% and 9%, respectively. It is necessary to encourage surgeons to constantly avoid situations that increase the chance of causing a BDI. An example of such a circumstance is a patient who presents with a severely inflamed gallbladder, in which case the surgeon is advised to consider a two-stage treatment. The first stage would be to "cool down" the gallbladder with antibiotics and/or percutaneous or operative drainage. Thereafter, in the second stage, an elective cholecystectomy can be performed 4-6 weeks later. There are different diagnostic methods used to determine the presence of a BDI. In case a BDI is suspected during cholecystectomy, intraoperative cholangiography can be used to determine the type of injury. An unsuspected BDI may manifest with complications in the immediate post-operative period, or months to year later with symptoms secondary to cholestasis.

The Strasberg Classification categorizes BDI from A through E. In type A through D, the defining characteristic is the intact communication between the intrahepatic ducts and the duodenum; in contrast, with Type E injuries this communication is lost.

The goals of biliary reconstruction are: to provide definitive internal biliary drainage, to ensure long term anastomotic patency with low chance of stricture, and to avoid major post-operative complications such as bile leak, sepsis, organ failure and death.

* Corresponding author: Adnan Alseidi, MD EdM, P: (206)341-1908, F: (206)341-0048, Adnan.Alseidi@ vmmc. org.

I. Introduction

Among the most challenging patients for surgeons are those with bile duct injuries (BDIs). BDI is associated with substantial morbidity, impaired quality of life and mortality. [1-4] Morbidity following BDI is reported to be as high as 47% and mortality anywhere from 1.7% to 9%. [1, 5, 6] Morbidity and mortality is related not only to the severity of the bile duct injury and any associated bowel injury, but also to delays in management, inadequate management or complications directly related to failed repair. Failed repairs can result in post-operative peritonitis, biliary sepsis, or anastomotic stricture which can result in long term recurrent cholangitis, biliary cirrhosis and death. Numerous studies have noted that the level of BDI correlates with surgical outcome, with worse outcomes occurring more frequently in patients with higher levels of BDI. [7-9]

The focus of this chapter is to identify situations and conditions which may increase the incidence of BDI and provide strategies for their prevention. The unfortunate reality is that BDI can be caused by any surgeon, at any time, and in any environment. Preventative measures should always be employed where the risk of BDI is increased. Sound judgment, knowledge and management are necessary to avoid BDI in patients at risk. Once a BDI has occurred, recognition--preferably intra-operatively but also post-operatively--will decrease the chances of significant complications such as organ failure, sepsis or death. Successful outcomes require swift recognition and the knowledge of appropriate management pathways.

Table 1. Strasberg Classification of Bile Duct Injury

Type of Injury	Description	Examples	Treatment	Presentation	
A	bile leak from a transected minor duct or cystic duct that does not disturb the continuity with the common bile duct	transected small duct of Luschka from gallbladder fossa or cystic duct leak	clip or ligate if operated upon or endoscopic stenting	(1)pain, (2)fever, (3)sepsis, (4)mild hyperbilirubinemia, (5)biloma or biliary ascites, (6) possible peritonitis	maintains continuity between the central biliary tree and duodenum
B	ligation of aberrant right posterior sector duct or aberrant segment duct VI or VII	occlusion of aberrant right hepatic duct using a clip	observation initially	(1) asymptomatic elevation in AST, ALT and alkaline phosphatase with normal bilirubin (2) late presentation as pain or segmental cholangitis in obstructed liver segment (3) liver atrophy of proximal liver segment or right posterior sector (4) compensatory hypertrophy of left lobe or right anterior	

Type of Injury	Description	Examples	Treatment	Presentation	
C	bile leak from a duct not in communication with the common bile duct	transection of an aberrant right posterior sector or segment duct	ligation, drainage only or RY hepaticojejunostomy	same as A injury	
D	lateral injury to major ducts of the extrahepatic biliary tree	laceration or tear of the CHD, necrosis of lateral bile duct wall from cautery	primary repair, T-tube or RY hepaticojejunostomy	same as A injury	
E1	CHD stricture or occlussion > 2cm below the biliary bifurcation	resection/abaltion with cautery; stenosis above the cystic duct junction with at least 2 cm of CHD before the bifurcation	RY hepaticojejunostomy Bilateral hepaticojejunostomy, or right hemihepatectomywith left hepaticojejunostomy if serious vascular injury to R lobe	obstructive jaundice if total occlussion and no leak. Signs and symptoms similar to Class A, C, D if leak present from proximal duct(s)	disruption between major biliary tree and duodenum
E2	CHD stricture/ occlussion within 2 cm of the biliary bifurcation	resection/abaltion with cautery; stenosis above the cystic duct junction with less than 2 cm of CHD before the bifurcation			
E3	Injury to common hepatic duct and biliary confluence with preservation of the back wall	resection/abaltion with cautery; stenosis at the bifurcation of the right and left hepatic ducts resulting in no CHD			
E4	Injury to the confluence including the back wall resulting in the loss of communication between right and left hepatic ducts	resection/abaltion with cautery of the CHD including the bifurcation			
E5	common hepatic duct and right duct injury	resection/abaltion with cautery the hepatic duct along with injury to abberant right duct			

Surgeons may encounter a patient with BDI through a variety of avenues. They may create a BDI themselves, they may be called to the operating room by a colleague who has made an injury, or they may inherit a patient transferred to their care from an outside facility or through their hospital's emergency room. This chapter provides a guide for the surgeon on how to avoid a BDI, the workup of patients suspected of having a BDI (both intra-operatively and post-operatively), and the immediate management of patients with BDIs (Figure 1a-c). The guiding principles discussed herein are provided while keeping in mind the complexity of the problem as it tends to merge variable patient, surgeon, and setting-specific factors.

II. Epidemiology and Background

Background: The Strasberg Classification System

There are a number of systems that have been used to classify BDIs. Such systems are important for understanding how the injury occurred, for management decisions and for long term reporting of outcomes. Of the various methods used to classify BDI, we recommend the Strasberg Classification because it provides a reasonable approach to treatment based upon the type of injury. [10] The Strasberg classification organizes BDIs using key features and will be used in this chapter to help direct the physician in a predetermined care pathway.

The Strasberg Classification categorizes BDI from A through E (Figure 2, Table 1). Type A through D injuries include leaks, lateral injuries, occlusions and transected minor ducts. The defining characteristic of these injuries is the intact communication between the intrahepatic ducts and the duodenum. However, this communication is lost in Type E injuries, which are further subclassified into $E_1 - E_5$. Each of these subcategories is indicative of a loss of direct communication between the intrahepatic ducts and the duodenum. This separation of the liver from the duodenum can be due to duct stenosis, complete occlusion of the duct or loss of ductal tissue as a consequence of resection. E_2, E_3 and E_4 injuries are the most common type of BDIs that occur during laparoscopic cholecystectomy. [10,11]

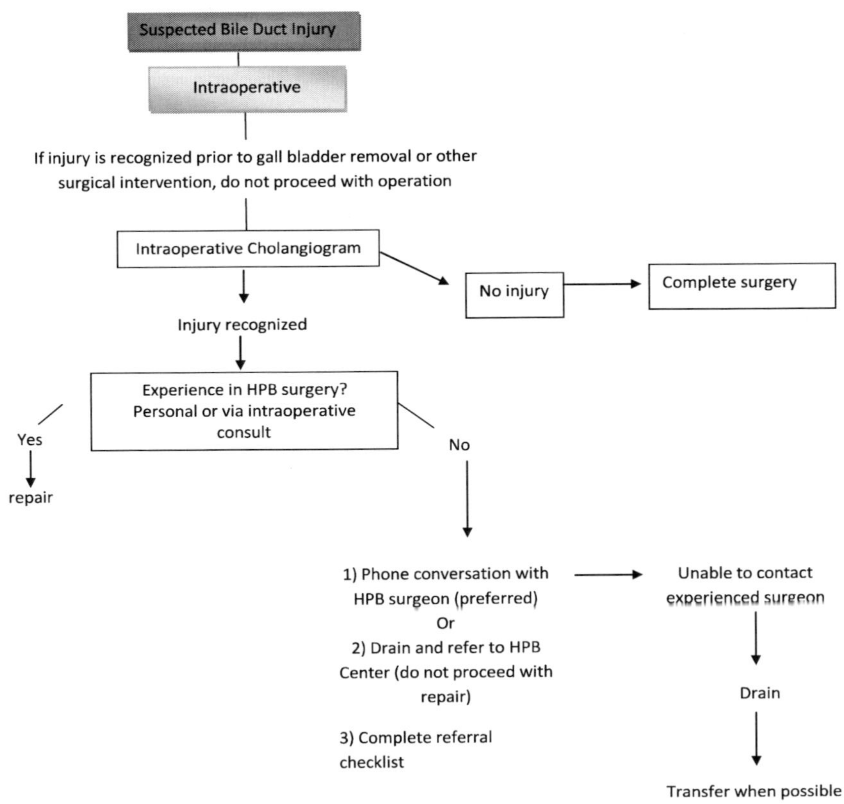

(a)

Figure 1. (Continued).

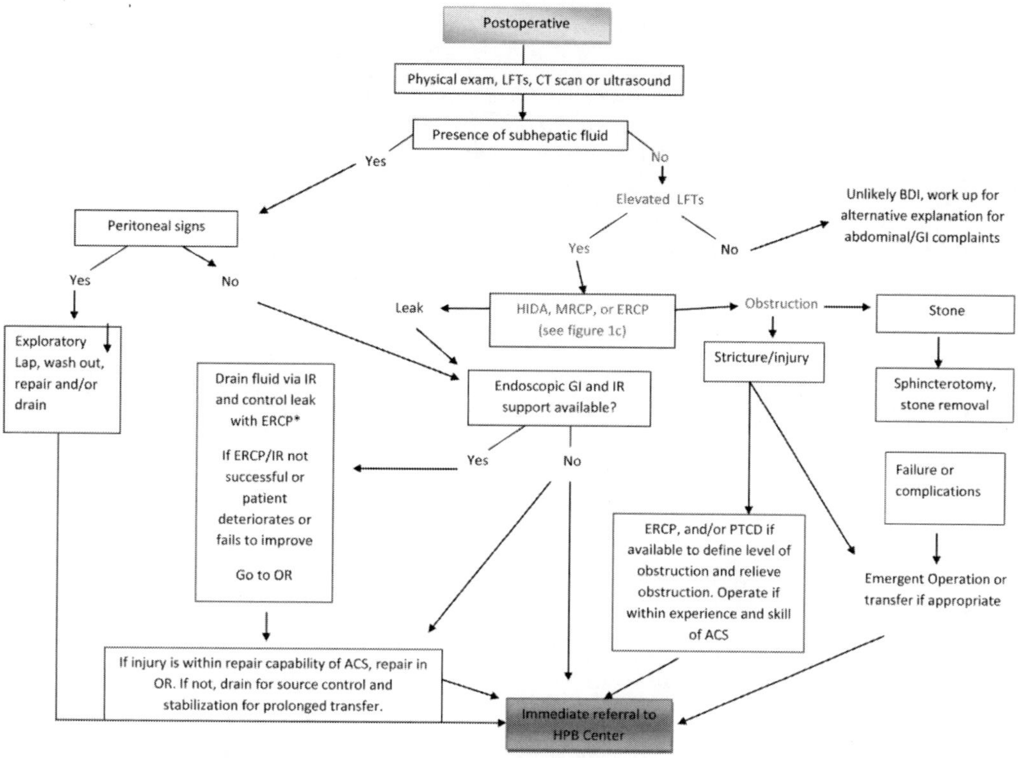

(b)

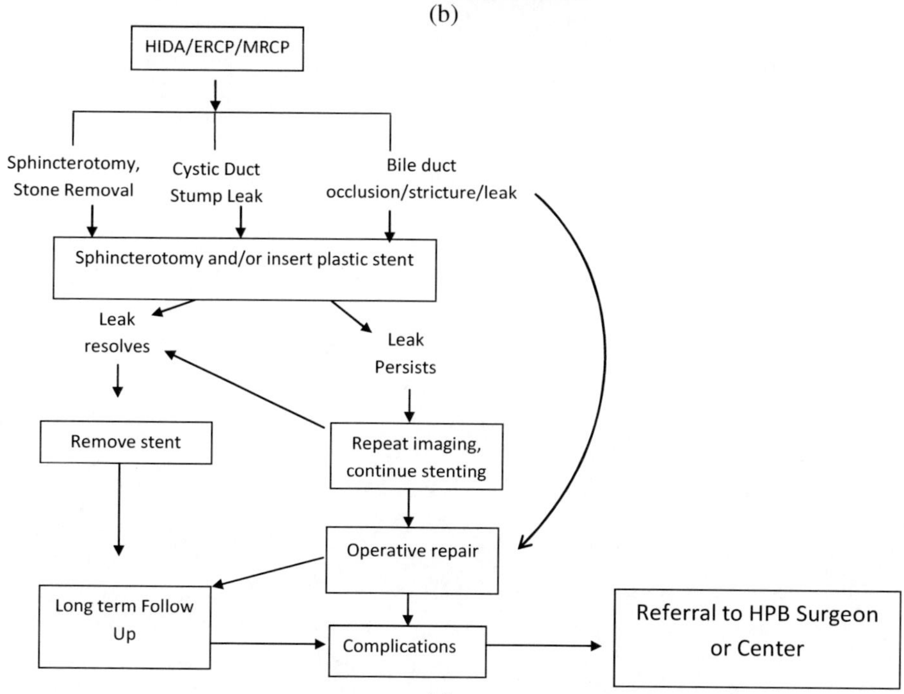

(c)

Figure 1. Algorithm for management of suspicion of BDI.

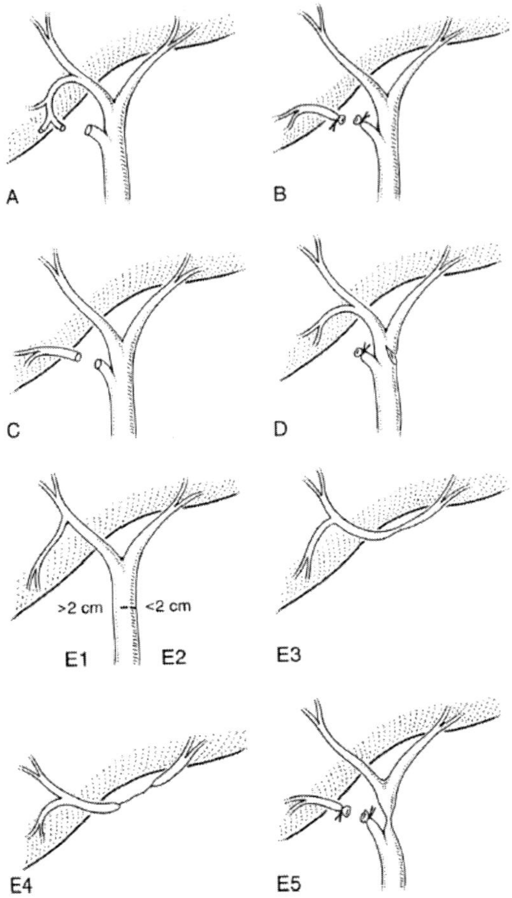

Figure 2. The Strasberg Classification System for Biliary Injury.

Etiology, Incidence, & Pathogenesis

Iatrogenic injury through operative trauma is the main cause of BDI, accounting for 96% of all BDIs. Injuries arise through mechanical causes or anatomic misidentification. Mechanical causes of BDI range from direct injury via inadvertent transection, excision, or clip application, to indirect injury caused by excessive traction or cautery. Anatomic misidentification is commonly associated with mistaking the common bile duct for the cystic duct or an aberrant duct, which has been termed the "Classic Injury." [12] Any operation performed in the right upper quadrant of the abdomen poses a risk for BDI. Procedures such as gastrectomy, pancreatectomy, hepatic resection, or exploration of the common bile duct (via endoscopic, laparoscopic, interventional transhepatic, or open approach) have been implicated in BDIs. However, the highest risk procedure for operative biliary injury is cholecystectomy, with the laparoscopic approach being the leading cause. [13]

Laparoscopic cholecystectomy is known to provide many benefits, namely less pain postoperatively, earlier return of bowel function, fewer cosmetic defects, shorter length of hospital stay, earlier return to full activity, and decreased overall cost in comparison to open cholecystectomy. [14-16] However, the incidence of BDI has dramatically increased with the adoption of laparoscopy as the method of choice for gallbladder removal. The traditional open approach to cholecystectomy demonstrated a stable 0.16-0.2% rate of BDI. [10,17] This is in stark contrast to more recent data suggesting the incidence of BDIs resulting from laparoscopic cholecystectomy to be between 0.3-0.7%. [18] Moreover, according to two recent studies, these injuries are often more complex Strasberg Class E (Table 1). [11, 19]

The relative low incidence of BDI during cholecystectomy is magnified by the volume of cholecystectomies performed nationally. In the United States, there are approximately 750,000 cholecystectomies performed every year, making it the most common abdominal operation. [18] This number reflects not only the burden of gallstone disease in the US population, but also places the onus on surgeons to recreate a procedure with exceptional high standards and to practice preventive methods to avoid BDIs. Given the high volume of cholecystectomy and incidence of biliary injury, it is estimated that between 2,250 and 5,250 bile duct injuries occur each year.

III. Avoidance

Avoidance of BDIs requires a change in the way a surgeon manages cholecystitis prior to operating, and how he/she manages a suspicion of BDI once in the operating room. Dr. Steven Strasberg has stressed the importance of "changing the culture of cholecystectomy" as a means to teach surgeons how to reduce BDIs during cholecystectomy. [20,21] He encourages surgeons to constantly assess methods of avoiding situations that increase the chance of causing a BDI. An example of such a circumstance is a patient presenting with a severely inflamed gallbladder. In such settings, cholecystostomy tube and antibiotics may be a safer option. [22-24] While retrospective studies have concluded that operating on a severely inflamed gallbladder may be safe, these were uniformly underpowered to assess BDIs. In such a setting, BDI is much more likely and a surgeon should consider drainage procedures as part of the treatment pathway. [20,21,25]

A surgeon practicing by the "culture of safety" should preoperatively review a patient's imaging and clinical presentation with the question of safety in mind. If imaging reveals a severely inflamed gallbladder, the surgeon is advised to consider a two-stage treatment of the disease process. The first stage would be to cool down the gallbladder with antibiotics plus or minus drainage of the gallbladder either percutaneously, laparoscopically, or via a mini laparotomy depending on the setting and availability of resources and expertise. The second stage, an elective cholecystectomy, would then be performed 4-6 weeks later. Within the "culture of safety," rushing to the operating room for a cholecystectomy is almost never necessary.

IV. Prevention

In the operating room, achieving the "critical view of safety" prior to duct or artery transection is universally recognized as the safest and most appropriate manner of avoiding BDI (Figure 3). [10, 26-28] Unfortunately, the critical view of safety cannot be safely obtained in a significant percentage of patients because inflammation, bleeding or anatomic variations which precludes safe dissection at the neck of the gallbladder. At this juncture, the surgeon may wisely choose to convert to a two-stage process (as discussed in the section above) and proceed only with a cholecystostomy tube. Alternatively, if the surgeon chooses to proceed with cholecystectomy, he/she should adopt alternative techniques for addressing the gallbladder disease and the inability to obtain the critical view of safety. Such techniques include early cholangiography through the gallbladder, and asking for assistance from another experienced surgeon. [29] Conversion to an open procedure is also another very helpful technique in such a setting, however it should not be viewed as an error-proof or injury-free approach. In fact, BDI often occur after conversion to an open approach and may result in a higher level injury. The act of converting is not necessarily protective against BDI; rather, it is the approach the surgeon takes after conversion that results in a safer procedure. The surgeon, once converted to open, is advised to employee techniques such as partial cholecystectomy, fundus- first approach, and open cholangiography to further assist in obtaining the critical view of safety. The key avoidance technique is to avoid dissection within the porta hepatis when inflammation exists. In addition, the gallbladder is often obliterated with no plane of separation from the cystic plate of the liver; under these circumstances the surgeon is advised to leave the back wall of the gallbladder intact and perform a partial cholecystectomy. Surgeons who are inexperienced in such open techniques may be advised to proceed with a two-phase approach and perform only a cholecystostomy tube. Failure to employ these techniques and proceed with dissection with unclear anatomy or inability to achieve a clear critical view of safety is ill- advised and increases the risk of causing a BDI.

Bile duct injury prevention, once in the operating room, is also aided by maintaining a high degree of vigilance and not ignoring any deviation from the norm or any suspicion of BDI. A surgeon must pause and systematically evaluate the situation as soon as a suspicion for BDI becomes apparent. Intraoperative prevention and vigilance towards avoiding increasing the level of the BDI once it occurs will be later discussed.

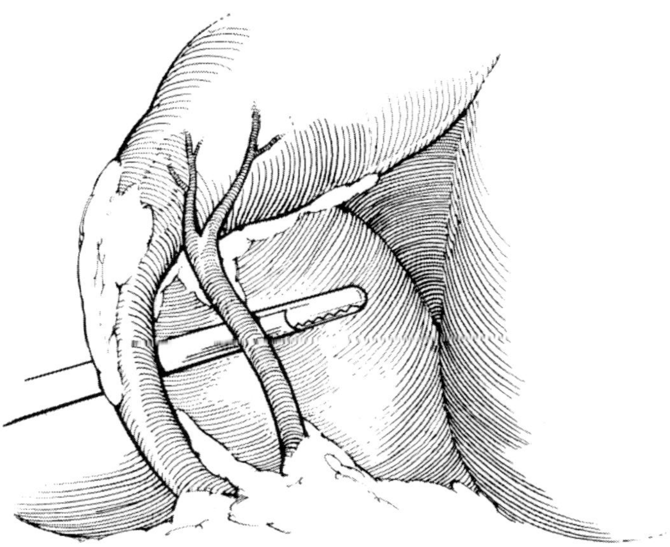

Figure 3. The Critical View of Safety.

V. Clinical Presentation

Approximately 20-30% of BDIs are appreciated during the index operation. [10,30,31] The type of injury and the surgical approach used are factors in predicting early or late recognition. Major injuries to the main bile duct (types D and E) are identified intraoperatively one-quarter to one-half of the time. [10,32] Type A and B injuries, however, being more subtle in nature, are rarely identified during the index operation.[10] The timing of recognition also differs in open versus laparoscopic cases. As may be expected, open cases that result in biliary injury are more likely to be appreciated during the index operation than those that occur during laparoscopic procedures. [32]

A BDI should be suspected or placed high in the differential diagnosis of any patient following a recent operation in the right upper quadrant who presents in one of two ways. The first is with elevation of liver function tests. More specifically, total bilirubin and alkaline phosphatase levels will incrementally elevate beyond the patient's normal levels if obstruction is proximal to biliary injury. The second presentation is due to symptoms caused by bilious drainage within the peritoneal cavity, such as fevers, chills, and abdominal pain. These symptoms can result from a self-contained biloma or bile peritonitis in the peritoneal cavity from diffuse biliary ascites.

Patient Characteristics

The demographics of patients who sustain BDI tend to mirror those that require procedures on or around the biliary tree. A 2005 report compiled patient, institutional, and outcome characteristics from 1991-2000 on patients who required reconstruction after sustaining a BDI resulting from laparoscopic cholecystectomy. [3] This series found that about 2/3 of injuries occur in female patients with an age range of 40-75 years. A common misconception is that most patient with BDI present via the emergency department. The fact is that only about 35% of patients with BDI present through the ED while 61% present in other medical settings (clinics, offices) and a small proportion (2.5%) are transferred from other institutions. [3] Emergency cholecystectomy is associated with a higher rate of BDI (57%) compared to elective surgeries (31.8%). Upon discharge, the majority of patients with BDI (74.9%) are routed home while 19.6% were transferred to short-term hospitals or skilled nursing facilities. [3]

VI. Bile Duct Injury Diagnosis & Patient Management

It is important to note that proper management of BDI starts prior to definitive diagnosis of an injury. Ignoring the suspicion of BDI is in fact often the main cause in patient deterioration, and often cause for medico-legal complications (see section on litigation). The surgeon is advised to treat any deviation in a patient's expected postoperative recovery (a rapid return to normal function) as a potential BDI until proven otherwise.

Suspicion of BDI can occur intraoperatively (surgeon's intuition, presence of bile, unexpected anatomy) or postoperatively. The exact management pathway a surgeon follows when such suspicion arises is influenced heavily by several factors: surgeon factors (his/her experience level), setting factors (resources at hand including interventional radiology and gastroenterologic support), and patient factors (patient stability and comorbidity and patient and family wishes). This section, and the algorithm presented in Figure 1a-c should help the surgeon navigate these variables to achieve a favorable outcome. Any surgeon that is in the position of having to manage BDIs is encouraged to understand these factors and assess their personal ability, their facility's resources, their local and regional resources, and their comfort level with managing BDI repair. The surgeon should develop a management plan for addressing BDI that is specific to their situation and ensures the best possible recovery of the patient.

VI-A. Intraoperative BDI Suspicion (Figure 1a)

Bile duct injury avoidance extends into the operating room before and after suspicion of injury. Intraoperatively, the avoidance of BDI starts by halting further progression of the operation once a suspicion of BDI exists. Oftentimes progression results in worse injury due to the surgeon being in the wrong plane and, in the attempt to reenter the correct plane, can cause biliary or vascular structural injuries. Thus, as soon as a BDI is suspected intraoperatively, the procedure should stop and management of the possible injury begins.

In such a setting, the surgeon is advised to employ methods to better define the anatomy, such as intraoperative cholangiography (IOC) or asking for a second surgeon to scrub in and assist in the assessment and management of the injury. A properly performed IOC that clearly shows all parts of the biliary tree (duodenum, CBD, CHD, CD, right anterior section, right posterior section, and left liver) should reassure the surgeon to proceed with the procedure. An IOC that is not complete, i.e. does not show all parts listed, can easily be misinterpreted and the surgeon is advised not to ignore his/her suspicion and utilize techniques to complete the IOC (see section on Cholangiography) or ask for a second opinion. He/she may also request a formal radiology read of an IOC if there is any doubt about biliary or hepatic anatomy.

If a BDI is demonstrated, then the expertise of the operating surgeon or other in-house surgeon for managing BDI dictates the next step in management. It is important to note that BDIs occur across a spectrum and while expertise and skill may exist to manage low bile duct injuries (Strasberg A, D, E_1), high injuries (Strasberg E_2-E_4), posterior sector duct injuries (Strasberg B, C, E_5) [33-35] and/or vasculobiliary injuries [36, 37] require a different set of expertise and hepatobiliary capability that typically does not exist except in specialized hepatobiliary units.

In the event that repair of a particular BDI is beyond the surgeon's or hospital's ability, immediate telephone contact with a HPB referral surgeon or center is advised to ensure optimal patient outcome. This is best accomplished immediately from the operating room. Again, these referral patterns are best established in advance. If immediate phone conversation is not possible, the surgeon is advised not to proceed but rather establish good drainage of the injury. It is important to speak with the family and patient and refer the patient with all documentation, images, and ensure surgeon-surgeon phone conversation in a timely manner. The use of a referral check list (Table 2) is recommended to avoid errors of omission and affect a safe transfer to a higher level of care hospital and HPB surgeon.

Table 2. Transfer Check List

☐ Communicate with patient and key family members rational and need for transfer
☐ Name of receiving physicians and hospital
☐ Medical records/chart
☐ Key laboratory tests
☐ Current medications
☐ Brief note on physical/physiologic status
☐ patient cognition, awareness of situation
☐ urine output
☐ IV access
☐ drains-clearly label, secure
☐ pain control plan
☐ All pertinent imaging studies on a disk
☐ Operative note
☐ Define the biliary injury as understood
☐ Hand drawn figure portraying injury/anatomy and position of drains
☐ Cholangiograms
☐ send intraoperative digital picture if possible
☐ Surgeon to surgeon communication
☐ before transfer
☐ follow up communication plan

If the type of BDI lends itself to immediate intraoperative repair, i.e. absence of a vascular injury and the presence of sufficient surgical expertise, such repair should proceed based on best standards for such injury. In this situation, the surgeon is advised to leave the operating room, if safe, in order to inform the patient's family or whomever has accompanied them to the hospital, that an injury has occurred and additional surgery is going to occur in an effort to repair the injury. Immediate disclosure to the patient about the nature of the injury and repair should occur as soon as the patient is awake and alert. Caution is advised in ignoring an injury to the right hepatic artery or an accessory right hepatic artery or in underestimating the level of injury because immediate repair in such setting may result in poor long-term outcomes. [5,38,39]

VI-B. Postoperative Suspicion of BDI (Figure 1b)

The surgeon may be confronted with a patient with complications of BDI in the immediate post-operative period or months to years after a previous right upper quadrant operation. Patients presenting in the immediate post-operative period (e.g. less than 30 days) will usually give a history of never having felt well with signs of acute illness. The evaluation and management of these patients is discussed in detail below. In contrast, patients who present with injury months or years later usually have an insidious onset of symptoms related to an underlying bile duct stricture, which manifests in the form of abdominal pain, jaundice and/or cholangitis. These strictures may be secondary to an unrecognized injury made at the time of operation related to a clip or thermal damage to the bile duct. Alternatively, a bile duct stricture may have evolved following bile duct injury that was addressed in the immediate post-operative period from reoperation, endoscopic or percutaneous management. These patients should be referred to a surgeon and/or endoscopist experienced in the management of biliary strictures. Discussion of these patients is beyond the scope of this chapter and the interested reader can read about the approach. [40-42]

As stated previously, suspicion of BDI should occur when any patient undergoing right upper quadrant surgery complains of abdominal problems in the early post-operative period or has an unexpected post-operative course. A prompt and thorough evaluation of these patients to exclude BDI is indicated. This evaluation should include physical examination, laboratory studies (to include liver function tests), and abdominal imaging. While this evaluation is being initiated, the patient should be resuscitated and broad spectrum antibiotics initiated. An important early step in the evaluation process of a presumed BDI is for the surgeon to determine if the patient has an active bile leak as part of their biliary injury or if they have a ligated or clipped duct without a leak. This is important because if a bile leak exists, surgical site control of the leak becomes the next priority (see section on Source Control). If a leak does not exist, the management follows a different pathway (Figure 1b).

Abdominal imaging is best achieved by either ultrasound or CT scan. If ultrasound is performed, the sonographer should be asked to interrogate the arterial and portal venous flow to the right lobe of the liver as well. In many patients, ileus, obesity or intestinal gas may prevent clear views of the subhepatic or subdiaphragmatic spaces by ultrasound. For this reason, an abdominal/pelvic CT scan with intravenous and oral contrast provides the most information because it can identify fluid collections anywhere in the abdomen as well as provide anatomic detailed information about the critical structures in the porta hepatis as well as integrity of arterial and portal blood supply to the liver. However, intravenous contrast should not be given to a patient if they are dehydrated or have an elevated creatinine.

A bile leak will usually lead to diffuse ascites or loculated fluid collections. It is important to note that patients with an active leak with large amounts of bile in their peritoneal cavity may have little to no tenderness while others with a small amount of bile in the peritoneal cavity may have peritoneal irritation. The absence of peritoneal signs on examination does not exclude a major bile leak and the surgeon should not be lulled into complacency regarding the potential dire consequences of an active bile leak. An active bile leak that is walled off from the peritoneal cavity (usually in the subhepatic or subdiaphragmatic spaces) often is not accompanied by abdominal tenderness. It is important to remember that many patients with a biliary leak from BDI can also have partial or complete obstruction of other segments of their biliary tree.

If no fluid collections or ascites is found on CT or ultrasound, and the patient has normal liver function tests, BDI is probably not the cause of the patient's symptoms and physical findings. In such circumstances, alternative causes of the patient's complaints need to be further investigated. Alternatively, if no fluid collections or ascites are found on CT or ultrasound and the patient is jaundiced, or has elevated liver function tests, then it is presumed that the patient has biliary obstruction (follow red text in Figure 1b). The most common cause of obstruction in the post-operative period include a retained common bile duct stone or an inadvertently clipped common or hepatic bile duct. A HIDA scan or ERCP can confirm the presence of obstruction and also exclude with confidence a bile leak. ERCP, if available, is the diagnostic test of choice as it can not only identify the point of obstruction, but also because it can be therapeutic by relieving obstruction through removal of a stone or placement of a stent across a partially clipped but intact duct.

With an understanding of how BDIs occur, experienced HPB surgeons can usually predict the type of BDI a patient has after reviewing only the operative report, the CT or ultrasound and lab studies, and noting the presence, number and position of clips on abdominal radiographs or CT scan. This knowledge and understanding is also important for the surgeon evaluating and managing patients with BDIs because it can alert them to specific types of BDI that they may elect not to explore in favor of early referral. A number of typical scenarios are provided to serve as examples of how various BDIs present in Table 5.

Understanding some important physiologic facts can help the surgeon properly interpret liver function tests in the setting of BDI. A mild elevation in bilirubin (<3mg/dl) with otherwise normal LFTs or minimally elevated LFTs can result from bile in the peritoneal cavity. Marked elevation in serum bilirubin and clinical jaundice usually occurs only with complete bile duct obstruction. If one-half of the liver is not obstructed, marked jaundice usually does not develop. However, serum alkaline phosphatase will become elevated with obstruction of just one single liver segment.

Source Control of Bile Leak

Once the presence or absence of a fluid collection and biliary obstruction is determined, the surgeon needs to use his/her judgment as to the next best course of action depending upon a number of factors: his/her experience and comfort level of dealing with a bile duct injury, the physiologic condition of the patient, availability of resources, and availability and time necessary for transfer to a tertiary center that can provide multidisciplinary HPB care. The inexperienced surgeon should not endeavor to repair any bile duct injury laparoscopically unless it is an easily identified cystic duct leak. Likewise, the inexperienced surgeon should not dissect in the porta hepatis in an effort to identify an injured bile duct for they could cause further damage and/or bleeding.

The principle goal of the acute care surgeon at the time of laparoscopic exploration is to achieve source control of the leak as a means to stabilize the patient. Secondary goals of exploration are to identify the source and nature of the bile leak. We recommend that patients with diffuse intra-abdominal fluid collections accompanied with physical signs of peritonitis, or systemic toxicity be explored urgently once they are reasonably resuscitated. This is important, even if the surgeon is not experienced in surgically correcting bile duct injury for two reasons. First, the goal of exploration is drainage of bile collections, peritoneal toilet and surgical site control of the leaking bile duct(s). This is thoroughly and rapidly accomplished with exploration of the abdomen. Secondly, abdominal exploration is the best way to identify and treat a hollow viscous injury, which frequently accompanies biliary injury [43] and can be difficult to distinguish from BDI. In fact, a duodenal or small bowel perforation can be misinterpreted as a bile duct injury and these injuries are not effectively managed with percutaneous drainage. In addition, failure to recognize, drain and control a hollow viscus injury in a timely manner (e.g. < 24 hrs) is associated with substantially increased risk of death.

Abdominal exploration can be initiated safely via a laparoscopic approach and is preferred in patients who were initially operated upon laparoscopically. The rationale for starting abdominal exploration laparoscopically occurs when the patient is found to have a simple cystic duct leak or type D injury that can be managed without laparotomy. An additional justification for laparoscopic exploration occurs when the surgeon chooses not to repair the BDI and only drain it externally. Drainage is easily and rapidly accomplished and spares the patient the morbidity of a laparotomy incision just prior to hospital transfer. If for any reason effective irrigation and drainage of the peritoneal cavity and a leaking bile duct cannot be accomplished laparoscopically, or if hollow viscus injury not confidently ruled out, the surgeon should proceed to laparotomy. This approach eliminates the devastating consequences of a missed bowel injury, rapidly stabilizes the patient by eliminating bile peritonitis and reduces the probability of the patient developing SIRS or organ failure as they are being prepared for transfer to a tertiary care center. If the hospital and acute care surgeon lack the ability to safely perform emergent laparoscopy or laparotomy, immediate contact and transfer to a higher level of care is advised.

Classification of Injury

Once a patient is resuscitated, stable, and adequately drained, an effort to classify the type and level of BDI should be performed via ERCP, MRCP or PTC. This is a critical step in the management of any BDI because bile leakage from a Strasberg Class A, B or C injury may be easily and appropriately managed by the acute care surgeon whereas a higher injury at or above the bifurcation may be beyond the capabilities of the surgeon and/or hospital. Even an experienced HPB surgeon must try to understand the level and complexity of a bile duct injury prior to operation so that an appropriate and safe reconstructive operation can be planned and carried out.

While uncommon, a small bile leak can exist without a large fluid collection being detected by imaging. Therefore, if BDI is suspected for any reason, even in the absence of intra-abdominal fluid collections a HIDA scan, MRCP, ERCP, or PTC can be obtained-preferably in that order (from least invasive to most invasive, see Figure 1c). If adjunct biliary imaging is not available and hence the nature and location of the injury cannot be determined preoperatively, the acute care surgeon must decide if the patient is stable for transport to a higher level of care or if emergent damage control laparotomy is warranted first as a means of stabilization prior to transport.

The type of bile duct injury encountered coupled with the surgeon's experience and judgment will dictate if the injury can be definitively managed at the time of exploration (e.g. simple cystic duct leak or small laceration of common bile duct) or if definitive repair should be deferred such as Strasberg Class E or vasculobiliary injury. Based on the type of injury identified, the center specific pathways should define the best method of management. This may be endoscopic management (i.e. stent), percutaneous or surgical management if expertise and resources allow. Again, patients with a BDI at or above the biliary bifurcation, vasculobiliary injury, or who fail to respond to resuscitation should be immediately transferred to a center where multidisciplinary expertise exists in HPB disease.

VI-C. Cholangiography

Intraoperative cholangiography is an essential tool in the surgeon's arsenal, and he/she is advised to know the exact ability of their operating room in advance. [18,44] The ability to have live fluoroscopy is essential. Further, the ability to replay the fluoroscopy run is very helpful and essential for accurate determination of the presence BDI and level of injury. [45]

The surgeon needs to also be comfortable in utilizing techniques that allow for better visualization of proximal ducts. These techniques are often necessary in patients with a history of sphincterotomy where obtaining enough intrabiliary contrast pressure to view intrahepatic ducts can be challenging.

The surgeon should not accept an incomplete cholangiogram as sufficient to alleviate suspicion of BDI. An improperly read cholangiogram in the presence of a BDI is a common phenomenon primarily because the cholangiogram is incomplete. A complete IOC must include visualization of the CBD, CHD, CD, left-sided intrahepatic ducts, and right anterior and posterior section ducts. It must also show passage of contrast into duodenum. Adjunct techniques to achieve a complete cholangiogram may be needed, including: manipulating patient positioning; clamping the distal bile duct to facilitate proximal filling; using a smaller syringe to obtain higher injection pressure; using balloon occlusion in the duct (with the ability to inject proximal and distal to the balloon); needle cholangiography via the common bile duct; duct irrigation with saline; and use of sphincter relaxants such as glucagon. Cholangiographic pictures and cine loops obtained intraoperatively are critically important information to transfer to the surgeon who ultimately manages the repair. If immediate surgical repair is not performed at the time of the index operation, subsequent cholangiography can be performed via the subhepatic drains once they are well walled off from the abdominal cavity or via percutaneous transhepatic drainage.

VI- D. Repair Goals

The goals of biliary reconstruction are to provide definitive internal biliary drainage, to ensure long term anastomotic patency with low chance of stricture, and to avoid major post-operative complications such as bile leak, sepsis, organ failure and death. To achieve these goals, surgeons repairing BDIs should possess appropriate knowledge about biliary anatomy and injury, exercise solid judgment with respect to the timing of repair, the choice of repair and possess sufficient experience and technical skill in biliary surgery. [9,11,19,31,46,47] A surgeon who elects not to repair a BDI still plays a pivotal role in achieving the best possible outcome for the patient by timely diagnosis, stabilization through surgical site control, and early referral.

Basic Principles of Bile Duct Injury Repair

There are no set rules in BDI repair. However, there are general principles that a surgeon should follow as a means to achieve the best possible outcomes for the patient with BDI (see Tables 3 and 4). Optimal clinical outcomes of BDI repair begins with appropriate timing of the repair. The timing of surgical repair must always be individualized and will vary from patient to patient. [9,19,46,48] As discussed earlier, the best possible outcome is achieved if a BDI is recognized at the time it occurs and repaired during the same operation. [46,49] Unfortunately for most patients, the BDI is not recognized at the time it occurs and the patient subsequently presents in the post-operative period. When an experienced HPB surgeon is confronted with a patient several days after BDI has occurred, he/she has to evaluate and use their judgment if an early versus a late repair should be performed. There is no high level medical evidence to support one approach over the other though many reports have shown that delayed repair results in excellent outcomes. [48] In fact, it is not realistic to perform a prospective, controlled, randomized trial to solve this question because of the variations in patients' anatomy, inflammatory response, and type of injury. However, some basic criteria for proceeding with immediate repair are offered in Table 3 while other criteria for delaying repair are listed in Table 4.

Patients satisfying the criteria for early repair (e.g. within 2-4 days of injury) can have excellent long term outcomes when repaired by experienced HPB surgeons. [50,51] However, when a patient satisfying these criteria is explored early and found to have significant inflammation of the porta hepatis and/or of their intestines or an unexpected vasculobiliary injury, long term results of repair are less satisfactory and post-operative complications are high. [36, 39, 52] Under such circumstances the surgeon must decide to risk repair and accept a high rate of early and late failure or to delay repair, typically for 6 weeks to 3 months. This is a critically important decision that requires keen judgment and experience. [2, 8, 31, 41, 47, 48, 51] If the surgeon decides not to repair a BDI at initial laparotomy, then the right upper quadrant should be adequately drained via trans-abdominal drains placed in the subhepatic space.

Table 3. Conditions for Going Ahead with Bile Duct Repair

- Physiologically stable
- No systemic or localized infection
- No significant edema of the bile duct or intestine
- Absence of concomitant major vascular injury
- Minimal or well controlled medical comorbidities
- Complete cholangiography of all liver segments obtained

Table 4. Surgical Check List for Considering Emergent Repair

The following guidelines can serve as a surgical check list for the surgeon who is faced with the challenge of repairing a bile duct. A yes answer to any of these questions is grounds for not performing repair, delaying repair or transferring the patient to an experienced surgeon in biliary repair.

- Is there systemic or intraabdominal sepsis?
- Is the patient hemodynamically unstable ?
- Is there significant inflammation in the porta hepatis or bowel wall edema?
- Is the level of injury at or above the bifurcation (Strasberg E2 or higher).
- Is there a right posterior sector duct injury?
- Is there significant thermal injury to the bile duct close to the bifurcation or to any of the sector ducts?
- Are the orifices of the hepatic duct or sector ducts < 3 mm?
- Is there evidence of concomitant vascular injury, such as ligation of the right or an accessory right hepatic artery?
- Is the surgeon unable to delineate all liver segments with cholangiography?
- Is the surgeon not able to identify healthy proximal hepatic duct below the bifurcation with good blood supply that is at least 5 mm in diameter?

Table 5. Typical Presentation Scenarios of Bile Duct Injury and the Suggested Management

Scenario 1. Marked elevation in bilirubin, alkaline phosphatase, AST, ALT No peritoneal fluid seen on imaging. No peritoneal irritation or abdominal guarding. Additional clips are seen in midline than cannot be explained if just the cystic duct and cystic artery were ligated. Clips positioned along the same vertical axis should be suspected to be on the common bile duct and hepatic ducts. Possibilities: 1) obstruction from stone; 2) clip completely across bile duct (E1, E2) or right and left ducts (E4) with no bile duct transection; 3) complete transection of duct with complete occlusion of proximal biliary system (any E).
Scenario 2. Mild elevation in liver function tests (bilirubin <3, and near normal alkaline phosphatase) with abdominal fluid present. Abdominal tenderness may or may not be present Possibilities: Strasberg A, D, C or any E if one side of liver is not occluded.
Scenario 3. Mild elevation in AST, ALT, bili (<3). Moderate elevation in alkaline phosphatase. No fluid observed on CT. No leak demonstrated by HIDA with intact flow into small bowel. ERCP shows no obstruction or bile leak and is commonly interpreted as normal by endoscopist and radiologist. However, failure to fill a right posterior sector or segment VI or VII ducts is a partially clipped or unclipped transected right posterior sector duct (see Figure 3). Probable: Strasberg B. Diagnosis confirmed by absence of right posterior sector or segmental ducts on ERCP, differential perfusion of right posterior segments VI or VII or right posterior section on a four phase CT scan, cholangiography filling right posterior sector ducts without filling of common bile duct.
Scenario 4. High bile duct injury suspected or observed. Decreased perfusion to the right hemi-liver during the arterial phase of CT, or enhanced perfusion to the right hemi liver during the portal venous phase of CT scan is indirect evidence of right hepatic arterial ligation. Marked elevation in AST, ALT without elevation in bilirubin shortly after operation. Possibility: vasculobiliary injury.

Also, when a patient has high biliary transection (e.g. Strasberg E_2-E_4), or very small ducts in whom percutaneous transhepatic catheters have not yet been placed, the orifices of the transected ducts can be cannulated with small pediatric feeding catheters (usually 5F) which are secured to the edge of the transected duct and then exteriorized. These catheters can subsequently be used to obtain cholangiograms to help delineate the patient's biliary anatomy and to serve as guides for future biliary reconstruction.

Additional subhepatic drainage is always indicated in these patients because even with ductal cannulation and drainage, bile will leak around these catheters into the subhepatic space.

Patients with localized intra-abdominal or systemic sepsis or hemodynamic instability within the first few days of a BDI should not undergo early repair. Management should be centered around and limited to achieving source control thorough external drainage of all collections, as well as controlling sepsis and correcting organ dysfunction. Effective trans-abdominal drainage via two large (at least #15F) soft silastic round closed suction drains is perhaps the most important thing that an surgeon can and should ensure as a means of stabilizing the patient should he/she decide to transfer them to a higher level of care. Round drains are preferred over flat drains because they are more easily exchanged over a guide wire and replaced with pigtail catheters should the need arise.

One drain is placed in the sub diaphragmatic space and right colonic gutter and the other in the sub hepatic space; both exit posterior laterally through the abdominal wall. Patients rarely become systemically ill when external biliary diversion is managed by trans-abdominal drains and usually promptly improve. Subhepatic drains, while providing early safe and effective drainage of intra-abdominal biliary leaks should ideally not be kept in place long term because of the risk for eroding into bowel loops and causing biliary-enteric cutaneous fistulae. [43] This however is not something that the acute care surgeon will usually have to deal with but rather rests with the surgeon managing delayed repair.

When complete biliary intestinal disconnection exists as occurs with complete transection or ligation of the hepatic or common bile duct (Strasberg E), external biliary drainage is ultimately best managed via a percutaneous transhepatic biliary drainage (PTBD) tube. Such drains can traverse the opening of the transected biliary tree and even drain the sub hepatic space. Complete biliary diversion creates a special physiologic situation that the surgeon can play an important role in managing through placing a GJ or feeding jejunostomy tube at the time of initial exploration.

This is important for patients who must be repaired in a delayed manner so that bile collected through their PTBD catheters can be fed through a feeding tube into their proximal small bowel. Bile should not be fed through a G tube or placed down a NG tube because it can cause bile gastritis; it must be placed into the duodenum or farther downstream. (See section on post-operative complications for the importance of bile refeeding).

Austere Environments

Surgeons in a remote or isolated setting may find themselves in a circumstance where the patient has a suspected BDI, no interventional radiology support, no gastroenterology support, and the inability to transfer the patient due to lack of immediate resources. In such a setting, appropriate source control and drainage is the primary goal. The secondary goal, when safe and feasible, is operative repair using the principles discussed earlier. Definitive repair in the presence of widespread contamination, severe inflammation, sepsis, or patient instability has rather poor outcomes and should not be contemplated.

If the patient is found to have a complete biliary disconnection with total biliary diversion, and is subject to prolonged external drainage (e.g. months) then the surgeon should give consideration to bile refeeding. This can be accomplished by placing a feeding jejunostomy tube at the time of laparotomy or via a nasoduodenal feeding tube post operatively. Once the patient is stable, they can be transferred to a higher level of care.

References

[1] Flum, DR; Cheadle, A; Prela, C; Dellinger, EP; Chan, L. Bile duct injury during cholecystectomy and survival in medicare beneficiaries. *JAMA*, 2003, 290(16), 2168-2173.

[2] Walsh, RM; Henderson, JM; Vogt, DP; Brown, N. Long-term outcome of biliary reconstruction for bile duct injuries from laparoscopic cholecystectomies. *Surgery*, 2007, 142(4), 450-456.

[3] Dolan, JP; Diggs, BS; Sheppard, BC; Hunter, JG. Ten-year trend in the national volume of bile duct injuries requiring operative repair. *Surg Endosc*, 2005, 19(7), 967-973.

[4] Melton, GB; Lillemoe, KD; Cameron, JL; Sauter, PA; Coleman, J; Yeo, CJ. Major bile duct injuries associated with laparoscopic cholecystectomy: effect of surgical repair on quality of life. *Ann Surg*, 2002, 235(6), 888-895.

[5] Buell, JF; Cronin, DC; Funaki, B; et al. Devastating and fatal complications associated with combined vascular and bile duct injuries during cholecystectomy. *Arch Surg*, 2002, 137(6), 703-708.

[6] Sicklick, JK; Camp, MS; Lillemoe, KD; et al. Surgical management of bile duct injuries sustained during laparoscopic cholecystectomy: perioperative results in, 200 patients. *Ann Surg*, 2005, 241(5), 786-792.

[7] Johnson, SR; Koehler, A; Pennington, LK; Hanto, DW. Long-term results of surgical repair of bile duct injuries following laparoscopic cholecystectomy. *Surgery*, 2000, 128(4), 668-677.

[8] Mercado, MA; Chan, C; Orozco, H; et al. Prognostic implications of preserved bile duct confluence after iatrogenic injury. *Hepatogastroenterology*, 2005, 52(61), 40-44.

[9] Mercado, MA. Early versus late repair of bile duct injuries. *Surg Endosc*, 2006, 20(11), 1644-1647.

[10] Strasberg, SM; Hertl, M; Soper, NJ. An analysis of the problem of biliary injury during laparoscopic cholecystectomy. *J Am Coll Surg*, 1995, 180(1), 101-125.

[11] Winslow, ER; Fialkowski, EA; Linehan, DC; Hawkins, WG; Picus, DD; Strasberg SM. “Sideways”: results of repair of biliary injuries using a policy of side-to-side hepatico-jejunostomy. *Ann Surg*, 2009, 249(3), 426-434.

[12] Davidoff, AM; Pappas, TN; Murray, EA; et al. Mechanisms of major biliary injury during laparoscopic cholecystectomy. *Ann Surg*, 1992, 215(3), 196-202.

[13] Lillemoe, KD; Melton, GB; Cameron, JL; et al. Postoperative bile duct strictures: management and outcome in the, 1990s. *Ann Surg*, 2000, 232(3), 430-441.

[14] Barkun, JS; Barkun, AN; Sampalis, JS; et al. Randomised controlled trial of laparoscopic versus mini cholecystectomy. The McGill Gallstone Treatment Group. *Lancet*, 1992, 340(8828), 1116-1119.

[15] Bass, EB; Pitt, HA; Lillemoe KD. Cost-effectiveness of laparoscopic cholecystectomy versus open cholecystectomy. *Am J Surg*, 1993, 165(4), 466-471.

[16] Soper, NJ; Barteau, JA; Clayman, RV; Ashley, SW; Dunnegan DL. Comparison of early postoperative results for laparoscopic versus standard open cholecystectomy. *Surg Gynecol Obstet*, 1992, 174(2), 114-118.

[17] Adamsen, S; Hansen, OH; Funch-Jensen, P; Schulze, S; Stage, JG; Wara, P. Bile duct injury during laparoscopic cholecystectomy: a prospective nationwide series. *J Am Coll Surg*, 1997, 184(6), 571-578.

[18] Flum, DR; Dellinger, EP; Cheadle, A; Chan, L; Koepsell, T. Intraoperative cholangiography and risk of common bile duct injury during cholecystectomy. *JAMA*, 2003, 289(13), 1639-1644.

[19] Perera, MT; Silva, MA; Hegab, B; et al. Specialist early and immediate repair of post-laparoscopic cholecystectomy bile duct injuries is associated with an improved long-term outcome. *Ann Surg*, 2011, 253(3), 553-560.

[20] Strasberg, SM. Biliary injury in laparoscopic surgery: part 1. Processes used in determination of standard of care in misidentification injuries. *J Am Coll Surg*, 2005, 201(4), 598-603.

[21] Strasberg, SM. Biliary injury in laparoscopic surgery: part 2. Changing the culture of cholecystectomy. *J Am Coll Surg*, 2005, 201(4), 604-611.

[22] Berber, E; Engle, KL; String, A; et al. Selective use of tube cholecystostomy with interval laparoscopic cholecystectomy in acute cholecystitis. *Arch Surg*, 2000, 135(3), 341-346.

[23] Borzellino, G; de MG; Ricci, F; Castaldini, G; Guglielmi, A; Cordiano, C. Emergency cholecystostomy and subsequent cholecystectomy for acute gallstone cholecystitis in the elderly. *Br J Surg*, 1999, 86(12), 1521-1525.

[24] Byrne, MF; Suhocki, P; Mitchell, RM; et al. Percutaneous cholecystostomy in patients with acute cholecystitis: experience of 45 patients at a US referral center. *J Am Coll Surg*, 2003, 197(2), 206-211.

[25] Halpin, V; Gupta, A. Acute cholecystitis. *Clin Evid* (Online), 2011, 2011.

[26] SAGES Guidelines for the Clinical Application of Laparoscopic Biliiary Tract Surgery., 2012. Ref Type: Online Source

[27] Yegiyants, S; Collins, JC. Operative strategy can reduce the incidence of major bile duct injury in laparoscopic cholecystectomy. *Am Surg*, 2008, 74(10), 985-987.

[28] Avgerinos, C; Kelgiorgi, D; Touloumis, Z; Baltatzi, L; Dervenis, C. One thousand laparoscopic cholecystectomies in a single surgical unit using the "critical view of safety" technique. *J Gastrointest Surg*, 2009, 13(3), 498-503.

[29] Strasberg, SM. Biliary injury in laparoscopic surgery: part 2. Changing the culture of cholecystectomy. *J Am Coll Surg*, 2005, 201(4), 604-611.

[30] Carroll, BJ; Birth, M; Phillips, EH. Common bile duct injuries during laparoscopic cholecystectomy that result in litigation. *Surg Endosc*, 1998, 12(4), 310-313.

[31] Lillemoe, KD. Current management of bile duct injury. *Br J Surg*, 2008, 95(4), 403-405.

[32] Russell, JC, Walsh, SJ, Mattie, AS; Lynch, JT. Bile duct injuries, 1989-1993. A statewide experience. Connecticut Laparoscopic Cholecystectomy Registry. *Arch Surg*, 1996, 131(4), 382-388.

[33] Lillemoe, KD; Petrofski, JA; Choti, MA; Venbrux, AC; Cameron, JL. Isolated right segmental hepatic duct injury: a diagnostic and therapeutic challenge. *J Gastrointest Surg*, 2000, 4(2), 168-177.

[34] Perera, MT; Monaco, A; Silva, MA; et al. Laparoscopic posterior sectoral bile duct injury: the emerging role of nonoperative management with improved long-term results after delayed diagnosis. *Surg Endosc*, 2011, 25(8), 2684-2691.

[35] Mazer, LM; Tapper, EB; Sarmiento, JM. Non-operative management of right posterior sectoral duct injury following laparoscopic cholecystectomy. *J Gastrointest Surg*, 2011, 15(7), 1237-1242.

[36] Strasberg, SM; Helton, WS. An analytical review of vasculobiliary injury in laparoscopic and open cholecystectomy. *HPB* (Oxford), 2011, 13(1), 1-14.

[37] Pulitano, C; Parks, RW; Ireland, H; Wigmore, SJ; Garden, OJ. Impact of concomitant arterial injury on the outcome of laparoscopic bile duct injury. *Am J Surg*, 2011, 201(2), 238-244.

[38] Strasberg, SM. Error traps and vasculo-biliary injury in laparoscopic and open cholecystectomy. *J Hepatobiliary Pancreat Surg*, 2008, 15(3), 284-292.

[39] Koffron, A; Ferrario, M; Parsons, W; Nemcek, A; Saker, M; Abecassis, M. Failed primary management of iatrogenic biliary injury: incidence and significance of concomitant hepatic arterial disruption. *Surgery*, 2001, 130(4), 722-728.

[40] Hepp, J. Hepaticojejunostomy using the left biliary trunk for iatrogenic biliary lesions: the French connection. *World J Surg*, 1985, 9(3), 507-511.

[41] Mercado, MA; Chan, C; Orozco, H; Tielve, M; Hinojosa, CA. Acute bile duct injury. The need for a high repair. *Surg Endosc*, 2003, 17(9), 1351-1355.

[42] Jarnagin, W; Blumgart, LH. Blumgart's Surgery of the Liver, Pancreas and Biliary Tract. 5th Edition ed. Elsevier Saunders, 2012.

[43] Mercado, MA; Chan, C; Orozco, H; et al. Iatrogenic intestinal injury concomitant to iatrogenic bile duct injury: the second component. *Curr Surg*, 2004, 61(4), 380-385.

[44] Fletcher, DR; Hobbs, MS; Tan, P,; et al. Complications of cholecystectomy: risks of the laparoscopic approach and protective effects of operative cholangiography: a population-based study. *Ann Surg*, 1999, 229(4), 449-457.

[45] Carroll, BJ; Friedman, RL; Liberman, MA; Phillips, EH. Routine cholangiography reduces sequelae of common bile duct injuries. *Surg Endosc*, 1996, 10(12), 1194-1197.

[46] Stewart, L; Way, LW. Bile duct injuries during laparoscopic cholecystectomy. Factors that influence the results of treatment. *Arch Surg*, 1995, 130(10), 1123-1128.

[47] Chapman, WC; Abecassis, M; Jarnagin, W; Mulvihill, S; Strasberg, SM. Bile duct injuries 12 years after the introduction of laparoscopic cholecystectomy. *J Gastrointest Surg*, 2003, 7(3), 412-416.

[48] Strasberg, SM; Picus, DD; Drebin, JA. Results of a new strategy for reconstruction of biliary injuries having an isolated right-sided component. *J Gastrointest Surg*, 2001, 5(3), 266-274.

[49] Stewart, L; Way, LW. Laparoscopic bile duct injuries: timing of surgical repair does not influence success rate. A multivariate analysis of factors influencing surgical outcomes. *HPB* (Oxford), 2009, 11(6), 516-522.

[50] Wudel, LJ Jr; Wright, JK; Pinson, CW; et al. Bile duct injury following laparoscopic cholecystectomy: a cause for continued concern. *Am Surg*, 2001, 67(6), 557-563.

[51] Mercado, MA; Franssen, B; Dominguez, I; et al. Transition from a low: to a high-volume centre for bile duct repair: changes in technique and improved outcome. *HPB* (Oxford), 2011, 13(11), 767-773.

[52] Stewart, L; Robinson, TN; Lee, CM; Liu, K; Whang, K; Way, LW. Right hepatic artery injury associated with laparoscopic bile duct injury: incidence, mechanism, and consequences. *J Gastrointest Surg*, 2004, 8(5), 523-530.

In: Bile Duct
Editor: Miguel Ángel Mercado

ISBN: 978-1-63321-771-3

Chapter 12

Ampullary Tumors and Tumor Like Lesions: Histological Classification, Diagnosis and Surgical Treatment

Wenqing Cao MD[1]*, Kate L. Forssell MD[2], Dylan R. Nieman MD, PhD[3], Danielle Marino MD[2] and Jiangzhou Yu MD, PhD[1]

[1]Department of Pathology and Laboratory Medicine,
Gastrointestinal and Liver Pathology,
University of Rochester Medical Center, Rochester, NY
[2]Department of Medicine, Gastroenterology and Hepatology Division,
University of Rochester Medical Center, Rochester, NY
[3]Department of Surgery, University of Rochester Medical Center, NY

Abstract

The ampulla of Vater is a complex region adjoined by three distinct anatomic structures: common bile duct, pancreatic duct and duodenum. This region is lined by mixed intestinal, foveolar and pancreaticobiliary-type epithelium. Adenomas and adenocarcinomas are the predominant primary ampullary tumors. Neuroendocrine tumors, comprised of low grade neuroendocrine tumors (carcinoids) and high grade neuroendocrine carcinomas, are rare. Benign tumor-like lesions constitute a heterogeneous group of entities that includes primary sclerosing cholangitis, recurrent pyogenic cholangitis, inflammatory myofibroblastic tumor, and recently recognized autoimmune pancreatitis and IgG4-related sclerosing cholangitis. Stricture and obstructive jaundice are the most common presentations in ampullary tumors and tumor-like lesions. Despite the advances in imaging techniques, discriminating ampullary carcinoma from benign tumors and tumor-like conditions is still challenging. Differentiating IgG4-related sclerosing cholangitis from primary sclerosing cholangitis

* Corresponding author.

and cholangiocarcinoma is particularly important, as IgG4-related sclerosing cholangitis is often responsive to steroid treatment. Immunohistochemical stains can be helpful for histological diagnosis and staging, but they have limitations. The current classification system for ampullary carcinoma has limited value for predicting prognosis. Recent studies have suggested that histological differentiation (intestinal type vs pancreaticobiliary type) and sub-location (intra-AMP, AMP-ductal, peri-AMP-duodenal and AC-not otherwise specified) of ampullary carcinoma have prognostic significance. The treatment for benign tumors and tumor-like lesions is mainly endoscopic local resection. Pancreaticoduodenectomy is the most appropriate resectional procedure for large adenomas and early stage ampullary carcinomas, whereas stent or surgical palliation may be offered for late stage, unresectable cancers. In this review, we describe ampullary tumors and tumor-like lesions, and summarize different histological classification systems for ampullary carcinoma. We also address the challenges in discriminating malignant and benign ampullary lesions, and introduce the potential biomarkers for early diagnosis and predicting prognosis. In the meantime, the classical and emerging surgical treatment approaches will be illustrated.

1. Anatomy of the Ampulla of Vater

The ampulla of Vater is composed of the confluence of the biliary, pancreatic, and digestive tracts and marks the transition from embryologic foregut to midgut. The ampulla includes the junction of the common bile duct and the pancreatic duct, the surrounding sphincter of Oddi, the fenestra choledochae (window in the duodenal wall), and duodenal papilla. While the arrangement of these intersections has some variability, there are common and predictable structural relationships that can be appreciated to facilitate endoscopic identification of anatomy and safe intervention.

The predominant anatomical variant, present in approximately 60% of cases, involves a common channel up to 8 mm in length resulting from the confluence of the common bile duct and the main pancreatic duct (Figure 1 A). [1] The labeling of this common channel as an "ampulla" (flask-like dilated duct) may in fact be a historical misnomer resulting from an early artifact of dissection since in the vast majority of studied cases there is no dilatation. [2] The second most common variant (38%) does not include any common channel, with the junction of the biliary and pancreatic tracts occurring at the apex of the papilla. Approximately 2% of cases demonstrate separate duodenal openings for the biliary and pancreatic drainage.

The location of the ampulla is predominantly on the postero-medial aspect of the descending second portion of the duodenum (75%), though can occur along the horizontal third portion of the duodenum to the right of the superior mesenteric axis (25%). [3] In the former scenario, the pancreatic duct is inferior and anterior to the common bile duct, and in the latter the duct is left or medial to the common bile duct. These relationships aid in the selective endoscopic cannulation of the appropriate ducts.

The sphincter of Oddi, the regulator of biliary and pancreatic drainage that allows for intermittent biliary drainage, originates separately from the duodenal musculature from the periductal mesenchyme and later becomes incorporated into the duodenal wall. [3] Anatomic studies suggest that there are components specific to the common channel which are contained within the papilla and the duodenal wall, and components specific to the common bile duct and pancreatic duct which extend outside of the duodenal wall. [1] Functionally, the sphincter can be thought of as consisting of an extramural occlusive zone, an intramural infundibulum, and an intra-luminal zone contained in the papilla which is amenable to safe sphincterotomy. [4]

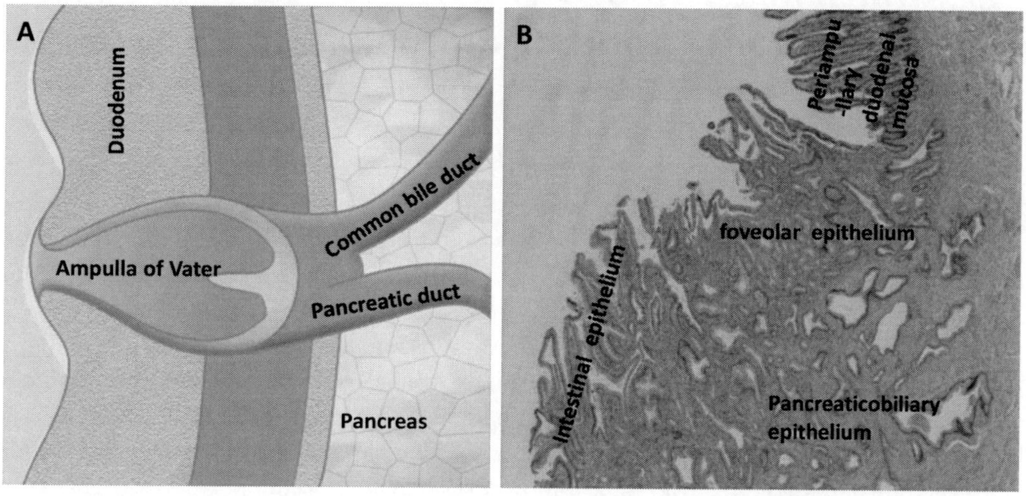

Figure 1. Anatomy and histology of the ampulla of Vater. A. Anatomic location of the ampulla of Vater: adjoined by distal common bile duct, main pancreatic duct and the duodenum. B. Ampullary mucosa: lined by mixed intestinal, foveolar, and pancreaticobiliary epithelium. (H&E staining, original magnification X 20).

The fenestra choledocha, or duodenal window, which surrounds and incorporates the sphincteric complex is a quadrilateral orifice in the wall of the duodenum roughly 5 to 7 mm per side formed by the separation of the deep circular muscle fibers proximally and distally, and superficial longitudinal muscle fibers anteriorly and posteriorly. [1] This window is usually located along the postero-medial wall of the duodenum with the common bile duct entering at an acute angle of approximately thirty degrees and the pancreatic duct closer to horizontal, joining inferior and anterior to the bile duct at an angle of about sixty degrees. Of note, the geometries of the tethering muscle fibers of the duodenal wall result in a lesser density of fibers behind the papilla where mucosal diverticula of the duodenal window may develop. [5]

The duodenal papilla itself is a mucosal prominence of five to ten millimeters in size amidst circular duodenal folds. It typically is situated between a transverse hood and one or more inferior longitudinal folds which serve as useful landmarks as they are the only vertical structures in the duodenal mucosa. In some patients, a lesser duodenal papilla is present several centimeters above the greater papilla and drains only pancreatic secretions from a patent accessory pancreatic duct of Santorini. [6] In the case of pancreas divisum, where dorsal and ventral pancreatic ducts have not fused, the lesser papilla may drain the entire dorsal pancreas.

The arterial blood supply to the ampulla includes contributions from the posterior and superior pancreaticoduodenal arch, the ventral commissural arch, and the anterior and inferior pancreaticoduodenal arch, the latter two of which participate in the juxtapapillary submucosal plexus. [7] The arteries of the duodenal wall run in a horizontal direction and consequently, duodenotomies near the ampulla should be performed horizontally. The lymphatic drainage of the ampulla is the same as that of the right pancreas.

2. Ampullary Tumors and Tumor-Like Lesions: Clinical Presentations, Diagnosis and Endoscopic Management

Tumors of the ampulla of Vater are uncommon. The estimated incidence in the United States is 3,000 cases per year, with a reported prevalence of 0.04% to 0.12% in autopsy series. [8] They account for 6 to 10% of periampullary tumors (a group including pancreatic, duodenal and distal bile duct tumors). [9] Over 95% of ampullary tumors are either adenomas or adenocarcinomas. [10] Carcinoid tumors account for another 3% of ampullary tumors. The remaining 2% includes a wide variety of exceedingly rare neoplasms including: malignant neuroendocrine tumor, gastrointestinal stromal tumor (GIST), hamartoma, follicular lymphoma, signet cell carcinoma, Paneth cell carcinoma and mucinous (colloid) carcinoma. Also included ion the differential for an ampullary lesion should be metastatic cancer (breast, kidney, and melanoma) or local invasion from pancreatic or duodenal adenocarcinoma. Finally, there are a few entities that can present as a stricture/mass but are not neoplasms, including primary sclerosing cholangitis and IgG4-associated sclerosing cholangitis. IgG4-associated sclerosing cholangitis is an important entity to recognize as this is responsive to steroids and, therefore, treatable without resection.

2.1. Adenoma

Ampullary adenomas are benign neoplasms arising from the mucosa. They account for less than 10% of all neoplasms of the ampulla of Vater, although they are, by far, the most common benign neoplasm. They can occur sporadically, or in the context of familial polyposis syndromes such as Familial Adenomatous Polyposis (FAP) and its variant, Gardner syndrome. Although they are classified as benign lesions, they have the potential to undergo malignant transformation, following the adenoma-to-carcinoma pathway. [11] Neoplastic transformation of intestinal mucosa occurs more commonly near the ampulla than any other area; probably because the epithelium of the ampulla of Vater is exposed to a mix of pancreatic, intestinal secretions and bile. [12] The incidence of transformation to carcinoma is estimated to range from 25-85% for sporadic adenomas. It has been demonstrated that there is a correlation between the degree of preoperative dysplasia and potential for malignant transformation. Sporadic adenomas are most commonly diagnosed in the sixth to seventh decade of life, and are rarely found in those younger than 40. Although sporadic adenomas are uncommon, an estimated 50-100 % of patients with FAP will manifest adenomatous changes in their ampulla. [8] These lesions tend to occur at a younger age and endoscopic screening programs are recommended in these patients.

2.2. Adenocarcinoma

Ampullary adenocarcinoma represents 2% of all GI malignancies and 20% of all tumors of the extrahepatic biliary tree. [13] Similar to the adenoma, they are more common later in life, typically diagnosed in the seventh decade (unless the patient has a familial polyposis syndrome). There is a described slight male to female predominance, 1.48: 1. [14] FAP is an important risk factor for ampullary carcinoma. Among patients with FAP, ampullary adenocarcinoma is the second most common cause of death (after colorectal cancer). There has also been shown to be a higher incidence of ampullary carcinoma in patients with neurofibromatosis type I [15] and in patients with chronic liver fluke infection. [(14]) Compared to distal bile duct carcinomas and pancreatic adenocarcinomas, ampullary adenocarcinomas have a significantly better prognosis. The five-year survival rates of patients with resected ampullary carcinoma are reported to be 37-68%, [16-18] significantly better than that with resected pancreatic cancer and bile duct cancer (10-30%). The favorable prognosis of ampullary adenocarcinoma is thought to be at least partially due to early presentation of obstructive symptoms such as jaundice. However, tumor biology may also be an explanation for the relatively good prognosis of this disease.

2.3. Neuroendocrine Tumor

Neuroendocrine tumors (NETs) of the ampulla of Vater are rare and represent approximately 2% of ampullary tumors, [19] 10% of duodenal region NETs, and less than 1% of all GI NETs.[(20] Data in the literature really only exists as case reports with few reviews. There is some discussion about a rising incidence seen in the literature recently. [21] Autopsy studies have shown that up to 10% of patients have carcinoid micronests in the minor and major ampullas. [22] Carcinoid syndrome associated with ampullary carcinoid tumors is rare, described in only 2.8% of cases. [21] It has been estimated that metastases are present in over 50% of cases, even with small tumors < 2 cm in size. [23] Based on this data, it is generally recommended that NET of the ampulla of Vater be surgically resected if possible.

2.4. IgG4-Associated Cholangitis and Primary Sclerosing Cholangitis

Several diseases of the bile duct can present with biliary duct strictures that can occur anywhere along the biliary tree. Two such entities are IgG4 associated cholangitis (IAC) and primary sclerosing cholangitis (PSC). IAC refers to the biliary manifestations of IgG4-related systemic disease which is associated with elevated IgG4 levels in the blood and deposition of IgG4 in other organs (including the pancreas). IAC is much more common in males and typically presents in the sixth or seventh decade with obstructive jaundice, weight loss, abdominal pain or steatorrhea. [24] Typically, on imaging, a stricture is found, often mimicking pancreatic head adenocarcinoma or cholangiocarcinoma depending upon the location of the stricture. Evaluation with an Endoscopic Retrograde Cholangio-Pancreatography (ERCP) for a cholangiogram, as well as biopsies of the ampulla or bile duct typically yields the diagnosis, but this is not infrequently mistaken for malignancy. It is an important diagnosis to recognize, as although inflammatory fibrosis may damage and stricture the biliary duct, the process typically responds to steroid therapy. PSC is also an inflammatory biliary process of unclear etiology resulting in str-icturing of the bile ducts. The strictures are typically multifocal and progressive over time. [25] It is typically associated with inflammatory bowel disease (up to 90% patients are found to have ulcerative colitis)[(26]) and those diagnosed with PSC should undergo a colonoscopy if the IBD diagnosis has not already been established. Approximately half of patients with PSC are asymptomatic and are found to have abnormal liver function tests on routine testing. They most commonly have an elevated alkaline phosphatase with otherwise normal liver function tests. Subsequent biliary imaging with either cross sectional studies or endoscopic cholangiography can show inflammation and saccular dilations of the bile duct, giving a "beaded" appearance of the bile duct. If the diagnosis is still not certain, liver biopsy can be performed, although it is not routinely recommended or frequently necessary to establish a diagnosis. [(26]) Patients with PSC have a lifetime risk of 10 to 15 percent of developing cholangiocarcinoma. The disease is progressive and there is no recommended medical therapy. If a dominant stricture is present, endoscopic dilation or stenting can be considered. The treatment of choice for advanced disease is now liver transplantation.

2.5. Clinical Presentations

Despite different underlying pathophysiology, the presenting symptoms for the majority of ampullary tumors are very similar. Some patients are asymptomatic, with lesions found either through screening endoscopies or incidentally through endoscopy or cross-sectional imaging done for the evaluation of unrelated symptoms. When symptoms are present, they typically reflect obstruction of the bile duct or, less commonly, the pancreatic duct. The most common presenting symptom is jaundice, which has been found to occur in up to 80% of patients with ampullary adenomas and ampullary carcinomas, and in two thirds of carcinoid patients. Biliary colic, nausea, vomiting and weight loss are other common symptoms. Multiple other symptoms are possible, including cholangitis, abdominal pain, weight loss, pancreatitis, occult or overt gastrointestinal bleeding or diarrhea secondary to fat malabsorption. 15-30% of patients also have concurrent choledocholithiasis at the time of their diagnosis due to chronic cholestasis. [8] A classic (but rare) finding described secondary to ampullary adenocarcinoma is "silver stools" which arise from acholicalcoholic stools mixed with blood from chronic upper gastrointestinal bleeding of the tumor. Due to their anatomic location at the opening of the bile duct, ampullary tumors tend to cause symptoms earlier than other tumors at the choledochoduodenal junction (pancreatic, duodenal) and, therefore, are typically diagnosed earlier. As a result of this earlier detection, there is significantly improved survival than with other related lesions in this area.

2.6. Diagnosis

Typically, ampullary masses are diagnosed based on their endoscopic appearance and biopsy results. Endoscopically, adenomas or other benign entities tend to be soft and polypoid, whereas firm, indurated, or ulcerated lesions are more concerning for malignancy. Diagnosis cannot sufficiently be made based on endoscopic appearance alone, and biopsies are a necessity. ERCP is perhaps the most important diagnostic test given the ability for direct visualization and biopsy of the ampulla using the side viewing duodenoscope, as well as the ability to obtain brushings from the bile duct and to provide therapeutic sphincterotomy or stent placement.

Non-endoscopic tests which visualize the biliary tree have been discussed as diagnostic modalities, including Magnetic Resonance Cholangio-Pancreatography (MRCP) and Percutaneous Transhepatic Cholangiography (PTC), but they do not have the same clinical utility as ERCP due to poor visualization of the ampulla and inability to biopsy the lesion if found. In a patient with symptoms of obstruction who is high risk for an endoscopic procedure, MRCP can be considered as an initial test, but typically this will need to be followed by an ERCP to allow for biopsy of any lesion found. ERCP has been found to be highly accurate in identifying the presence of even small ampullary lesions [27] and remains the initial diagnostic test of choice.

Endoscopic ultrasound (EUS) can also be considered as an initial test as it has been found to be as accurate as ERCP; however it does not provide the same therapeutic effect as ERCP and, thus, is most typically reserved for staging diagnosed malignancies or evaluating for occult pancreatic tumors when a biliary stricture is found.

Ampullary carcinomas have been described based on their endoscopic appearance. They are divided into three subtypes: intramural protruding (intraampullary), extramural protruding (periampullary) and ulcerating (ampullary). The latter carries the worst prognosis as this is typically diagnosed at a later stage and is most commonly associated with positive lymph nodes. [14] Carcinoid or neuroendocrine tumors are frequently submucosal and difficult to identify. They are infrequently associated with ulceration on the mucosal surface. EUS can be used to aid in the diagnosis of these submucosal ampullary lesions. It is important to note that diagnosis of an ampullary lesion cannot sufficiently be made based on endoscopic appearance alone, and biopsies are a necessity. However, even forceps biopsy in ERCP does have limitations.

Ampullary biopsies are highly subject to sampling error. Autopsy studies have shown that ampullary adenomas are at risk for harboring foci of dysplasia and carcinoma, and normal appearing ampullas can harbor islands of neuroendocrine tissue. The clinical relevance of undetected neuroendocrine tissue is unclear, but that of adenocarcinoma is quite important. In the literature, it has been described that 15-50% of excised ampullary adenomas harbor foci of adenocarcinoma. [8] False-negative biopsy results are not uncommon, and have been found to occur in 25 to 60% of patients with the eventual diagnosis of adenocarcinoma. [8] Thus, absence of carcinoma in a biopsy of an adenoma does not rule out malignancy. Methods have been described to try and improve the accuracy of biopsies including more samples taken at the time of the procedure and biopsies taken 48 hours after sphincterotomy. The only way to be completely sure that no malignancy is present is to completely resect the adenoma or perform endoscopic ampullectomy.

Further imaging can be helpful after diagnosis of malignancy to stage the tumor by evaluating for the presence of local spread or nodal and distal metastases. EUS has been found to be superior to CT, MRI and transabdominal ultrasound for tumor staging. [28, 29] EUS has been described to have an accuracy of 80-90% in detecting local tumor invasion. [30] However, MRI is superior to EUS for nodal staging and CT and PET scans can detect metastases not seen on EUS. If there is a high clinical suspicion of malignancy despite a benign diagnosis on biopsy, EUS can also be helpful in detecting invasive carcinoma. A specialized form of EUS, IntradDuctal UltrasSound (IDUS), has been evaluated in the literature. In two2 studies, this was more accurate in staging tumor spread than conventional EUS. However, this is considered a more cumbersome test and is not available at all centers, so its role in diagnosis remains unclear. [10]

Of note, there is no data to support a role for serum tumor markers in the diagnosis of ampullary adenomas. Serologic diagnosis of carcinoid tumors is beyond the scope of this chapter, but can be an adjunct to endoscopic diagnosis of this entity.

2.7. Endoscopic Treatment

If an ampullary lesion is benign, there is no current consensus on which lesions should be removed and which should be kept under surveillance. [31] If the adenoma is small and the patient does not have FAP, surveillance can be considered. However, larger lesions are riskier given the possibility that they may harbor a focus of malignancy, and thus should be removed. Unlike pancreatic carcinomas, 77 to 88% of ampullary carcinomas are resectable at the time of diagnosis. [32]

There are two methods of removal for ampullary lesions; endoscopic or surgical. The traditional manner of treating an ampullary lesion is surgical resection. However, endoscopic ampullectomy is another option. Certain factors are important to consider when deciding if a lesion should be removed endoscopically or surgically. Presence of malignancy typically means a patient should proceed with surgical resection. Endoscopic removal of adenocarcinoma has been described in non-surgical candidates but is not routinely recommended. [31]

Size is also important, and although there are no definitive guidelines, typically lesions greater than or equal to 4-5 cm should proceed to surgery, as larger lesions are at higher risk for harboring malignant tissue. High grade dysplasia in an adenoma is not a contraindication for endoscopic resection, but other factors should be evaluated prior to deciding on endoscopic resection. Studies have suggested that some endoscopic features including firmness, friability, ulceration and lack of lift on submucosal injection are all indications of possible malignancy and such lesions should be considered for surgical removal even if biopsies are benign. [33]

3. Pathology

The Ampulla of Vater is a complex region adjoined by three different anatomic structures: common bile duct, pancreatic duct and duodenum. It is lined by three different types of epithelium: the duodenal surface is lined by intestinal epithelium; the papilla of Vater shows transitional features of foveolar-like mucosa with scattered goblet cells; the ampullary ducts are lined by pancreaticobiliary type epithelium (Figure 1 B). A heterogeneous group of tumors and tumor-like lesions may arise from this small region.

3.1. Benign Ampullary Tumors

Adenoma

Grossly, ampullary adenomas are exophytic, papillary/granular or flat in appearance ranging from 0.3 to 3.5cm in diameter (Figure 2 A). They are classified as tubular, tubulovillous or villous adenoma based on the histologic growth pattern. Villous adenomas tend to be larger and more likely to harbor high grade dysplasia and carcinoma.

Microscopically, ampullary adenomas are subclassified as intestinal type and pancreaticobiliary type. Intestinal type low grade adenomas show variably complex glands with elongated pencil-shaped and stratified nuclei (Figure 2 B), whereas high grade adenomas show complex and cribriform architecture, pleomorphic nuclei, prominent nucleoli, and loss of polarity (Figure 2 C). Scattered goblet cells and luminal necrotic debris may be present. Pancreaticobiliary type adenomas usually demonstrate high grade morphology with complex arborizing papillae, nuclear pleomorphism and eosinophilic cytoplasm (Figure 2 D).

There are molecular similarities and differences between sporadic adenomas and FAP-related adenomas. For example, inactivating mutations of both APC alleles is thought to be necessary for the development of adenomas in FAP, [(34]) whereas in sporadic adenomas, the frequency of somatic *APC* mutation is only 17% and the site of somatic *APC* mutation is different. [35] KRAS mutations are observed in both settings, but more frequently in sporadic ampullary adenomas (28.6%-44%) than FAP-related adenomas (17%). [36, 37] BRAF mutations are rare in both sporadic and FAP-related adenomas. [37] Microsatellite instability (MSI) is found in 10% of sporadic adenomas [(38]). Interestingly, Wagner et al. [37] evaluated molecular features of 22 duodenal nonampullary adenomas, 9 sporadic ampullary adenomas and 12 FAP-related adenomas using combined immunohistochemical and molecular approaches. They found no differences in Wnt signaling pathway (beta-catenin, APC), MAP kinase pathway (KRAS, BRAF) and DNA repair mechanisms (MSI) among the groups. [37] In their series, none of the sporadic adenomas or FAP adenomas showed MSI-H, three of the FAP-related adenomas showed MSI-L. [37].

Similar to colonic adenomas, ampullary adenomas are precursor lesions to adenocarcinomas following the adenoma-carcinoma sequence. [11] Adenoma components have been found in 16.7-91% of ampullary carcinoma cases. [14, 39] Importantly, in about 30-60% of biopsied adenomas, invasive carcinomas are detected in resection specimens. [(39, 40]) It is critical to diagnose or predict adenocarcinoma in the biopsy sample since the treatment of choice for pure ampullary adenoma is endoscopic ampullectomy, whereas the standard treatment for carcinoma is surgical pancreaticoduodenectomy (Whipple's procedure). [31] The clinical and histological features of ampullary tumors have been studied to help diagnose carcinoma in biopsy samples, but the results are controversial. Some studies show that tumor size >1cm appears to correlate with malignant potential. [41] Others claim that tumor size is not a reliable criterion since 9-40% of carcinomas are less than 1cm, and 25% of carcinomas have a diameter of 1-1.5cm. [18, 39]. Kim et al. [40] evaluatedstudied a total of 91 biopsied adenoma resection cases and studied clinical, laboratory, radiologic and pathologic factors that may predict the risk of carcinoma. Univariate analysis revealed some radiologic features (papilla enlargement on CT, duct dilatation on imaging) as well as laboratory findings (bilirubin >2 mg/dl, aspartate aminotransferase >40IU/L, alanine aminotransferase > 40IU/L, and alkaline phosphatase >90U/L) were associated with malignancy in patients more than 65 years old. Furthermore, they found that high grade dysplasia and ductal dilatation were significant predictors of malignancy in ampullary adenomas. [40] Intraoperative frozen sectioning is frequently used to help identify carcinoma during surgery. The estimated diagnostic accuracy for preoperative biopsy and intraoperative frozen sectioning is 79% and 84% respectively. [42]

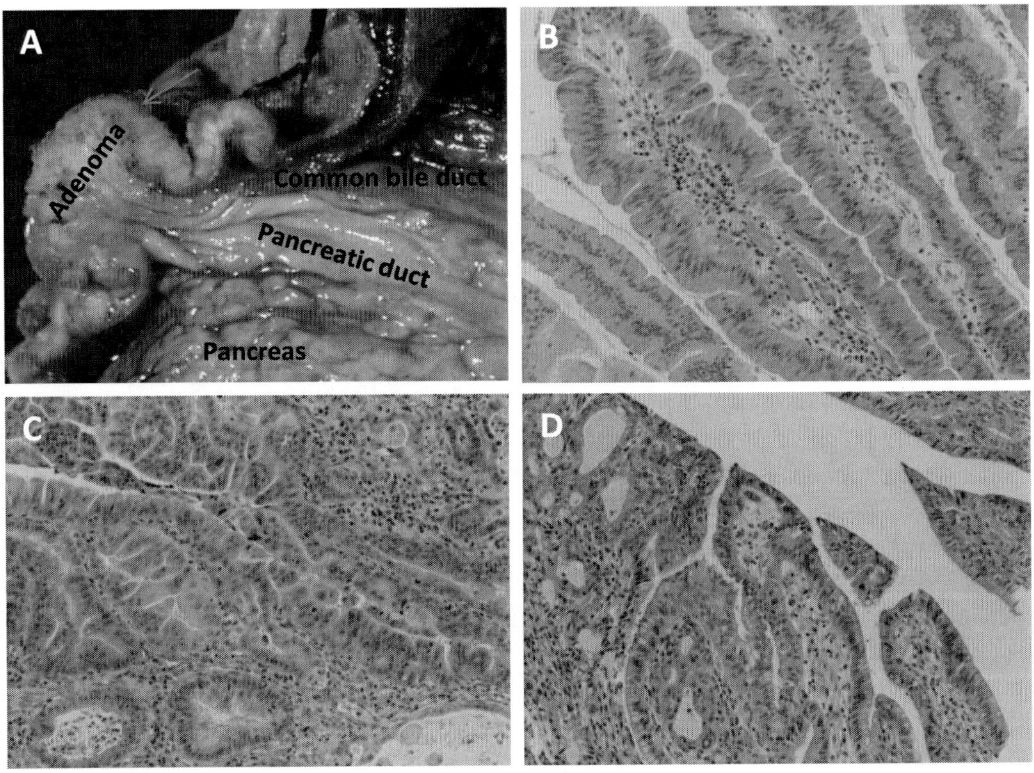

Figure 2. Ampullary adenoma. A. Gross appearance of an ampullary adenoma and its relationship with common bile duct and pancreatic duct. B. Intestinal type adenoma with low grade dysplasia. C. Intestinal type adenoma with high grade dysplasia. D. Pancreaticobiliary type adenoma. (H&E staining, original magnification X200).

Adenomyoma

Ampullary adenomyoma, also called adneomyomatous hyperplasia, is a benign lesion that can cause long term biliary obstruction. [43] Clinically it mimics adenoma or adenocarcinoma. Grossly, it is white, firm, and usually 0.5cm or more (1-3cm). Microscopically, it is characterized by lobules of ducts and ductules with interlacing bundles of smooth muscle surrounded by fibroblastic proliferation. Immunophenotypically, the epithelial areas are positive for CK7 and negative for CK20, similar to pancreaticobiliary epithelium. The hyperplastic myofibroblastic cells express smooth muscle actin. The clinical characteristics suggest an either reactive and/or malformative nature of the lesion.

Gangliocytic Paraganglioma

Gangliocytic paragangliomas are rare tumors that are mainly (>90%) periampullary or located at the second portion of the duodenum. [44] These are submucosal tumors that may appear sessile or polypoid. Histologically, the tumor is triphasic with various amounts of epithelioid cells with endocrine growth pattern, spindle Schwan-like cells, and ganglion cells. Immunohistochemically, epithelioid cells are positive for pancreatic polypeptide and somatostatin, spindle cells are positive for S100, and ganglion cells are positive for synaptophysin, chromgranin, neuron specific enolase and somatostatin. The differential diagnosis includes carcinoid tumor, ganglioneuroma and paraganglioma.

The majority of gangliocytic paragangliomas follow a benign course, although rare cases with regional lymph node metastasis have been reported. [45]

Other Benign Ampullary Tumors

Other benign ampullary tumors that have been described mostly in case reports include pancreatic and gastric heterotopia, and a variety of mesenchymal tumors such as leiomyoma, hemangiolymphangioma, gastrointestinal stromal tumor (GIST), and granular cell tumor. Endoscopic biopsies are usually required for definitive diagnosis.

3.2. Malignant Ampullary Tumors

Adenocarcinoma

Most malignant neoplasms of the ampulla of Vater are adenocarcinomas. Grossly, ampullary adenocarcinomas may be polypoid or ulcerating (Figure 3 A). They are often small (less than 2cm), although larger carcinomas up to 7.5cm in diameter have been reported. The tumors invade through the sphincter of Oddi into the adjacent duodenal wall and pancreas. Lymph node metastasis can occur at early stages. In one study, about 20% of stage I tumors and 40-50% of tumors greater than 1.5cm have lymph node metastasis. [18]

Histologically, ampullary adenocarcinomas are further subclassified into intestinal type (50-80%) and pancreaticobiliary type (15-20%). [12, 14] Rare cases with mixed intestinal and pancreaticobiliary types are also present. The intestinal type ampullary adenocarcinomas resemble colonic adenocarcinomas. They are composed of individual and cribriform glands with moderate desmoplastic stroma. Scattered goblet cells and Paneth cells may be seen in better differentiated tumors. Abundant luminal necrosis is common (Figure 3 B). The nuclei are elongated and pseudostratified with moderate to marked pleomorphism. Extracellular mucin pools may be present in less than 50% of the tumor. In contrast, pancreaticobiliary type adenocarcinomas often contain well-formed individual glands associated with marked desmoplastic stroma (Figure 3 C). The glands are lined by a single layer of columnar/cuboidal cells with round uniform nuclei, resembling pancreatic ductal adenocarcinoma. Papillary, cribriform and single cell growth may be present. The mixed type adenocarcinoma contains both intestinal and pancreaticobiliary components, each component comprising greater than 10% of the tumor.

Immunohistochemically, intestinal type adenocarcinomas are characterized as positive for CK20, MUC2 and CDX2, and negative for CK7 and CK17. Pancreaticobiliary type adenocarcinomas generally express CK7, CK17 and MUC1 with a lack of CK20 and CDX2 expression. [46-48]

Data have suggested ampullary adenocarcinomas share molecular analogies with both colorectal and pancreatic cancers. KRAS mutations are early events and present in 25-67% of ampullary adenocarcinomas. [49-51] The frequency of KRAS mutation is similar to colorectal adenocarcinoma (50%) but significantly lower than pancreatic carcinoma (95%).

The pattern of KRAS mutations is thought to be closer to colorectal adenocarcinoma [50] in some studies but not others [49]. Interestingly, in one large study of 277 patients (170 pancreatic adenocarcinomas and 107 ampullary adenocarcinomas), KRAS mutation is found to be an independent prognostic marker of shorter five-year survival and overall survival in patients with ampullary adenocarcinoma but not in patients with pancreatic adenocarcinoma [49]. BRAF mutations are uncommon in ampullary adenomas and adenocarcinomas (6-10%).[36, 49] APC gene mutation is rare in pancreatic adenocarcinomas but can be found in 64% of FAP-related ampullary adenocarcinomas and 17-47% of sporadic ampullary adenocarcinomas. [37, 52] SMAD4 mutations are found in 50% of ampullary carcinomas, suggesting SMAD4 is a major factor in ampullary cancer development. [53] P53 mutations are found in 32% of early and 53% of advanced ampullary carcinomas, suggesting the role of p53 in carcinogenesis. [50] Abnormal mismatch repair protein expression occurs in 6-10% ampullary carcinoma, [38, 54] less frequently than in colorectal adenocarcinomas (15%).Most of the studies on molecular alterations in ampullary adenocarcinoma did not specify different subtypes. A recent study tested molecular features of intestinal like and pancreaticobiliary like groups, and found no significant difference between the two groups in the prevalence of mutations of KRAS, BRAF, PIK3CA genes, or MSI phenotype. [55] More recently, Demeure et al., [56] used whole genome sequencing to analyze the genome of a resected ampullary adenocarcinoma and whole blood. They found KRAS and SMAD4 mutations, and focal deletion of the PTEN gene in this patient. The data not only suggests ampullary carcinomas are cancers distinct from common bile duct or pancreatic carcinomas, but also provide molecular evidence of therapeutic relevance of dual mTOR/PI3K inhibitors in these tumors.

A diagnosis of ampullary carcinoma generally requires clinical evaluation, endoscopic staging and histologic confirmation. The histologic diagnosis of carcinomas can be challenging in small ampullary biopsies. This is mostly due to small sample size, crushing artifact, frequent mixed inflammation and overlapping histologic features of reactive and neoplastic changes. [57] Studies have tried to use immunohistochemical markers to help with histologic diagnosis. P53 and ki-67 cannot reliably differentiate reactive changes from adenoma and carcinoma. [57, 58] Insulin-like growth factor II mRNA binding protein 3 (IMP3) has been found useful in differentiating many benign and malignant tumors including bile duct carcinomas. [59] In bile duct carcinomas, positive IMP3 is reported in 50-77% of the cancer cases. [59, 60] However, focal IMP3 staining is frequently observed. Therefore a positive IMP3 staining may be helpful, but a negative staining does not rule out malignancy. A combination of several markers has been studied to increased sensitivity and specificity. Levy et al. [60] studied the expression of a panel of IMP3, S100P and Von Hipple-Lindau product (pVHL) in 72 endoscopic bile duct biopsies including 40 adenocarcinomas and 32 benign bile duct mucosae. They found 70% of the carcinomas showed a S100P+/IMP3+/pVHL pattern, 15% with a S100P+/IMP3-/pVHL- pattern, and 5% with a S100P-/IMP3+/pVHL- pattern. The data suggests a combination of these three markers may help distinguish adenocarcinoma from reactive epithelial changes. Baumhoer et al. [61] studied CD24, S100A, and p-cadherin in resection specimens of 177 ampullary carcinomas, 114 adenomas and 152 normal mucosa. They found strong CD24 staining in 19% of carcinomas but only in 6% of normal mucosae and in 0% of adenomas. They also observed strong S100A staining in 11% of adenomas and in 32% of carcinomas but virtually no staining in normal mucosae. Positive membranous p-cadherin was found in 40% of adenomas and 60% of carcinomas but 7% normal mucosae. They claimed CD24, but not others may be helpful in differentiating adenoma from carcinoma. A recent study by Zakharov et al. [57] evaluated diagnostic values of HMGA1, HMGA2, p53, and β-catenin in 48 ampullary and distal bile duct biopsies. Expression of HMGA1 was found in 21% of samples with reactive atypia, 42% of adenomas and 91% of adenocarcinomas. HMGA2 was positive in 14% samples with reactive atypia, 42% of adenomas and 86% of adenocarcinomas. More interestingly, combined HMGA1 and HMGA2 positivity was seen in 80% of adenocarcinomas, but in 0% of adenomas and in 8% of samples with reactive atypia. They concluded that HMGA1 and HMGA2 may serve as markers to discriminate between adenocarcinoma, adenoma and reactive atypia. [57]

The current WHO system (2010) classifies ampullary carcinomas as tumors of the ampullary region and stages the tumors based on the depth of invasion. Pathologic stage T1 tumors are tumors confined to the ampulla of Vater or sphincter of Oddi. Tumors invading duodenal wall and pancreas are stage T2 and T3 respectively. Tumors that involve peripancreatic tissue are stage T4. It has been argued that the term "ampullary carcinoma" lacks a precise definition and the current classification and staging system is not well defined, with a lack of reproducibility. [62] For example, substaging of small papillary cancers as T1a, T1b and T1c does not exist in ampullary cancers. Furthermore, the definitions for peripancreatic soft tissue, common bile duct involvement and vascular involvement are vague, making stage T3 highly subjective. [62] The current staging system also has limited value in separating ampullary carcinomas into different prognostic groups and therefore it is not useful in selecting patients for appropriate adjuvant therapy and interpreting clinical trials. [63] Several subclassification systems of ampullary carcinomas have been proposed.

Several studies have attempted to subclassify ampullary carcinomas according to the location and compartment in which the tumor arises: periampullary tumors grow predominantly towards the duodenal lumen; intra-ampullary tumors grow internally; and mixed-type tumors demonstrate ulcerative or fungating patterns. [19, 64, 65] Recent studies have suggested that the sub-location of ampullary carcinoma also has prognostic significance.

By correlating gross and microscopic features, Adsay et al. [62] classified ampullary carcinomas into four distinct subtypes: 1. Intra-ampullary papillary-tubular neoplasm with invasion (*Intra-AMP*, 25%); 2. Ampullary-ductal (*AMP-ductal,* 15%); 3. Periampullary-duodenal (*Peri-AMP-Duodenal,* 5%); and 4. Ampullary-not otherwise classified (*AC-NOS,* 55%). The tumors in different subtypes demonstrate different demographic, gross and histologic features, and prognosis. Peri-AMP-duodenal tumors are the largest (mean size, 4.7cm), show exophytic ulcero-fungating growth, and are typically intestinal histologic type. They have the highest risk of lymph node metastasis (50%) and intermediate prognosis (3-year survival, 69%). AMP-ductal tumors, on the other hand, are the smallest (mean size 1.9cm), usually forming a stricture or sclerotic and plaque-like thickening of the ductal wall. The histologic features of these tumors are more likely to be pancreaticobiliary type. Although they carry the worst prognosis among the groups (3-year survival, 41%), the AMP-ductal tumors show significantly better prognosis when compared to ordinary pancreatic ductal adenocarcinoma (3-year survival, 11%, $p<0.001$). The gross and histologic features of intra-AMPamp subtype tumors closely resemble intraductal papillary mucinous neoplasm (IPMN) of the pancreas, in which the tumors show predominantly papillary intraductal growth with minimal invasion. These tumors are commonly found in men, are predominantly of a lower TNM stage (85%, T1/2, and 72% N0), and carry the best prognosis among the four groups (3-year survival, 73%). This classification system requires proper grossing technique and appreciation of histo-anatomic subtleties of this complex region.

Recent publications emphasize the importance of pathogenesis and histologic differentiation of ampullary carcinomas, and subclassify ampullary adenocarcinomas into two distinct groups (intestinal and pancreaticobiliary groups), based on histomorphology, [12, 14, 46, 66], molecular characteristics, [47, 61, 63] and gene expression profile. [55] The tumors in these two groups not only have different histologic features, but also appear to develop from different epithelia through different signaling pathways, show different gene and protein profiles, and demonstrate dissimilar prognosis. The intestinal type tumors histologically resemble colonic adenocarcinoma. Wnt signaling appears to be important in cancer development. The genes that are significantly upregulated in the intestinal type of tumor include intestinal-associated markers such as meprin A alpha, guanylate cyclase 2C, glycoprotein A33 and CDX1. The proteomic profiling of this group show increased expression of β-catenin and E-Cadherin (suggesting activation of the Wnt signaling pathway), and both total and phosphor-c-MYC. [55] In contrast, pancreaticobiliary type tumors are morphologically closer to pancreatic adenocarcinoma. The development of this type of tumor involves NOTCH signaling pathway. MUC1, a pancreaticobiliary mucin, was found to be upregulated in this group. At the protein level, the markers for several kinase signaling pathways are elevated, including PI3K-AKT, RAS-RAF-MEK-ERK, and JAK-STAT pathways. [55]

Another study tried to define clinically relevant histomolecular phenotypes of ampullary adenocarcinomas. [(63]) In their training cohort and two validation cohorts, ampullary adenocarcinomas were subclassified into two groups based on histomolecular phenotype: pancreaticobiliary type (CDX2 negative, MUC1 positive) and intestinal type (CDX2 positive, MUC1 negative). In all three cohorts, pancreaticobiliary type tumors had significantly worse median overall survival (11.9-30.9 months) compared to intestinal type tumors (67-115.5 months). In addition, the authors found that the presence of CDX2 and lack of MUC1 are significant factors that predict better prognosis. Furthermore, using combined histomolecular phenotype and lymph node status, they subdivided ampullary adenocarcinomas into three distinct prognostic groups: the group of patients with histomolecular non-pancreaticobiliary type (intestinal) and no lymph node involvement had an excellent prognosis (five-year survival 87.5%); the group of patients with histomolecular pancreaticobiliary type and lymph node involvement had poor prognosis (five-year survival 20%); and the remaining patients (nodal positive, non-pancreaticobiliary type and nodal negative pancreaticobiliary type) had intermediate prognosis (five-year survival 47%). The authors claimed that this classification is important in ampullary adenocarcinoma, as it may determine treatment and select appropriate patients for adjuvant chemotherapy. [63]

Uncommon carcinomas

Mucinous carcinomas comprise less than 10% of ampullary carcinomas. By definition, these are tumors with extracellular mucin pools that occupy greater than 50% of the tumor (Figure 3 D). The gross appearance of the tumor is mucoid and gelatinous. Most mucinous carcinomas arise from intestinal adenomas and show intestinal immunophenotype (positive for CK20, MUC2 and CDX2).

Signet ring cell carcinomas are rare in the ampulla of Vater. The tumor cells are infiltrative and individually arranged into single files or small sheets. Intracellular mucin pushes the nucleus to the side giving it a signet ring morphology. Nuclear atypia and mitotic figures are frequently seen. A signet ring cell component may be found in conventional adenocarcinoma but should occupy less than 50% of the tumor. A metastasis from other sites such as stomach, breast and pancreas must be excluded before a diagnosis of primary ampullary signet ring cell carcinoma is rendered.

Adenosquamous carcinomas are adenocarcinomas with at least 25% squamous differentiation. These tumors comprise 1-3% of all ampullary malignancies. The glandular areas demonstrate similar morphologic features as that in pancreaticobiliary type adenocarcinoma. The squamous areas contain nests and sheets of large polygonal cells with distinct cell borders, eosinophilic cytoplasm and prominent nucleoli. Keratin pearls and individual cells with keratinization are usually present.

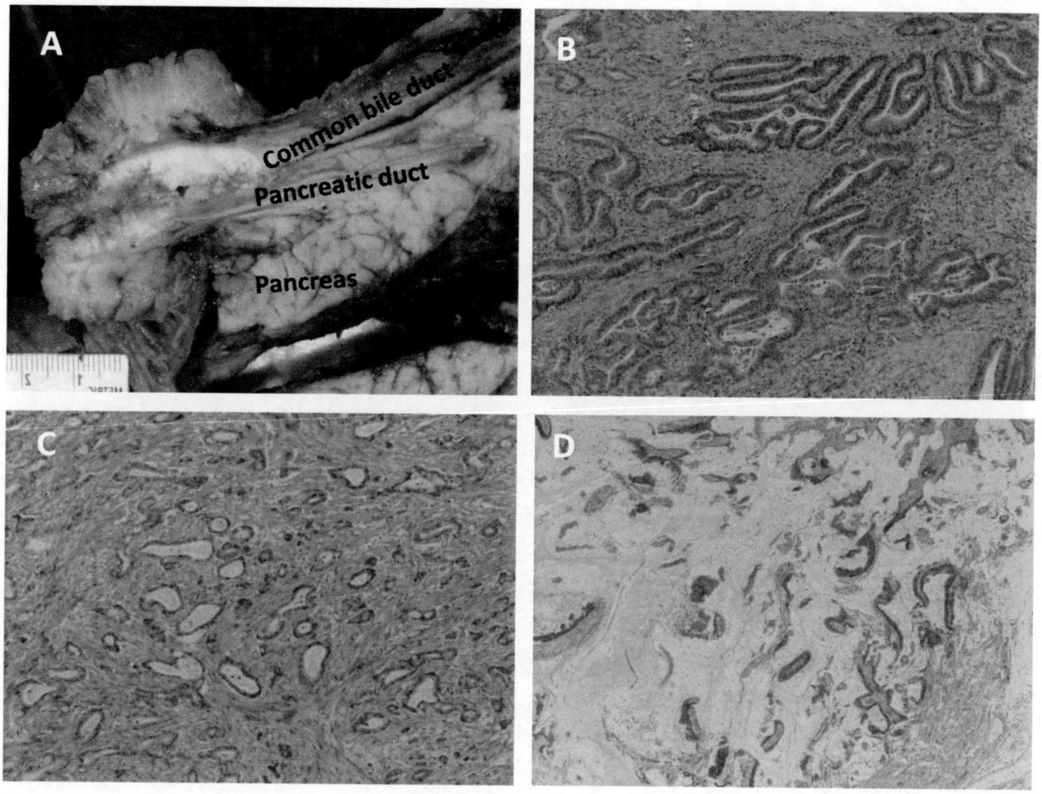

Figure 3. Ampullary carcinoma. A. Gross appearance of an ampullary carcinoma and its relationship with common bile duct and pancreatic duct. B. Intestinal type adenocarcinoma. C. Pancreaticobiliary type adenocarcinoma, with stromal desmoplasia. D. Mucinous carcinoma, >50% of the tumor is composed of mucin pools. (H&E staining, original magnification X100).

Neuroendocrine Neoplasm

Like neuroendocrine neoplasms in other parts of the GI tract, ampullary neuroendocrine neoplasms are classified into well differentiated NETs (carcinoids, 60%), and neuroendocrine carcinomas (large cell neuroendocrine carcinomas and small cell carcinomas, 40%). [19]

Grossly, a polypoid lesion or submucosal nodule/mass may be seen. Most ampullary NETs are solitary and nonfunctional. Somatostatin-producing nonfunctional glandular carcinoid tumors are common. Rare functional gastrinomas may be present. Neuroendocrine carcinomas are larger (mean size 3.05 cm) than carcinoids (mean size 1.76 cm) with more frequent nodal metastasis (62% versus 28.5%). [19] The five year survival rate of ampullary carcinoids is 82%, significantly higher than that of high grade neuroendocrine carcinomas, which is 15.7%. [19]

Histologically, well differentiated NETs show typical nested, acinar, and trabecular growth patterns. Somatostatinomas are gland forming carcinoid tumors showing tubular glands infiltrating fibrotic stroma. Psammoma bodies are characteristic in this type of tumor. The individual tumor cells of well differentiated NETs contain moderate amounts of pale to eosinophilic cytoplasm.

The nuclei are uniform with stippled chromatin. The ki-67 proliferative rate for well differentiated NETs is low (less than 20%). Mitotic rate is generally less than 10 mitotic figures per 10 high power fields; many are less than 1-2 mitosis per 10 high power fields. Necrosis is usually absent. Poorly differentiated endocrine carcinomas are uncommon. They include large cell neuroendocrine carcinomas and small cell carcinomas. Large cell neuroendocrine carcinomas contain large tumor cells with moderate amount of cytoplasm, round to oval shaped nuclei and often prominent nucleoli. The histologic features of small cell carcinomas resemble the small cell carcinomas of the lung: sheets of small and hyperchromatic cells with scant cytoplasm. Mitotic and apoptotic rates are high. Necrosis is commonly seen and can be extensive.

Immunohistochemically, NETs are positive for chromogranin and synaptophysin, although the staining of these markers is usually focal in poorly differentiated NETs. A diagnosis of small cell carcinoma can be made based on histology alone and does not require positive immunostaining. Case reports and single institute case series studies suggest NETs of the ampulla have more aggressive behavior and worse prognosis compared to duodenal NETs. A population-based study by Randle et al. ([20]) compared 120 ampullary NETs and 360 duodenal NETs in the Surveillance, Epidemiology, and End Results (SEER) cancer registry database. Compared to the duodenal NETs, the ampullary NETs are more commonly diagnosed at an earlier age (median age 62 vs 65 years) and in white patients (78% vs 67%). In surgically resected NETs, ampullary NETs are larger in size (median size 18mm vs 10mm), higher grade (poorly and undifferentiated 37.5% vs 6.6%), higher nodal metastasis (72.9% vs 48.4%), and more distant metastasis (11% vs 5.6%) [20]. In addition, the overall survival of patients with ampullary NETs is significantly worse than those with duodenal NETs (median overall survival 98 vs 143 months) [20]. The data suggests ampullary location is an independent predictor of worse prognosis in patients with proximal small bowel NETs.

Ampullary NETs can occur sporadically or in association with familial syndromes such as Neurofibromatosis type I (NF-1). In a review of ampullary NETs, 26% of ampullary NETs were found in NF-1 patients. [21]

Relles et al. [67] reported two cases and reviewed additional 74 periampullary tumors in NF-1 patients reported in the English literature since 1989. They found 47% of periampullary tumors in NF-1 are endocrine in origin, with 40% being reported as somatostatinoma, 6% as carcinoid, and 1% as malignant endocrine tumor. Somatostatinomas in NF-1 and non NF-1 patients share very similar clinical and histologic features except non-NF1 patients are less likely to have multihormone production (4.7% vs 16%). [68]

Other Malignant Tumors

Other primary malignant tumors that have been reported in the ampulla of Vater include lymphoma, rhabdomyosarcoma, Kaposi sarcoma and others. The pathologic features of these tumors are similar to those that arise in other anatomic locations.

In addition, ampullary involvement by adjacent cancers, particularly duodenal adenocarcinomas and pancreatic adenocarcinomas are not uncommon. Careful gross examination is critical in determination of the epicenter and primary site of origin of a tumor. In addition, microscopic identification of adenomatous component may be helpful in deciding where the tumor originated. Immunohistochemical and molecular studies are of limited value in determining the primary site of the tumor. Rare cases of metastatic melanoma and renal cell carcinoma to the ampulla of Vater have been reported in literature. [69]

3.3. Tumor-Like Lesions

Benign tumor- like lesions of the ampulla of Vater includes a group of nonneoplastic diseases that may clinically and/or histologically mimic malignancy.

Primary Sclerosing Cholangitis

Primary sclerosing cholangitis (PSC) represents an immune mediated chronic cholestatic liver and biliary tract disease of unknown etiology. [70, 71] It is characterized by progressive inflammation, fibrosis, strictures, and saccular dilatation the biliary tree. Associations of PSC with inflammatory bowel disease and cholangiocarcinoma have been observed. PSC often involves medium sized and/or large bile ducts but can also involve small bile ducts. Histologically, early stage PSC shows inflammation and concentric periductal (onion skin) fibrosis. The inflammatory infiltrates are composed predominantly of lymphocytes. Neutrophils may be abundant. Plasma cells and eosinophils are rare. As PSC progresses, biliary stricture, bile duct obliteration, scarring and loss may be present. Severe intrahepatic portal fibrosis leads to cirrhosis and liver failure. The median survival of PSA patients after diagnosis has been reported to be approximately 10-12 years. [70, 71] Currently, liver transplantation is the only potential curative treatment option in PSA patients with end stage liver disease. [70]

Autoimmune Pancreatitis and IgGg4-Related Sclerosing Cholangitis

Autoimmune pancreatitis and IgG4-related sclerosing cholangitis are both considered to be a part of systemic IgG4-related diseases (IgG4-RD) characterized by elevations in serum IgG4 concentrations, and a set of unique histologic features including lymphoplasmacytic infiltrate, storiform fibrosis, obliterative phlebitis and mild to moderate tissue eosinophilia. [72] It is very important to recognize this spectrum of disease as most of the IgG4-RD may present as mass lesion mimicking a malignancy. More importantly, many of the IgG4-RD cases can be treated effectively by steroid therapy.

Autoimmune pancreatitis, also named previously as chronic pancreatitis and inflammatory myofibroblastic tumor, presents with diffuse pancreatic enlargement (sausage pancreas) or a mass. Recent studies have suggested two types of autoimmune pancreatitis (AIP): type I and type II. [73, 74] Type I AIP is also called lymphoplasmacytic sclerosing pancreatitis. The histologic features of type I AIP include: dense infiltrating of plasma cells and lymphocytes, particularly periductal, storiform fibrosis, obliterative phlebitis, and abundant IgG4 positive plasma cells (greater than 10 IgG4 positive plasma cells per high power field). Type II AIP is also called idiopathic duct-centric pancreatitis. Characteristics of type II AIP include intraluminal and intraepithelial neutrophils in ducts and acini. Type II AIP often has none or very few IgG4 positive plasma cells and not associated with serum IgG4 elevation.

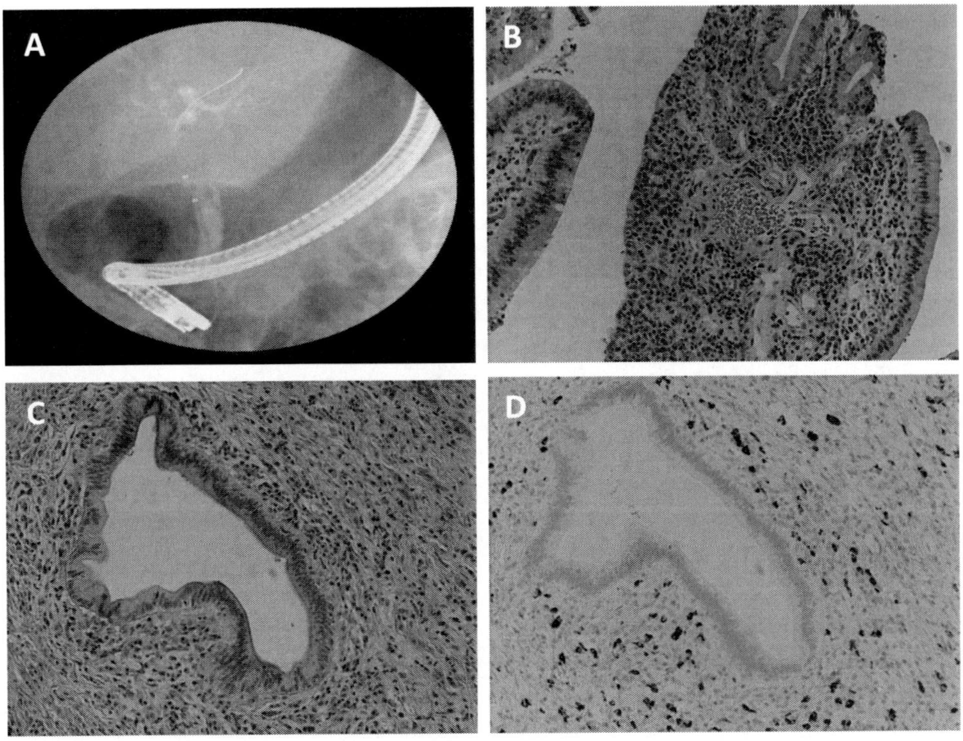

Figure 4. IgG4-associated sclerosing cholangitis. A. ERCP image. B. Ampullary mucosa with abundant plasma cells (H&E staining, original magnification X200). C. Periductal lymphoplasmacytic inflammation and fibrosis (H&E staining, original magnification X200). D. IgG4 positive plasma cells (Immunohistochemical staining, original magnification X200).

IgG4-related sclerosing cholangitis (IgG4-SC) is a recently recognized sclerosing cholangitis with unknown etiology associated with abundant infiltration of IgG4 positive cells. [75-78] IgG4-SC is frequently associated with type I AIP, although isolated IgG4-SC cases have been reported.

Bjornsson et al., first proposed the name IgG4 associated sclerosing (IAC) cholangitis for the patients who meet the diagnostic criteria of PSC but seem to have better prognosis and often associated with AIP. There are significant differences between PSC and IAC in clinical, biochemical, histopathologic features, treatment and prognosis. [75, 79, 80]. IAC patients are older and often present with obstructive jaundice whereas PSC patients are younger and rarely present with obstructive jaundice. IAC patients often have high serum IgG4 levels and characteristic histologic features: periductal lymphoplasmacytic infiltrate, obliterative phlebitis, and abundant IgG4 positive cells (Figure 4). The associations of PSC with IBD and cholangiocarcinoma are not observed in IAC patients. IAC patients are often responsive to steroid treatment whereas corticosteroids and other immunosuppressive agents are generally not effective in PSC patients. It is now well accepted that IgG4-SC is a distinct type of sclerosing cholangitis, in addition to primary sclerosing cholangitis and secondary sclerosing cholangitis. [76, 78]. Recently, the clinical diagnostic criteria for IgG4-SC have been established. [81]

The discrimination of IgG4-SC, PSC, and cholangiocarcinoma has become an important issue, as these diseases have very different treatment strategies and clinical outcomes. Although imaging and serologic examination are often used clinically to discriminate these conditions, in many cases, a pathologic diagnosis is necessary. Studies have been focused on using biopsy samples to confirm the diagnosis and direct the treatment. [82] Several studies have shown that the IgG4 immunohistochemical stain of biopsies from the ampulla of Vater and the distal bile duct is useful for diagnosing type I AIP and IgG4-SC. [77, 83, 84] In one study, when using a cut-off value of 10 IgG4 positive cells per high power field, the diagnostic sensitivity and specificity of the biopsies from ampulla and bile duct were 52% and 89%, and 52% and 96% respectively. [77] It should be noted that several recent studies have revealed raised serum IgG4 levels in 9-36% of PSC and pancreatic cancer patients. A recent study by Zhang et al. [85] found abundant IgG4 positive cells (>10 per high power field) in 23% of the explant livers with PSC. An elevation of IgG4 positive to IgG positive plasma cell ratio (great than 40%) has been suggested to help discriminate between IgG4-RD and other inflammatory conditions including chronic sclerosing sialadenitis, inflammatory pseudotumor of the lung and autoimmune pancreatitis. [86-88]

Secondary Sclerosing Cholangitis

Secondary causes of sclerosing cholangitis include diverse clinical conditions such as sclerosing cholangitis in critically ill patients, ischemic cholangiopathy, obstructive cholestasis caused by neoplasms, pancreatic disease or surgical (anastomotic) strictures, recurrent pyogenic cholangitis, and others. [70] It is necessary to rule out secondary cholangitis before a diagnosis of PSC or IgG4 cholangitis can be made. The histologic changes for secondary sclerosing cholangitis are usually nonspecific and include acute and chronic inflammation, fibrosis, and reactive epithelial changes. Clinical history and radiologic findings are essential for the diagnosis.

4. Surgical Treatment

Ampullary tumors can be surgically treated with endoscopic therapies, local excision, or pancreaticoduodenectomy depending on their potential for malignancy and the operative candidacy of the patient.

Pancreaticoduodenectomy

For a surgically fit patient with malignancy, pancreaticoduodenectomy remains the treatment of choice for curative oncologic therapy. First described by Whipple in 1935 [89], the procedure involves resection of the head of the pancreas, the gallbladder, the duodenum and proximal jejunum, all intervening ductal structures and surrounding lymphatic tissue, and reconstruction of the gastric, biliary, and pancreatic drainage to the jejunum. Classically, this resection included the pylorus and the gastric antrum with a roux-en-y jejunal reconstruction, though the operation may be performed with preservation of the pylorus. This offers the advantage of a faster operation, typically with one less anastomosis (no roux-en-y) as the gastrojejunostomy is performed in an end-to-side manner on the same jejunal loop as the pancreatic and biliary anastomoses. [90] Other benefits include less gastric "dumping" and post-operative weight loss, but critics argue pylorus preservation is associated with delayed gastric emptying in the early postoperative period and a less radical oncologic resection. Randomized control trials have shown minor differences in weight change and perioperative blood loss, but no meaningful differences in delayed gastric emptying, hospital length of stay, complication rates, or perioperative or long term mortality. [91, 92]

Even with advances in modern surgical and perioperative therapy, pancreatico-oduodenectomy still carries with it 2-5% perioperative mortality and 20-40% perioperative morbidity rates. [93] Studies have suggested there is a strong inverse correlation between the volume of pancreatic resections performed by individual surgeons and centers and the cost, length of hospital stay, complication and perioperative mortality rates. [94, 95] Pancreaticoduodenectomy remains the only therapeutic option currently available that offers the potential for oncologic cure for invasive malignancy.

Surgical Ampullectomy

For tumors with less potential for malignancy, or patients unable to tolerate such maximally invasive therapy, local resection can be accomplished via a transduodenal approach. Traditionally the duodenum is mobilized via a Kocher maneuver and a longitudinal duodenotomy is performed opposite the ampulla. A full thickness excision is performed with reimplantation of the common bile duct and pancreatic duct into the duodenal wall. Halsted first performed the procedure in 1899 proposing it as treatment for ampullary cancer [96] but local recurrence rates proved high. The role of ampullectomy for severe dysplasia, carcinoma in situ, [97] or even T1 lesions [98] continues to be debated, though it is generally reserved for benign disease or non-curative palliation given high local recurrence rate. [99] Given the 25-60% false negative rate of endoscopic biopsy [100-103] for adenocarcinoma, some caution against local resection even for suspected benign disease and advocate for pancreaticoduodenectomy. [104] Local excision is associated with a higher local recurrence rate [101, 105] than pancreaticoduodenectomy though is considerably less morbid.

Endoscopic Aampullectomy

Endoscopic therapies offer increasingly less invasive treatment options, including laser or thermal ablation or snare excision for resection of adenomas. [106]. Endoscopic ampullectomy is typically reserved for small, benign lesions. This is an en bloc resection, usually performed with a polypectomy snare on pulsed cutting and coagulation current

(Figure 5). Pancreatic and bile duct stents are usually placed to decrease the risk of biliary or pancreatic obstruction secondary to clot or edema.

Other adjunctive techniques, including submucosal saline injection and biliary or pancreatic sphincterotomy may enhance the technical success and decrease the complications of endoscopic ampullectomy.

Data is sparse on these relatively new modalities. Ablation is often accompanied by fibrosis and scarring so is customarily performed with sphincterotomy and stenting, and offers no pathological specimen to review for missed underlying carcinoma. This is generally reserved for palliation of obstruction in unresectable disease. Endoscopic snare resection offers the opportunity for histological review, but local adenomatous recurrence rates are as high as one in four, and sessile lesions may be technically challenging to remove. Ultimately, endoscopic interventions do not preclude eventual more radical resection and are finding an emerging role in the treatment of this disease process.

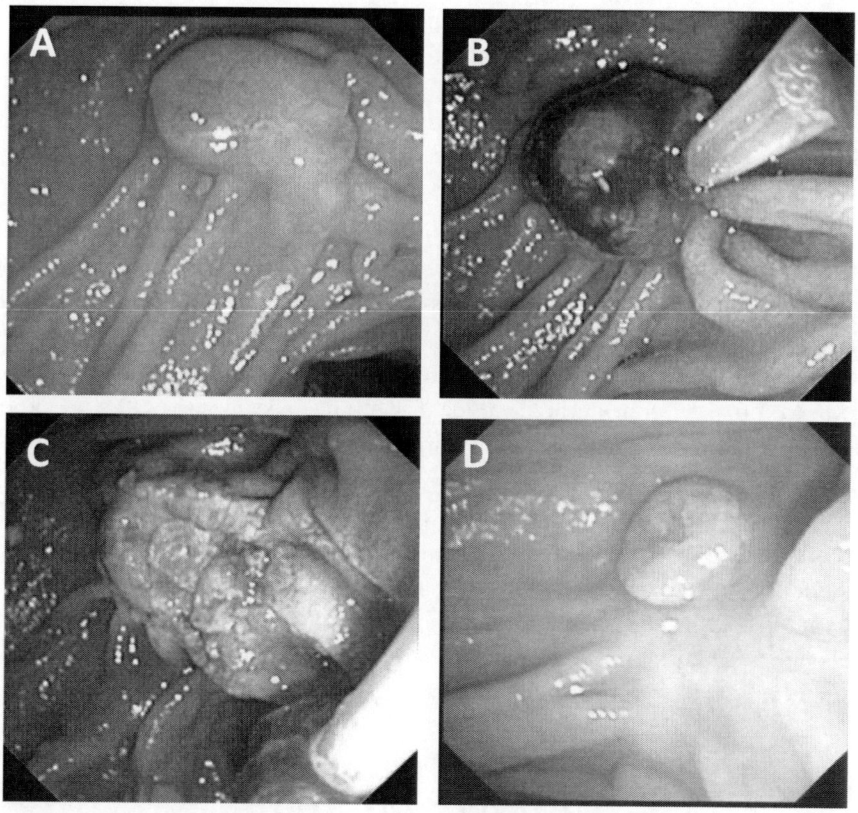

Figure 5. Endoscopic ampullectomy of an ampullary adenoma. A. Preresection appearance of the adenoma. B and C. Endoscopic resection. D. Postresection view of the ampullary region.

Palliative Interventions

For patients with identified metastatic malignancy at the time of diagnosis, palliative intervention is geared around relieving obstruction of biliary and gastric outflow, as well as ameliorating pain. Inoperable ampullary cancers frequently present as obstructive jaundice causing symptomatic pruritus, but may progress to hepatic failure from cholestasis and cholangitis. Relief of obstruction can be performed via endoscopic biliary stent placement or via surgical bypass.

While bypass is more durable, stent placement is considerably less invasive, and newer covered, self-expandable metal stents have shown increased patency rates with less subsequent interventions and less tumor ingrowth than prior prosthetics. [107] Respectively, endoscopic therapy typically involves fewer short term complications and shorter hospital stay, and surgical bypass involves fewer long term complications making it a better option for patients with longer predicted survival. [108] Surgical bypass is typically performed by resecting the gallbladder and dissecting the common hepatic duct back to the level of its bifurcation, dividing it there and performing a choledochojejunostomy to a roux limb.

As periampullary tumors progress, 30-50% of patients develop gastric outlet obstruction from either mechanical obstruction of the duodenum or poor motility associated with tumor infiltration of the celiac nerve plexus. [109] Mechanical obstruction may be avoided with surgical gastrojejunostomy performed at the time of choledochojejunostomy in a conventional "double bypass." Two randomized controlled trials have compared biliary bypass with and without prophylactic gastrojejunostomy and found no difference in perioperative outcomes, but a reduction in the rate of subsequent gastric outlet obstruction from 19% to 0%. [110, 111] As an alternative, duodenal stenting has shown promising early results, though data are still emerging.

With infiltration of the mesenteric or celiac nerve plexus comes visceral pain, usually located in the epigastrium and radiating to the back. If laparotomy is performed for surgical bypass, neurolytic celiac plexus blockade may be accomplished with the injection of 50% ethanol or 6% phenol under direct visualization on either side of the aorta at the level of the celiac axis. This can also be performed percutaneously with radiological guidance and has been shown to provide considerable relief for up to six months. [112] Thoracoscopic splanchnicectomy has also been described with excellent results. [113]

In summary, the surgical standard for proven malignancy or lesions with a high suspicion for malignancy and no evidence of metastasis is pancreaticoduodenectomy with or without pylorus preservation. For patients unable to tolerate such a large surgery, or for lesions with low suspicion for malignancy, surgical ampullectomy or endoscopic polyp resection are reasonable options, with the expectation of higher rates of local recurrence. For metastatic or unresectable tumors, palliative interventions target the relief of biliary obstruction, gastric outlet obstruction, and pain via surgical, endoscopic, or percutaneous means.

Acknowledgments

We thank Ms Meng Yu for her assistance with the figures.

Reference

[1] Papamiltiades M, Rettori R. [Muscular structure of choledocho-pancreato-duodenal juncture]. *Acta anatomica*. 1957;30(1-4):575-600.

[2] Marchal G, Hureau J. [Oddi's tumors (Vater's ampulomas)]. Journal de chirurgie. 1978;115(6-7):365-76.
[3] Avisse C, Flament JB, Delattre JF. Ampulla of Vater. Anatomic, embryologic, and surgical aspects. *The Surgical clinics of North America*. 2000;80(1):201-12.
[4] Barraya L, Pujol Soler R, Yvergneaux JP. [The region of Oddi's sphincter: millimetric anatomy]. *La Presse medicale*. 1971;79(55):2527-34.
[5] Egawa N, Anjiki H, Takuma K, Kamisawa T. Juxtapapillary duodenal diverticula and pancreatobiliary disease. *Digestive surgery*. 2010;27(2):105-9.
[6] Adda G, Hannoun L, Loygue J. Development of the human pancreas: variations and pathology. A tentative classification. *Anatomia clinica*. 1984;5(4):275-83.
[7] Donatini B. A systematic study of the vascularisation of the pancreas. *Surgical and radiologic anatomy: SRA*. 1990;12(3):173-80.
[8] Martin JA, Haber GB. Ampullary adenoma: clinical manifestations, diagnosis, and treatment. *Gastrointestinal endoscopy clinics of North America*. 2003;13(4):649-69.
[9] Patel R, Varadarajulu S, Wilcox CM. Endoscopic ampullectomy: techniques and outcomes. *Journal of clinical gastroenterology*. 2012;46(1):8-15.
[10] El H, II, Cote GA. Endoscopic diagnosis and management of ampullary lesions. *Gastrointestinal endoscopy clinics of North America*. 2013;23(1):95-109.
[11] Baker HL, Caldwell DW. Lesions of the ampulla of Vater. *Surgery*. 1947;21(4):523-31.
[12] Kimura W, Futakawa N, Zhao B. Neoplastic diseases of the papilla of Vater. *Journal of hepato-biliary-pancreatic surgery*. 2004;11(4):223-31.
[13] Ramfidis VS, Syrigos KN, Saif MW. Ampullary and periampullary adenocarcinoma: new challenges in management of recurrence. JOP: *Journal of the pancreas*. 2013;14(2):158-60.
[14] Fischer HP, Zhou H. Pathogenesis of carcinoma of the papilla of Vater. *Journal of* hepato-biliary-pancreatic surgery. *2004;11(5):301-9*.
[15] Costi R, Caruana P, Sarli L, Violi V, Roncoroni L, Bordi C. Ampullary adenocarcinoma in neurofibromatosis type 1. Case report and literature review. *Modern pathology: an official journal of the United States and Canadian Academy of Pathology*, Inc. 2001;14(11):1169-74.
[16] O'Connell JB, Maggard MA, Manunga J, Jr., Tomlinson JS, Reber HA, Ko CY, et al. Survival after resection of ampullary carcinoma: a national population-based study. *Annals of surgical oncology*. 2008;15(7):1820-7.
[17] Duffy JP, Hines OJ, Liu JH, Ko CY, Cortina G, Isacoff WH, et al. Improved survival for adenocarcinoma of the ampulla of Vater: fifty-five consecutive resections. *Archives of surgery* (Chicago, Ill: 1960). 2003;138(9):941-8; discussion 8-50.
[18] Yoon YS, Kim SW, Park SJ, Lee HS, Jang JY, Choi MG, et al. Clinicopathologic analysis of early ampullary cancers with a focus on the feasibility of ampullectomy. *Annals of surgery*. 2005;242(1):92-100.
[19] Albores-Saavedra J, Hart A, Chable-Montero F, Henson DE. Carcinoids and high-grade neuroendocrine carcinomas of the ampulla of vater: a comparative analysis of 139 cases from the surveillance, epidemiology, and end results program-a population based study. *Archives of pathology & laboratory medicine*. 2010;134(11):1692-6.
[20] Randle RW, Ahmed S, Newman NA, Clark CJ. Clinical Outcomes for Neuroendocrine Tumors of the Duodenum and Ampulla of Vater:A Population-Based Study. *Journal of*

gastrointestinal surgery : official journal of the Society for Surgery of the Alimentary Tract. 2013.

[21] Hartel M, Wente MN, Sido B, Friess H, Buchler MW. Carcinoid of the ampulla of Vater. *Journal of gastroenterology and hepatology*. 2005;20(5):676-81.

[22] Noda Y, Watanabe H, Iwafuchi M, Furuta K, Ishihara N, Satoh M, et al. Carcinoids and endocrine cell micronests of the minor and major duodenal papillae. Their incidence and characteristics. *Cancer*. 1992;70(7):1825-33.

[23] Poultsides GA, Frederick WA. Carcinoid of the ampulla of Vater: morphologic features and clinical implications. World journal of gastroenterology: *WJG*. 2006;12(43):7058-60.

[24] Ghazale A, Chari ST, Zhang L, Smyrk TC, Takahashi N, Levy MJ, et al. Immunoglobulin G4-associated cholangitis: clinical profile and response to therapy. *Gastroenterology*. 2008;134(3):706-15.

[25] Lee YM, Kaplan MM. Primary sclerosing cholangitis. *The New England journal of medicine*. 1995;332(14):924-33.

[26] Chapman R, Fevery J, Kalloo A, Nagorney DM, Boberg KM, Shneider B, et al. Diagnosis and management of primary sclerosing cholangitis. *Hepatology*. 2010;51(2):660-78.

[27] Desilets DJ, Dy RM, Ku PM, Hanson BL, Elton E, Mattia A, et al. Endoscopic management of tumors of the major duodenal papilla: Refined techniques to improve outcome and avoid complications. *Gastrointestinal endoscopy*. 2001;54(2):202-8.

[28] Schwarz M, Pauls S, Sokiranski R, Brambs HJ, Glasbrenner B, Adler G, et al. Is a preoperative multidiagnostic approach to predict surgical resectability of periampullary tumors still effective? *American journal of surgery*. 2001;182(3):243-9.

[29] Chen CH, Tseng LJ, Yang CC, Yeh YH, Mo LR. The accuracy of endoscopic ultrasound, endoscopic retrograde cholangiopancreatography, computed tomography, and transabdominal ultrasound in the detection and staging of primary ampullary tumors. *Hepato-gastroenterology*. 2001;48(42):1750-3.

[30] Puli SR, Singh S, Hagedorn CH, Reddy J, Olyaee M. Diagnostic accuracy of EUS for vascular invasion in pancreatic and periampullary cancers: a meta-analysis and systematic review. *Gastrointestinal endoscopy*. 2007;65(6):788-97.

[31] Standards of Practice C, Adler DG, Qureshi W, Davila R, Gan SI, Lichtenstein D, et al. The role of endoscopy in ampullary and duodenal adenomas. *Gastrointestinal endoscopy*. 2006;64(6):849-54.

[32] Talamini MA, Moesinger RC, Pitt HA, Sohn TA, Hruban RH, Lillemoe KD, et al. Adenocarcinoma of the ampulla of Vater. A 28-year experience. *Annals of surgery*. 1997;225(5):590-9; discussion 9-600.

[33] Cheng CL, Sherman S, Fogel EL, McHenry L, Watkins JL, Fukushima T, et al. Endoscopic snare papillectomy for tumors of the duodenal papillae. *Gastrointestinal endoscopy*. 2004;60(5):757-64.

[34] Lamlum H, Papadopoulou A, Ilyas M, Rowan A, Gillet C, Hanby A, et al. APC mutations are sufficient for the growth of early colorectal adenomas. *Proceedings of the National Academy of Sciences of the United States of America*. 2000;97(5):2225-8.

[35] Achille A, Scupoli MT, Magalini AR, Zamboni G, Romanelli MG, Orlandini S, et al. APC gene mutations and allelic losses in sporadic ampullary tumours: evidence of

genetic difference from tumours associated with familial adenomatous polyposis. International journal of cancer. *Journal international du cancer.* 1996;68(3):305-12.

[36] Schonleben F, Qiu W, Allendorf JD, Chabot JA, Remotti HE, Su GH. Molecular analysis of PIK3CA, BRAF, and RAS oncogenes in periampullary and ampullary adenomas and carcinomas. *Journal of gastrointestinal surgery: official journal of the Society for Surgery of the Alimentary Tract.* 2009;13(8):1510-6.

[37] Wagner PL, Chen YT, Yantiss RK. Immunohistochemical and molecular features of sporadic and FAP-associated duodenal adenomas of the ampullary and nonampullary mucosa. *The American journal of surgical pathology.* 2008;32(9):1388-95.

[38] Ruemmele P, Dietmaier W, Terracciano L, Tornillo L, Bataille F, Kaiser A, et al. Histopathologic features and microsatellite instability of cancers of the papilla of vater and their precursor lesions. *The American journal of surgical pathology.* 2009;33(5):691-704.

[39] Winter JM, Cameron JL, Olino K, Herman JM, de Jong MC, Hruban RH, et al. Clinicopathologic analysis of ampullary neoplasms in 450 patients: implications for surgical strategy and long-term prognosis. *Journal of gastrointestinal surgery: official journal of the Society for Surgery of the Alimentary Tract.* 2010;14(2):379-87.

[40] Kim HN, Kim KM, Shin JU, Lee JK, Lee KT, Lee KH, et al. Prediction of carcinoma after resection in subjects with ampullary adenomas on endoscopic biopsy. *Journal of clinical gastroenterology.* 2013;47(4):346-51.

[41] Hornick JR, Johnston FM, Simon PO, Younkin M, Chamberlin M, Mitchem JB, et al. A single-institution review of 157 patients presenting with benign and malignant tumors of the ampulla of Vater: management and outcomes. S*urgery.* 2011;150(2):169-76.

[42] Roggin KK, Yeh JJ, Ferrone CR, Riedel E, Gerdes H, Klimstra DS, et al. Limitations of ampullectomy in the treatment of nonfamilial ampullary neoplasms. *Annals of surgical oncology.* 2005;12(12):971-80.

[43] Handra-Luca A, Terris B, Couvelard A, Bonte H, Flejou JF. Adenomyoma and adenomyomatous hyperplasia of the Vaterian system: clinical, pathological, and new immunohistochemical features of 13 cases. *Modern pathology: an official journal of the United States and Canadian Academy of Pathology*, Inc. 2003;16(6):530-6.

[44] Burke AP, Helwig EB. Gangliocytic paraganglioma. *American journal of clinical pathology.* 1989;92(1):1-9.

[45] Hashimoto S, Kawasaki S, Matsuzawa K, Harada H, Makuuchi M. Gangliocytic paraganglioma of the papilla of Vater with regional lymph node metastasis. *The American journal of gastroenterology.* 1992;87(9):1216-8.

[46] Zhou H, Schaefer N, Wolff M, Fischer HP. Carcinoma of the ampulla of Vater: comparative histologic/immunohistochemical classification and follow-up. *The American journal of surgical pathology.* 2004;28(7):875-82.

[47] Chu PG, Schwarz RE, Lau SK, Yen Y, Weiss LM. Immunohistochemical staining in the diagnosis of pancreatobiliary and ampulla of Vater adenocarcinoma: application of CDX2, CK17, MUC1, and MUC2. *The American journal of surgical pathology.* 2005;29(3):359-67.

[48] Heinrich S, Clavien PA. Ampullary cancer. *Current opinion in gastroenterology.* 2010;26(3):280-5.

[49] Schultz NA, Roslind A, Christensen IJ, Horn T, Hogdall E, Pedersen LN, et al. Frequencies and prognostic role of KRAS and BRAF mutations in patients with localized pancreatic and ampullary adenocarcinomas. *Pancreas*. 2012;41(5):759-66.

[50] Esposito I, Friess H, Buchler MW. Carcinogenesis of cancer of the papilla and ampulla: pathophysiological facts and molecular biological mechanisms. Langenbeck's archives of surgery / *Deutsche Gesellschaft fur Chirurgie*. 2001;386(3):163-71.

[51] McCarthy DM, Hruban RH, Argani P, Howe JR, Conlon KC, Brennan MF, et al. Role of the DPC4 tumor suppressor gene in adenocarcinoma of the ampulla of Vater: analysis of 140 cases. *Modern pathology: an official journal of the United States and Canadian Academy of Pathology*, Inc. 2003;16(3):272-8.

[52] Wang LF, Hingorani SR, Tuveson DA. Detecting and diagnosing ampullary neoplasms. *Cancer biology & therapy*. 2004;3(7):657-9.

[53] Suto T, Sugai T, Habano W, Uesugi N, Kanno S, Saito K, et al. Allelotype analysis of the PTEN, Smad4 and DCC genes in biliary tract cancer. *Anticancer research*. 2002;22(3):1529-36.

[54] Agaram NP, Shia J, Tang LH, Klimstra DS. DNA mismatch repair deficiency in ampullary carcinoma: a morphologic and immunohistochemical study of 54 cases. *American journal of clinical pathology*. 2010;133(5):772-80.

[55] Overman MJ, Zhang J, Kopetz S, Davies M, Zhi-Qin J, Stemke-Hale K, et al. Gene expression profiling of ampullary carcinomas classifies ampullary carcinomas into biliary-like and intestinal-like subtypes that are prognostic of outcome. *PloS one*. 2013;8(6):e65144.

[56] Demeure MJ, Craig DW, Sinari S, Moses TM, Christoforides A, Dinh J, et al. Cancer of the ampulla of Vater: analysis of the whole genome sequence exposes a potential therapeutic vulnerability. *Genome medicine*. 2012;4(7):56.

[57] Zakharov V, Ren B, Ryan C, Cao W. Diagnostic value of HMGAs, p53 and beta-catenin in discriminating adenocarcinoma from adenoma or reactive atypia in ampulla and common bile duct biopsies. *Histopathology*. 2013;62(5):778-87.

[58] Takashima M, Ueki T, Nagai E, Yao T, Yamaguchi K, Tanaka M, et al. Carcinoma of the ampulla of Vater associated with or without adenoma: a clinicopathologic analysis of 198 cases with reference to p53 and Ki-67 immunohistochemical expressions. *Modern pathology: an official journal of the United States and Canadian Academy of Pathology,* Inc. 2000;13(12):1300-7.

[59] Riener MO, Fritzsche FR, Clavien PA, Pestalozzi BC, Probst-Hensch N, Jochum W, et al. IMP3 expression in lesions of the biliary tract: a marker for high-grade dysplasia and an independent prognostic factor in bile duct carcinomas. *Human pathology*. 2009;40(10):1377-83.

[60] Levy M, Lin F, Xu H, Dhall D, Spaulding BO, Wang HL. S100P, von Hippel-Lindau gene product, and IMP3 serve as a useful immunohistochemical panel in the diagnosis of adenocarcinoma on endoscopic bile duct biopsy. *Human pathology*. 2010;41(9):1210-9.

[61] Baumhoer D, Riener MO, Zlobec I, Tornillo L, Vogetseder A, Kristiansen G, et al. Expression of CD24, P-cadherin and S100A4 in tumors of the ampulla of Vater. *Modern pathology: an official journal of the United States and Canadian Academy of Pathology,* Inc. 2009;22(2):306-13.

[62] Adsay V, Ohike N, Tajiri T, Kim GE, Krasinskas A, Balci S, et al. Ampullary region carcinomas: definition and site specific classification with delineation of four clinicopathologically and prognostically distinct subsets in an analysis of 249 cases. *The American journal of surgical pathology*. 2012;36(11):1592-608.

[63] Chang DK, Jamieson NB, Johns AL, Scarlett CJ, Pajic M, Chou A, et al. Histomolecular phenotypes and outcome in adenocarcinoma of the ampulla of vater. *Journal of clinical oncology: official journal of the American Society of Clinical Oncology*. 2013;31(10):1348-56.

[64] Kayahara M, Ohta T. Gross appearance of the ampullary tumor predicts lymph node metastasis and outcome. *Digestive surgery*. 2010;27(2):127-31.

[65] Cubilla AL, Fitzgerald PJ. Surgical pathology aspects of cancer of the ampulla-head-of-pancreas region. *Monographs in pathology*. 1980;21:67-81.

[66] Westgaard A, Tafjord S, Farstad IN, Cvancarova M, Eide TJ, Mathisen O, et al. Pancreatobiliary versus intestinal histologic type of differentiation is an independent prognostic factor in resected periampullary adenocarcinoma. *BMC cancer*. 2008;8:170.

[67] Relles D, Baek J, Witkiewicz A, Yeo CJ. Periampullary and duodenal neoplasms in neurofibromatosis type 1: two cases and an updated 20-year review of the literature yielding 76 cases. *Journal of gastrointestinal surgery: official journal of the Society for Surgery of the Alimentary Tract*. 2010;14(6):1052-61.

[68] Cappelli C, Agosti B, Braga M, Cumetti D, Gandossi E, Rizzoni D, et al. Von Recklinghausen's neurofibromatosis associated with duodenal somatostatinoma. A case report and review of the literature. *Minerva endocrinologica*. 2004;29(1):19-24.

[69] Wente MN, Kleeff J, Esposito I, Hartel M, Muller MW, Frohlich BE, et al. Renal cancer cell metastasis into the pancreas: a single-center experience and overview of the literature. *Pancreas*. 2005;30(3):218-22.

[70] Krones E, Graziadei I, Trauner M, Fickert P. Evolving concepts in primary sclerosing cholangitis. *Liver international: official journal of the International Association for the Study of the Liver*. 2012;32(3):352-69.

[71] Bjornsson E, Chapman RW. Sclerosing cholangitis. *Current opinion in gastroenterology*. 2003;19(3):270-5.

[72] Mahajan VS, Mattoo H, Deshpande V, Pillai SS, Stone JH. IgG4-Related Disease. *Annual review of pathology*. 2013.

[73] Chari ST, Kloeppel G, Zhang L, Notohara K, Lerch MM, Shimosegawa T. Histopathologic and clinical subtypes of autoimmune pancreatitis: the honolulu consensus document. *Pancreatology: official journal of the International Association of Pancreatology*. 2010;10(6):664-72.

[74] Shimosegawa T, Chari ST, Frulloni L, Kamisawa T, Kawa S, Mino-Kenudson M, et al. International consensus diagnostic criteria for autoimmune pancreatitis: guidelines of the International Association of Pancreatology. *Pancreas*. 2011;40(3):352-8.

[75] Bjornsson E, Chari ST, Smyrk TC, Lindor K. Immunoglobulin G4 associated cholangitis: description of an emerging clinical entity based on review of the literature. *Hepatology*. 2007;45(6):1547-54.

[76] Okazaki K, Uchida K, Ikeura T, Takaoka M. Current concept and diagnosis of IgG4-related disease in the hepato-bilio-pancreatic system. *Journal of gastroenterology*. 2013;48(3):303-14.

[77] Kawakami H, Zen Y, Kuwatani M, Eto K, Haba S, Yamato H, et al. IgG4-related sclerosing cholangitis and autoimmune pancreatitis: histological assessment of biopsies from Vater's ampulla and the bile duct. *Journal of gastroenterology and hepatology*. 2010;25(10):1648-55.

[78] Nakazawa T, Naitoh I, Hayashi K, Miyabe K, Simizu S, Joh T. Diagnosis of IgG4-related sclerosing cholangitis. *World journal of gastroenterology: WJG*. 2013;19(43):7661-70.

[79] Nishino T, Oyama H, Hashimoto E, Toki F, Oi I, Kobayashi M, et al. Clinicopathological differentiation between sclerosing cholangitis with autoimmune pancreatitis and primary sclerosing cholangitis. *Journal of gastroenterology*. 2007;42(7):550-9.

[80] Nakazawa T, Ohara H, Sano H, Ando T, Aoki S, Kobayashi S, et al. Clinical differences between primary sclerosing cholangitis and sclerosing cholangitis with autoimmune pancreatitis. *Pancreas*. 2005;30(1):20-5.

[81] Ohara H, Okazaki K, Tsubouchi H, Inui K, Kawa S, Kamisawa T, et al. Clinical diagnostic criteria of IgG4-related sclerosing cholangitis 2012. *Journal of hepato-biliary-pancreatic sciences*. 2012;19(5):536-42.

[82] Hirano K, Fukushima N, Tada M, Isayama H, Mizuno S, Yamamoto K, et al. Diagnostic utility of biopsy specimens for autoimmune pancreatitis. *Journal of gastroenterology*. 2009;44(7):765-73.

[83] Kamisawa T, Tu Y, Egawa N, Tsuruta K, Okamoto A. A new diagnostic endoscopic tool for autoimmune pancreatitis. *Gastrointestinal endoscopy*. 2008;68(2):358-61.

[84] Kubota K, Kato S, Akiyama T, Yoneda M, Fujita K, Ogawa M, et al. Differentiating sclerosing cholangitis caused by autoimmune pancreatitis and primary sclerosing cholangitis according to endoscopic duodenal papillary features. *Gastrointestinal endoscopy*. 2008;68(6):1204-8.

[85] Zhang L, Lewis JT, Abraham SC, Smyrk TC, Leung S, Chari ST, et al. IgG4+ plasma cell infiltrates in liver explants with primary sclerosing cholangitis. *The American journal of surgical pathology*. 2010;34(1):88-94.

[86] Kitagawa S, Zen Y, Harada K, Sasaki M, Sato Y, Minato H, et al. Abundant IgG4-positive plasma cell infiltration characterizes chronic sclerosing sialadenitis (Kuttner's tumor). *The American journal of surgical pathology*. 2005;29(6):783-91.

[87] Sepehr A, Mino-Kenudson M, Ogawa F, Brugge WR, Deshpande V, Lauwers GY. IgG4+ to IgG+ plasma cells ratio of ampulla can help differentiate autoimmune pancreatitis from other "mass forming" pancreatic lesions. *The American journal of surgical pathology*. 2008;32(12):1770-9.

[88] Zen Y, Kitagawa S, Minato H, Kurumaya H, Katayanagi K, Masuda S, et al. IgG4-positive plasma cells in inflammatory pseudotumor (plasma cell granuloma) of the lung. *Human pathology*. 2005;36(7):710-7.

[89] Whipple AO, Parsons WB, Mullins CR. TREATMENT OF CARCINOMA OF THE AMPULLA OF VATER. *Annals of surgery*. 1935;102(4):763-79.

[90] Klinkenbijl JH, van der Schelling GP, Hop WC, van Pel R, Bruining HA, Jeekel J. The advantages of pylorus-preserving pancreatoduodenectomy in malignant disease of the pancreas and periampullary region. *Annals of surgery*. 1992;216(2):142-5.

[91] Seiler CA, Wagner M, Bachmann T, Redaelli CA, Schmied B, Uhl W, et al. Randomized clinical trial of pylorus-preserving duodenopancreatectomy versus

classical Whipple resection-long term results. *The British journal of surgery.* 2005;92(5):547-56.

[92] Tran KT, Smeenk HG, van Eijck CH, Kazemier G, Hop WC, Greve JW, et al. Pylorus preserving pancreaticoduodenectomy versus standard Whipple procedure: a prospective, randomized, multicenter analysis of 170 patients with pancreatic and periampullary tumors. *Annals of surgery.* 2004;240(5):738-45.

[93] Tarazi RY, Hermann RE, Vogt DP, Hoerr SO, Esselstyn CB, Jr., Cooperman AM, et al. Results of surgical treatment of periampullary tumors: a thirty-five-year experience. *Surgery.* 1986;100(4):716-23.

[94] Schmidt CM, Turrini O, Parikh P, House MG, Zyromski NJ, Nakeeb A, et al. Effect of hospital volume, surgeon experience, and surgeon volume on patient outcomes after pancreaticoduodenectomy: a single-institution experience. *Archives of surgery* (Chicago, Ill: 1960). 2010;145(7):634-40.

[95] Enomoto LM, Gusani NJ, Dillon PW, Hollenbeak CS. Impact of Surgeon and Hospital Volume on Mortality, Length of Stay, and Cost of Pancreaticoduodenectomy. *Journal of gastrointestinal surgery: official journal of the Society for Surgery of the Alimentary* Tract. 2013.

[96] Halstead WS. Contributions to the surgery of the bile passages, especially of the common bile duct. *Boston Med Surg J.* 1899;141:645-54.

[97] Beger HG, Treitschke F, Gansauge F, Harada N, Hiki N, Mattfeldt T. Tumor of the ampulla of Vater: experience with local or radical resection in 171 consecutively treated patients. *Archives of surgery* (Chicago, Ill : 1960). 1999;134(5):526-32.

[98] Rattner DW, Fernandez-del Castillo C, Brugge WR, Warshaw AL. Defining the criteria for local resection of ampullary neoplasms. *Archives of surgery* (Chicago, Ill : 1960). 1996;131(4):366-71.

[99] Zhong J, Palta M, Willett CG, McCall SJ, Bulusu A, Tyler DS, et al. The role of local excision in invasive adenocarcinoma of the ampulla of Vater. *Journal of gastrointestinal oncology.* 2013;4(1):8-13.

[100] Bjork KJ, Davis CJ, Nagorney DM, Mucha P, Jr. Duodenal villous tumors. *Archives of surgery* (Chicago, Ill : 1960). 1990;125(8):961-5.

[101] Galandiuk S, Hermann RE, Jagelman DG, Fazio VW, Sivak MV. Villous tumors of the duodenum. *Annals of surgery.* 1988;207(3):234-9.

[102] Sivak MV. Clinical and endoscopic aspects of tumors of the ampulla of Vater. *Endoscopy.* 1988;20 Suppl 1:211-7.

[103] Ryan DP, Schapiro RH, Warshaw AL. Villous tumors of the duodenum. *Annals of surgery.* 1986;203(3):301-6.

[104] Posner S, Colletti L, Knol J, Mulholland M, Eckhauser F. Safety and long-term efficacy of transduodenal excision for tumors of the ampulla of Vater. *Surgery.* 2000;128(4):694-701.

[105] Gertsch P, Matthews JB, Lerut J, Baer HU, Blumgart LH. The technique of papilloduodenectomy. *Surgery, gynecology & obstetrics.* 1990;170(3):254-6.

[106] Binmoeller KF, Boaventura S, Ramsperger K, Soehendra N. Endoscopic snare excision of benign adenomas of the papilla of Vater. *Gastrointestinal endoscopy.* 1993;39(2):127-31.

[107] Moss AC, Morris E, Mac Mathuna P. Palliative biliary stents for obstructing pancreatic carcinoma. *The Cochrane database of systematic reviews.* 2006(2):CD004200.

[108] Castano R, Lopes TL, Alvarez O, Calvo V, Luz LP, Artifon EL. Nitinol biliary stent versus surgery for palliation of distal malignant biliary obstruction. *Surgical endoscopy*. 2010;24(9):2092-8.

[109] Lillemoe KD. Palliative therapy for pancreatic cancer. *Surgical oncology clinics of North America*. 1998;7(1):199-216.

[110] Lillemoe KD, Cameron JL, Hardacre JM, Sohn TA, Sauter PK, Coleman J, et al. Is prophylactic gastrojejunostomy indicated for unresectable periampullary cancer? A prospective randomized trial. *Annals of surgery*. 1999;230(3):322-8; discussion 8-30.

[111] Van Heek NT, De Castro SM, van Eijck CH, van Geenen RC, Hesselink EJ, Breslau PJ, et al. The need for a prophylactic gastrojejunostomy for unresectable periampullary cancer: a prospective randomized multicenter trial with special focus on assessment of quality of life. *Annals of surgery*. 2003;238(6):894-902; discussion -5.

[112] Lillemoe KD, Cameron JL, Kaufman HS, Yeo CJ, Pitt HA, Sauter PK. Chemical splanchnicectomy in patients with unresectable pancreatic cancer. A prospective randomized trial. *Annals of surgery*. 1993;217(5):447-55; discussion 56-7.

[113] Ihse I, Zoucas E, Gyllstedt E, Lillo-Gil R, Andren-Sandberg A. Bilateral thoracoscopic splanchnicectomy: effects on pancreatic pain and function. *Annals of surgery*. 1999;230(6):785-90; discussion 90-1.

Editor Contact Information

Dr. Miguel Ángel Mercado, MD
National Institute of Medical Sciences and Nutrition
"Salvador Zubirán" Medical Association
E-mail: mercadiazma@yahoo.com

Index

A

B

C

D

E

F

G

H

I

N

O

P

Q

R

S

T

U

V